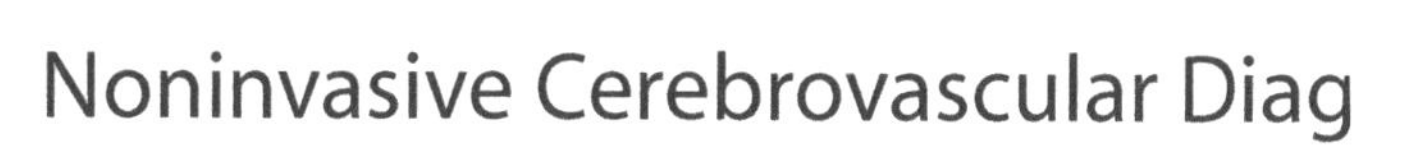
Noninvasive Cerebrovascular Diag

Ali F. AbuRahma · John J. Bergan
Editors

Noninvasive Cerebrovascular Diagnosis

Editors
Ali F. AbuRahma, MD, FACS, FRCS, RVT, RPVI
Professor
Chief, Vascular/Endovascular Surgery
Department of Surgery
Robert C. Byrd Health Sciences Center
West Virginia University
and
Medical Director, Vascular Laboratory
Co-Director, Vascular Center of Excellence
Charleston Area Medical Center
Charleston, WV, USA

John J. Bergan, MD, FACS, Hon FRCS
UCSD School of Medicine
La Jolla, CA
USA

ISBN 978-1-84882-956-5 e-ISBN 978-1-84882-957-2
DOI 10.1007/978-1-84882-957-2
Springer London Dordrecht Heidelberg New York

British Library Cataloguing in Publication Data
A catalogue record for this book is available from the British Library

Library of Congress Control Number: 2010920021

First published in 2000 as part of *Noninvasive Vascular Diagnosis*, edited by Ali F. AbuRahma and John J. Bergan, ISBN 1-85233-128-3, 2nd edition published 2007, ISBN 978-1-84628-446-5

Printed on acid-free paper

Springer is part of Springer Science+Business Media (www.springer.com)

Table of Contents

1 Overview of Cerebrovascular Disease

Ali F. AbuRahma

Stroke is the third leading cause of death in the United States, and the second leading cause of death for women in the United States. It is the cause of death in approximately 150,000 to 200,000 Americans annually. The morbidity of those who survive a stroke has a significant socioeconomic impact on our society. It is estimated that strokes account for the disability of two million Americans. The cost of medical bills, hospitalization, and rehabilitation was estimated to be around $40 billion in 1996.

It has been reported that 75% of patients suffering a stroke have surgically accessible extracranial vascular disease.[1] Ischemic strokes constitute 80–85% of all strokes, and the remaining 15–20% are caused by cerebral hemorrhage.[2,3] It has been estimated that ≥50% carotid stenosis may be responsible for up to 25% of all ischemic strokes. Large population studies using carotid ultrasound estimate the prevalence of ≥50% carotid artery stenosis to be 3–7%. This emphasizes the importance of early detection for stroke prevention.

Significant changes in our thinking and treatment of this disease have occurred over the past 50 years, but this has been a topic fraught with controversy since the first carotid endarterectomy was reported. Eastcott *et al.*[4] performed a carotid resection with reanastomosis of a diseased vessel in a patient who suffered a transient ischemic attack. This was published in 1954, but DeBakey[5] reported a successful performance of this procedure earlier.

Today, carotid endarterectomy is the most commonly performed vascular surgical procedure, however, it is still controversial. The debate over medical versus surgical treatment for carotid artery disease has been extensively analyzed in the medical literature over the past 10 years. The CASSANOVA, Asymptomatic Carotid Atherosclerosis Study (ACAS), Veteran's Administration (VA) Cooperative study, and Asymptomatic Carotid Surgery Trial (ACST) have looked at medical versus surgical therapy in asymptomatic carotid stenosis.[6–9] The VA Cooperative study, the North American Symptomatic Carotid Endarterectomy Trial Collaborators (NASCET) study, and the European Carotid Surgery Trialists' Collaborative Group (ECST) looked at symptomatic carotid disease.[10–12] Regardless of which criteria are used to determine whether operative intervention is warranted, a surgeon must stay within the accepted perioperative stroke rate of 3–7% (depending on indication) as recommended by the Ad Hoc Committee of the Stroke Council of the American Heart Association. What is generally agreed upon, however, is that early and accurate detection of stroke-prone patients remains one of the most important problems in medicine, since stroke has an immediate mortality of 20–25% within 30 days. Of the survivors of a first stroke, 25–50% will have an additional stroke.

Anatomy

The aortic arch gives off, from right to left, the innominate (brachiocephalic trunk), the left common carotid, and the subclavian arteries (Figure 1–1). The innominate artery passes beneath the left innominate vein before it branches into the right subclavian and the right common carotid arteries. The vertebral arteries branch off the subclavian arteries 2 or 3 cm from the arch, but many variations may occur (Figure 1–1). The left common carotid artery may arise from the innominate (bovine arch) in 16% of patients and cross to a relatively normal position on the left side. The left vertebral artery may arise directly from the aortic arch instead of from the left subclavian arteries (Figure 1–2). The right vertebral artery may arise as part of a trifurcation of the brachiocephalic trunk into subclavian, common carotid, and vertebral arteries (Figure 1–3). Occasionally, both subclavian arteries originate together as a single trunk off of the arch, or the right subclavian may arise distal to the left subclavian artery and cross to the right side.[13]

The common carotid arteries on each side travel in the carotid sheath up to the neck before branching into

A.F. Aburahma, J.J. Bergan (eds.), *Noninvasive Cerebrovascular Diagnosis*, DOI 10.1007/978-1-84882-957-2_1,

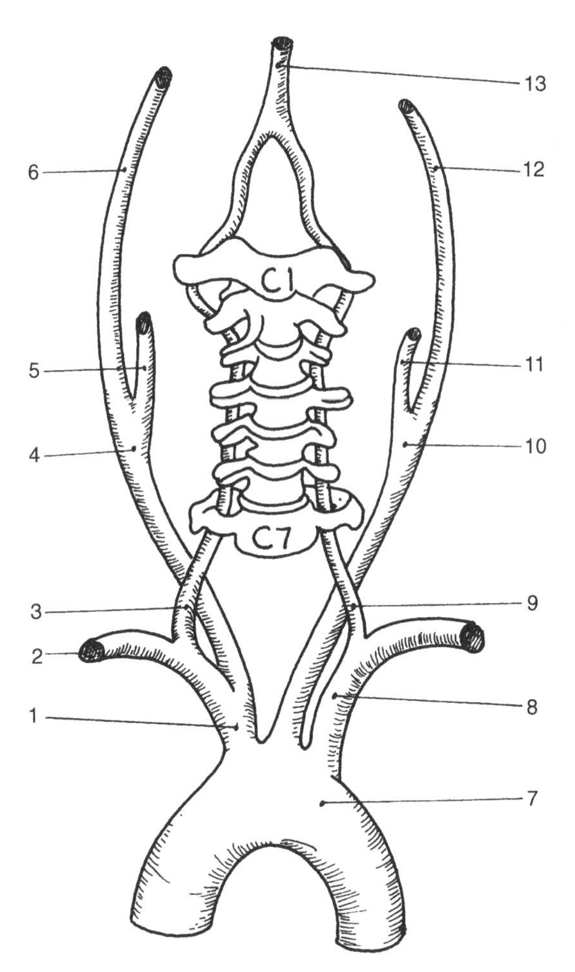

FIGURE 1–1. An illustration showing the aortic arch and its branches: (1) brachial-cephalic trunk, (2) right subclavian artery, (3) right vertebral artery, (4) right common carotid artery, (5) right external carotid artery, (6) right internal carotid artery, (7) aortic arch, (8) left subclavian artery, (9) left vertebral artery, (10) left common carotid artery, (11) left external carotid artery, (12) left internal carotid artery, (13) the basilar artery.

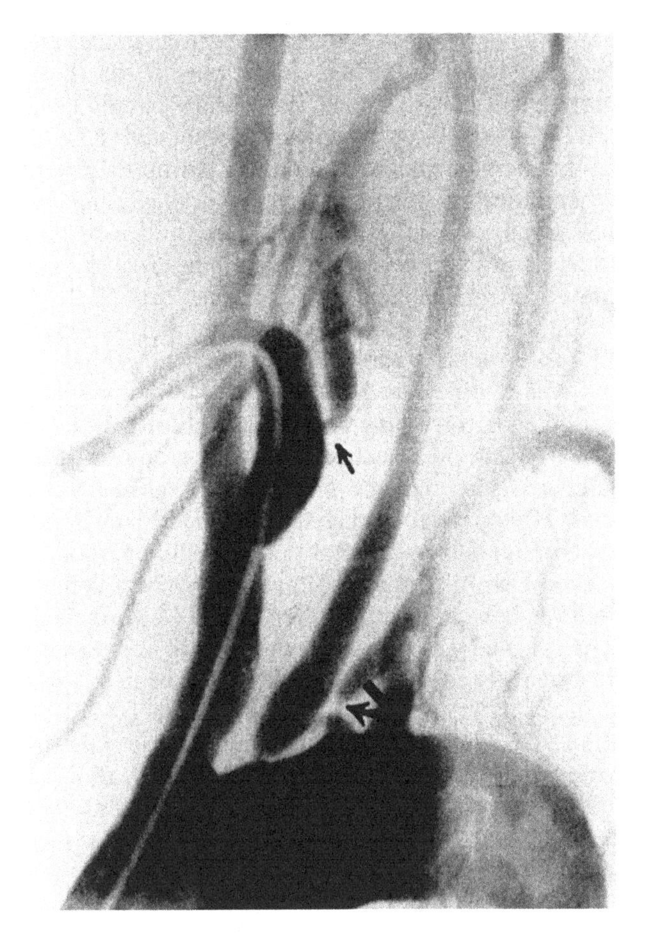

FIGURE 1–2. Arch aortogram showing the left vertebral artery originating from the arch of the aorta with tight stenosis at its origin (curved arrow) and the right vertebral artery (coming off the right subclavian artery) with a tight stenosis at its origin (straight arrow).

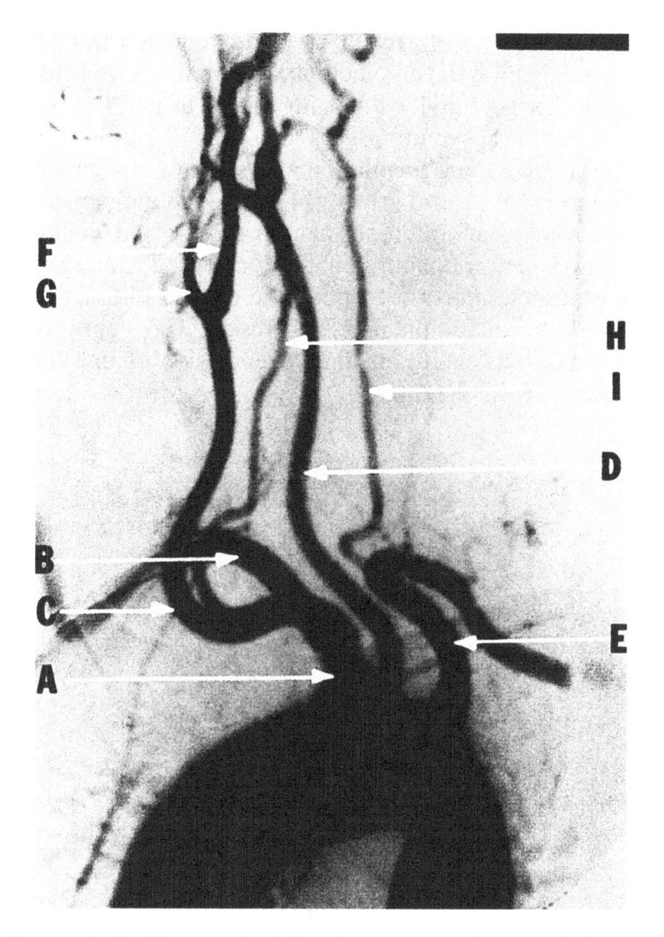

FIGURE 1–3. Abnormal origin of the vertebral artery (H) from the right common carotid artery (C) in a patient with a retroesophageal right subclavian artery (B). (Courtesy of Springer-Verlag, *Surgery of the Arteries to the Head*, 1992, by Ramon Berguer and Edouard Kieffer, eds.)

internal and external carotid arteries just below the level of the mandible. The external carotid artery supplies the face. Important branches of the external carotid artery include the superior thyroid, which can actually arise from the common carotid artery, and is important in that it accompanies the external branch of the superior laryngeal nerve, the ascending pharyngeal, and the lingual and occipital arteries that have a close association with the hypoglossal nerve (Figure 1–4). No branches of the internal carotid artery occur in the neck.

The carotid sinus, a baroreceptor, is located in the crotch of the bifurcation of the internal and external carotid artery. It is innervated by the nerve of Hering, which branches from the glossopharyngeal nerve. The carotid body is a very small structure that also lies in the crotch of the bifurcation and functions as a chemoreceptor, responding to low oxygen or high carbon dioxide levels in the blood. It is also innervated by the glossopharyngeal nerve via the nerve of Hering.

The corticotympanic artery and the artery to the pterygoid canal are branches of the internal carotid artery in its petrous portion. The cavernous, hypophyseal, semilunar, anterior meningeal, and ophthalmic arteries are branches of the cavernous portion of the internal carotid artery. The ophthalmic artery is clinically important since it communicates with the external carotid system, which is the basis of the periorbital Doppler study. The remaining branches of the internal carotid artery arise from the cerebral portion, i.e., the anterior and middle cerebral, posterior communicating, and chorioidal branches (Figure 1–5).

The vertebral artery leaves the subclavian artery and pushes upward through the foramina of the transverse processes of the cervical vertebrae into the cranium through the foramen magnum (Figure 1–6). The neck spinal branches enter the vertebral canal through the intervertebral foramen, and muscular branches are given off to the deep muscles of the neck. These latter branches anastomose with branches of the external carotid artery. Intracranially, the vertebral arteries give off the posterior inferior cerebellar and spinal arteries before they are united at the pontomedullary junction to form the basilar artery. The basilar artery terminates as the posterior cerebral artery after giving off the anterior inferior, superior cerebellar, pontine, and internal auditory arteries.

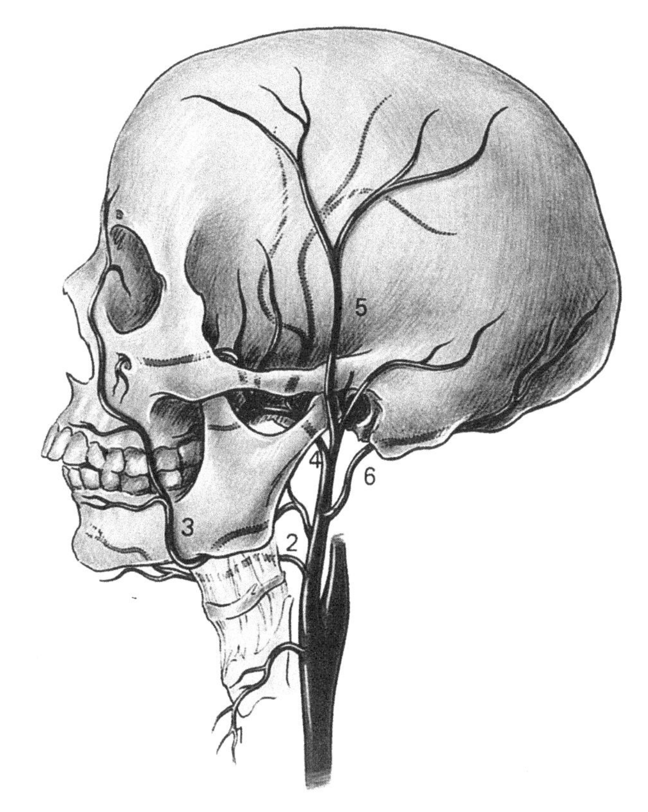

FIGURE 1–4. Main branches of the external carotid artery: (1) superior thyroid, (2) lingual, (3) facial, (4) internal maxillary artery, (5) superficial temporal artery, (6) occipital artery. (Courtesy of Springer-Verlag, *Surgery of the Arteries to the Head*, 1992, by Ramon Berguer and Edouard Kieffer, eds.)

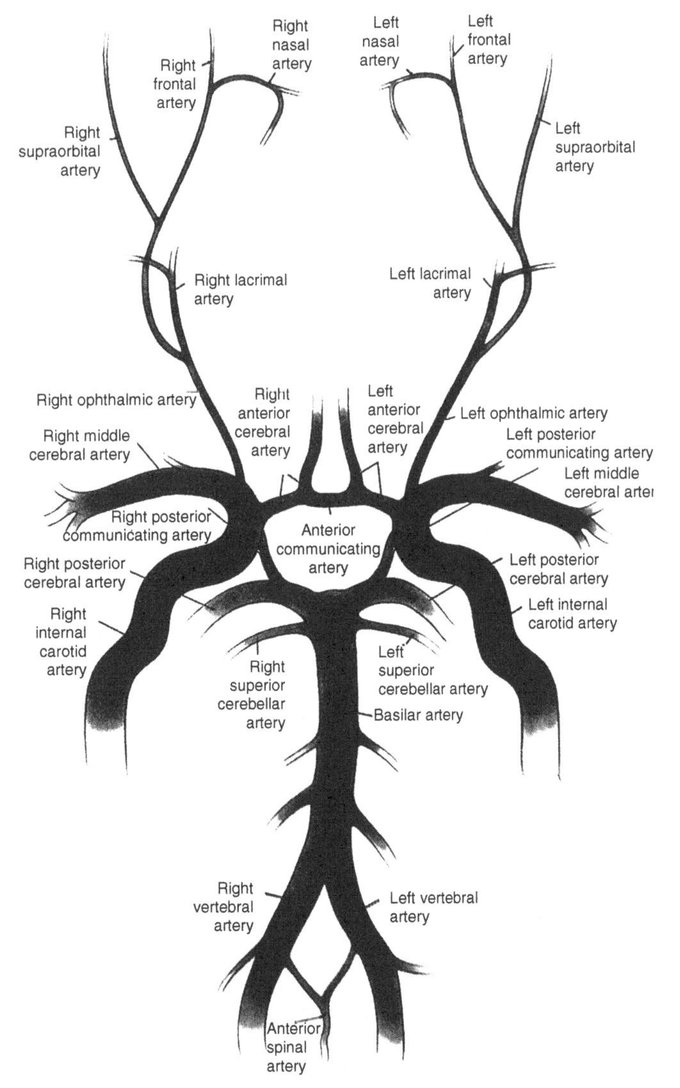

FIGURE 1–5. Major branches of the internal carotid artery (i.e., middle cerebral, anterior cerebral, posterior communicating, and ophthalmic artery) and vertebrobasilar arteries.

Blood flows through each internal carotid artery at about 350 ml/min, accounting for approximately 85% of the blood supply to the brain, and the vertebral arteries account for about 15% of the total blood supply to the brain.[14] Therefore, the carotid arteries, both from the standpoint of accessibility and functioning, become the system of importance for noninvasive testing.

Morphologic Variations of the Internal Carotid Artery

Tortuosity of the internal carotid artery (or loop) is generally defined as an S- or C-shaped elongation or curving in the course of the artery (Figure 1–7C). Coiling is a term used to describe an exaggerated, redundant S-shaped curve, or a complete circle, in the longitudinal axis of the artery (Figure 1–7A). Tortuosity and coiling are thought to be congenital developmental abnormalities that may become exaggerated with aging. They usually do not produce clinical symptoms.

Kinking is a sharp angulation with stenosis of segments of the internal carotid artery, (Figure 1–7B) and appears to be somewhat different than tortuosity and coiling. Kinking is less frequently bilateral and usually affects a few centimeters or more above the carotid bifurcation. Poststenotic dilatation may be present. Frequently, an atherosclerotic plaque on the concave side of the kink further narrows the lumen.

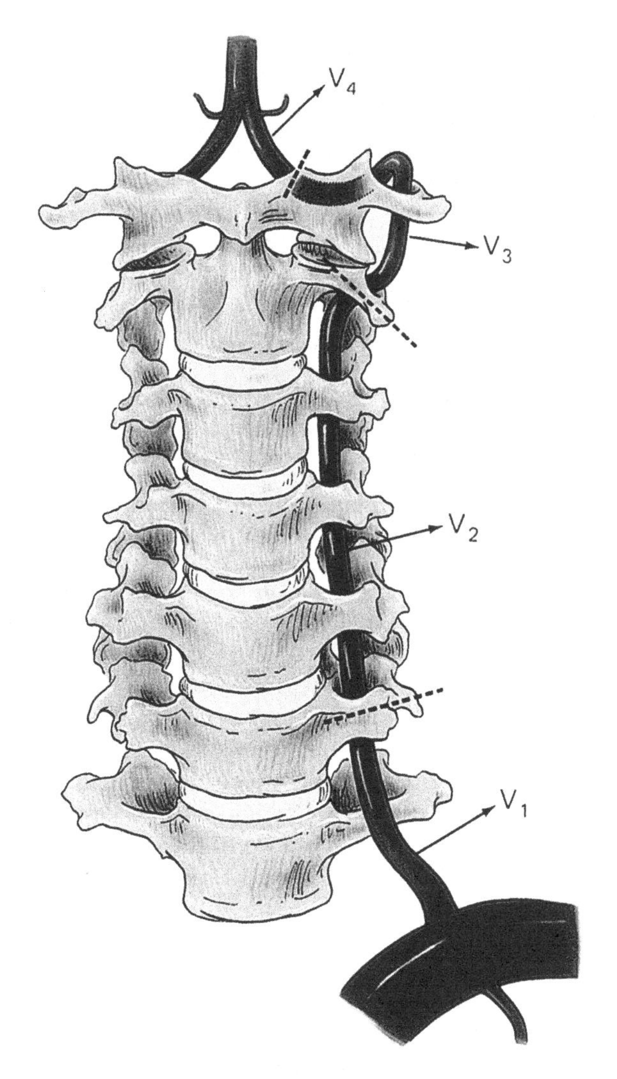

FIGURE 1–6. Relation of the vertebral artery and cervical spine. The dotted line indicates the level at which the vertebral artery becomes intradural. As noted, the vertebral artery is divided into four portions (V-1, V-2, V-3, and V-4). V-1 is the segment between its origin and the level where it enters the transverse process of the sixth cervical vertebra. V-2 is the segment of the artery through the foramina of the transverse processes of the cervical spines until the dotted line. V-3 is the segment between C-2 and C-1. V-4 is the segment prior to joining the other vertebral artery to form the basilar artery.

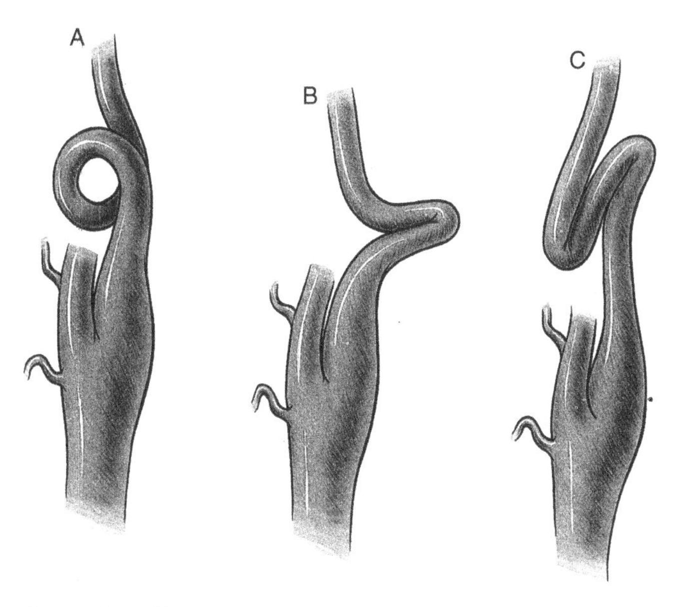

FIGURE 1–7. Three types of redundancy of the internal carotid artery. (A) Coil. (B) Kink. (C) Loop. (Courtesy of Springer Verlag, *Surgery of the Arteries to the Head*, 1992, Ramon Berguer and Edouard Kieffer, eds.)

Unlike tortuosity and coiling, kinking is thought to be an acquired abnormality, occurring mostly in older people in whom arteriosclerotic disease and hypertension are important factors. Changes in head and neck positions may produce cerebral ischemia in patients with carotid kinking, whereas tortuosity and coiling are usually asymptomatic.

Collateral Pathways

Single stenotic lesions may or may not produce carotid territory symptoms (hemispheric) or vertebrobasilar territory symptoms (nonhemispheric). The collateral system comes into play when resistance in the stenotic major artery is greater than the resistance in the smaller circulative collateral channel. As stenosis becomes more severe and the collateral channel arteries dilate in response to increased flow, the collateral channels will increase flow up to the point of capacity. It can then be seen that the more proximal the obstruction, the greater the potential for collateral pathways to exist. Proximal occlusion of the arteries arising from the aortic arch is, therefore, rarely associated with the stroke syndrome because of this collateral flow. Branches of each subclavian artery may anastomose with collaterals of the opposite subclavian artery and the branches of the external carotid system.

The subclavian steal syndrome[15] occurs with proximal subclavian occlusion and retrograde flow down the vertebral artery (Figures 1–8 and 1–9A). In innominate artery obstruction, the retrograde flow may be down to the carotid artery (Figure 1–9B). Therefore, vascular surgeons may use the mechanism of collateral flow in a constructive manner; a patient who has both a carotid stenosis and subclavian steal syndrome may be

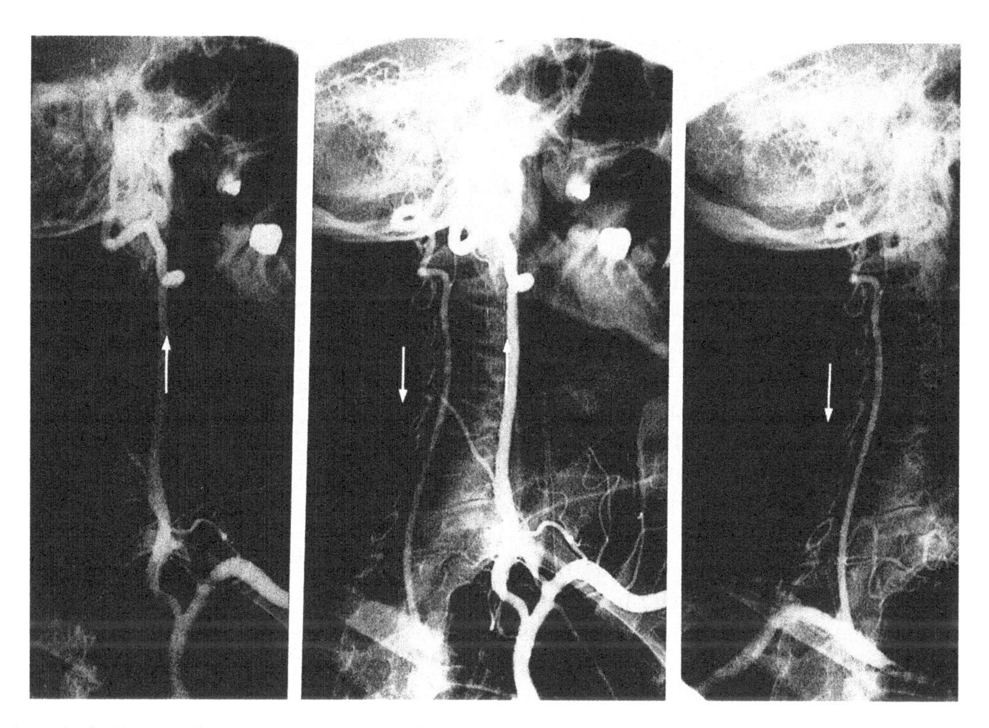

FIGURE 1–8. Right subclavian steal secondary to occlusion of the first segment of this artery. The left vertebral artery is filling from the left subclavian artery as seen on the left (arrow). In the middle, flow is seen retrograde in the right vertebral artery (arrow), and as seen on the right, the right subclavian artery is filling retrograde via the left vertebral artery. (Courtesy of Springer Verlag, *Surgery of the Arteries to the Head*, 1992, Ramon Berguer and Edouard Kieffer, eds.)

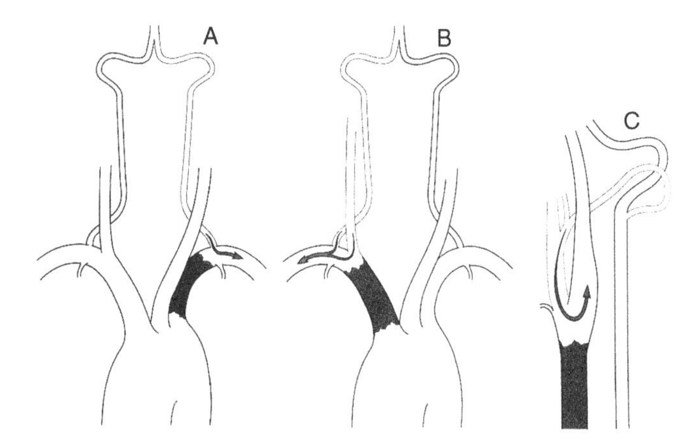

FIGURE 1–9. Three patterns of flow reversal. (A) Subclavian steal distal to an occluded left subclavian artery. (B) Reversal of flow in the carotid and vertebral arteries distal to an occluded innominate artery (innominate steal). (C) Reversal of flow in the occipital artery and proximal external carotid distal to an occluded common carotid artery (carotid steal). (Courtesy of Springer Verlag, *Surgery of the Arteries to the Head*, 1992, Ramon Berguer and Edouard Kieffer, eds.)

completely relieved of steal symptoms by carotid endarterectomy.

An interesting collateral pathway is the retrograde flow that may occur in the external carotid system by proximal occlusion of the common carotid artery (Figure 1–9C). Collateral flow to the internal carotid artery occurs by way of the ophthalmic artery or the Circle of Willis. Patients with a proximal internal carotid occlusion might have blood flow up the external carotid artery and retrograde through the supraorbital and frontal arteries into the ophthalmic artery and, finally, antegrade in the distal internal carotid artery and the Circle of Willis. This important pathway is the basis of the supraorbital Doppler cerebrovascular examination. Patients with proximal internal carotid occlusion and external carotid stenosis may be relieved of symptoms with correction of the external carotid occlusion, which alleviates symptoms of hypoperfusion.[16] Finally, emboli may course via the external carotid artery to the eye, producing amaurosis fugax in patients with a functional collateral pathway.[17]

The major collateral pathway, of course, is the Circle of Willis (Figures 1–10 and 1–11). This unique circle provides the major pathway between the internal carotid, the external carotid, and the vertebrobasilar systems. The Circle of Willis is anatomically complete in only one-third of patients, but it is physiologically adequate in around two-thirds of patients (Figure 1–12). Collateral arteries between the occipital branches of the external carotid arteries may bypass stenosis of the origin of both vertebral arteries and the muscular branches of the vertebral arteries (Figures 1–13, 1–14, and 1–15), or between the cervical branches of the thyrocervical trunk and vertebral

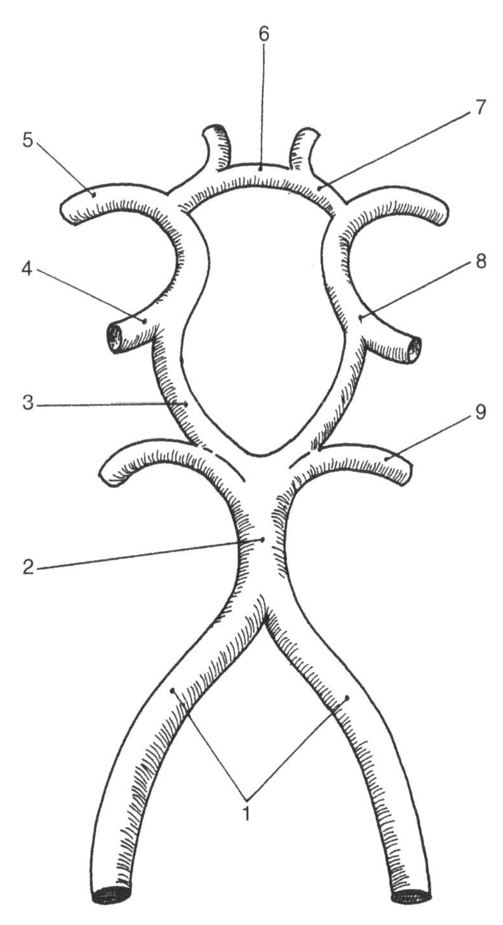

FIGURE 1–10. The Circle of Willis: (1) right and left vertebral arteries, (2) basilar artery, (3) right posterior communicating artery, (4) right internal carotid artery, (5) right middle cerebral artery, (6) anterior communicating artery, (7) left anterior cerebral artery, (8) left internal carotid artery, (9) left posterior cerebral artery.

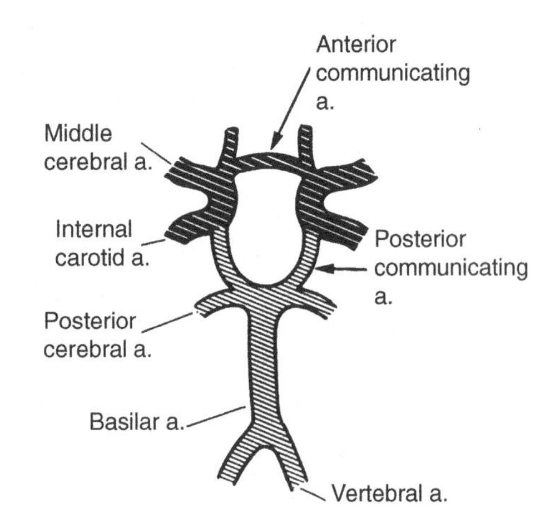

FIGURE 1–11. Circle of Willis showing the anterior cerebral circulation (shaded black) and the posterior circulation (shaded gray); a., artery.

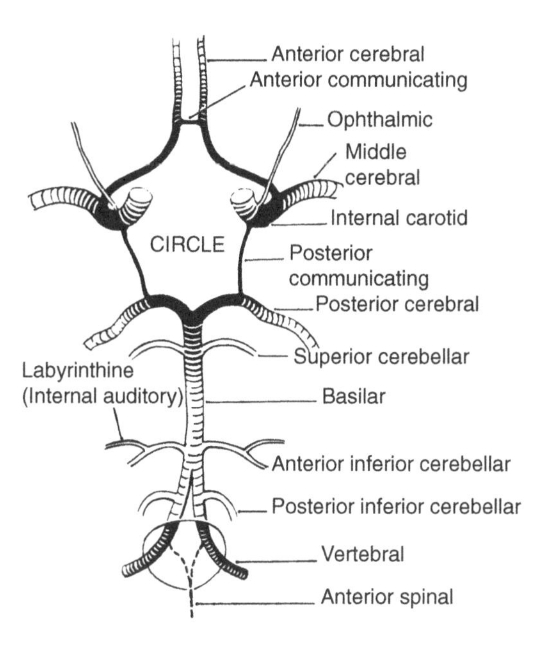

FIGURE 1–12. The Circle of Willis demonstrating rudimentary posterior communicating branches.

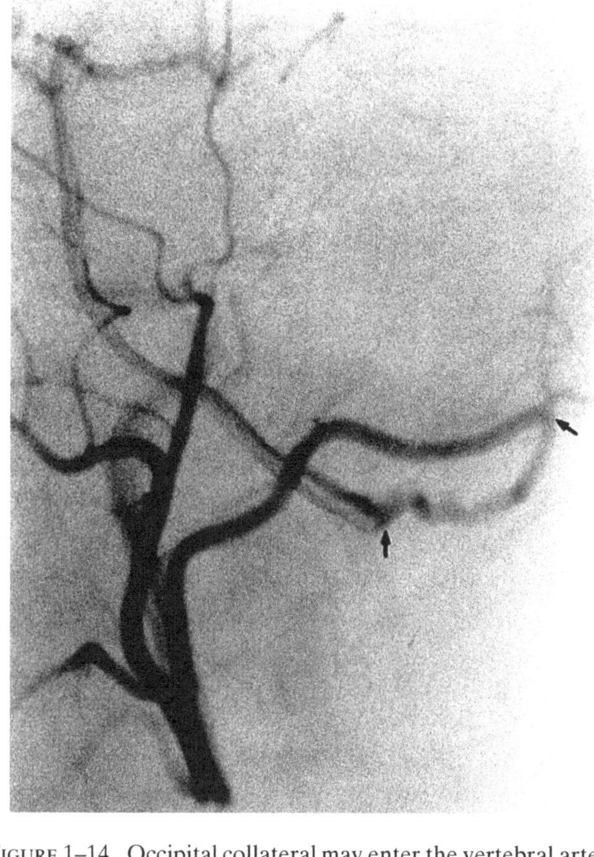

FIGURE 1–14. Occipital collateral may enter the vertebral artery at the level of C-1, as seen in this selective external carotid injection.

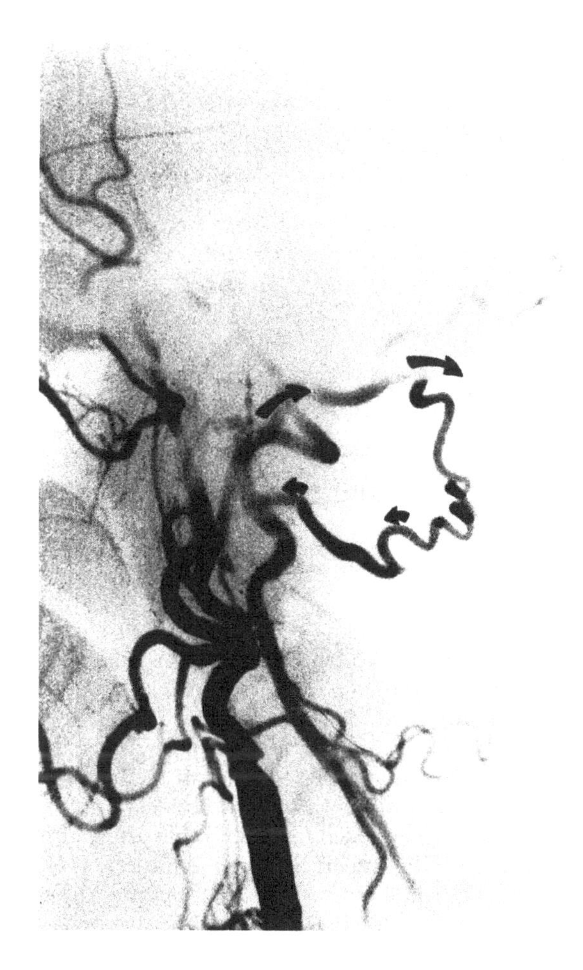

FIGURE 1–13. Occipital connection of the vertebral artery. In this patient with an occluded internal carotid artery, the collaterals from the occipital artery fill the vertebral artery anterograde toward the basilar artery and retrogradely toward the base of the neck, where the vertebral artery is occluded.

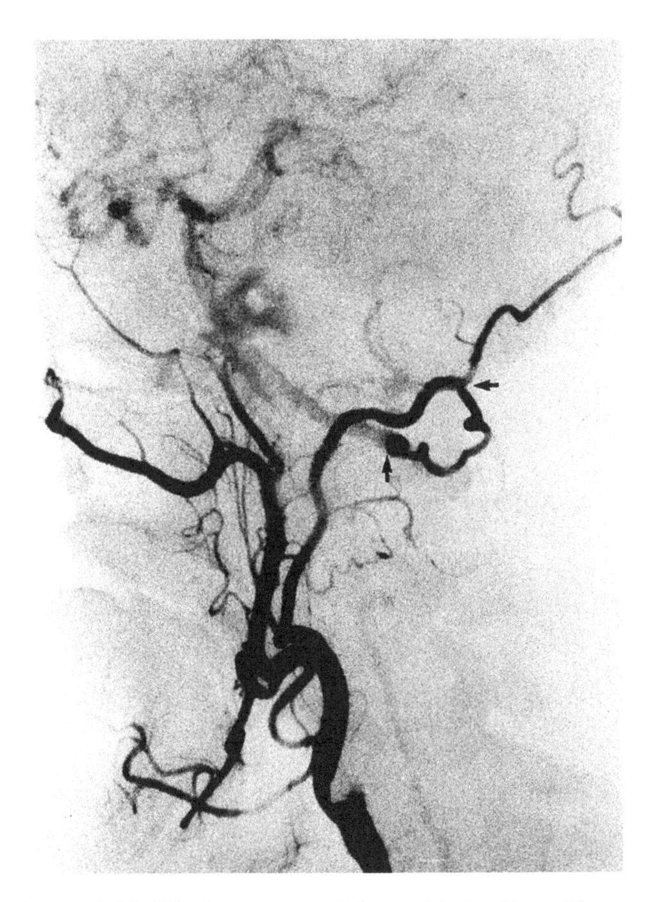

FIGURE 1–15. The importance of the occipital collateral is seen in this patient with an occluded internal carotid.

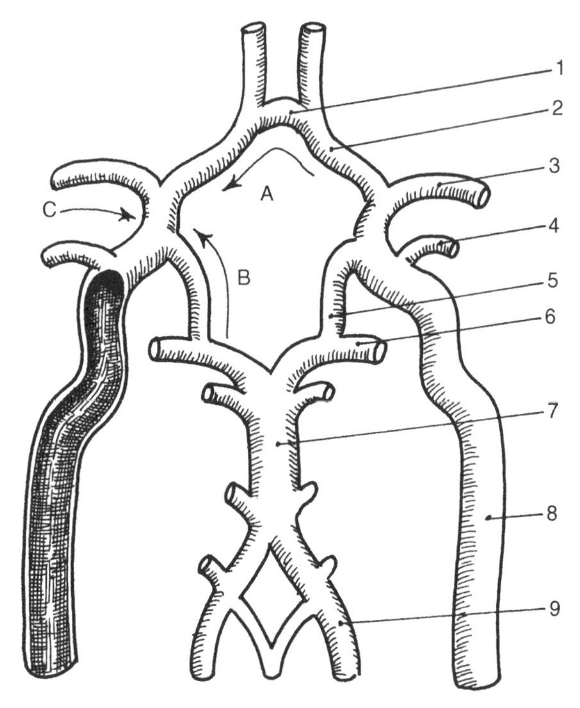

FIGURE 1–17. Illustration of a patient with an internal carotid artery occlusion. The flow to the corresponding cerebral hemisphere is maintained by flow from the opposite internal carotid artery (A), the vertebral basilar system (B), and the ophthalmic artery via the periorbital branches of the external carotid artery of the same side (C): (1) anterior communicating artery, (2) anterior cerebral artery, (3) middle cerebral artery, (4) ophthalmic artery, (5) posterior communicating artery, (6) posterior cerebral artery, (7) basilar artery, (8) internal carotid artery, (9) vertebral artery.

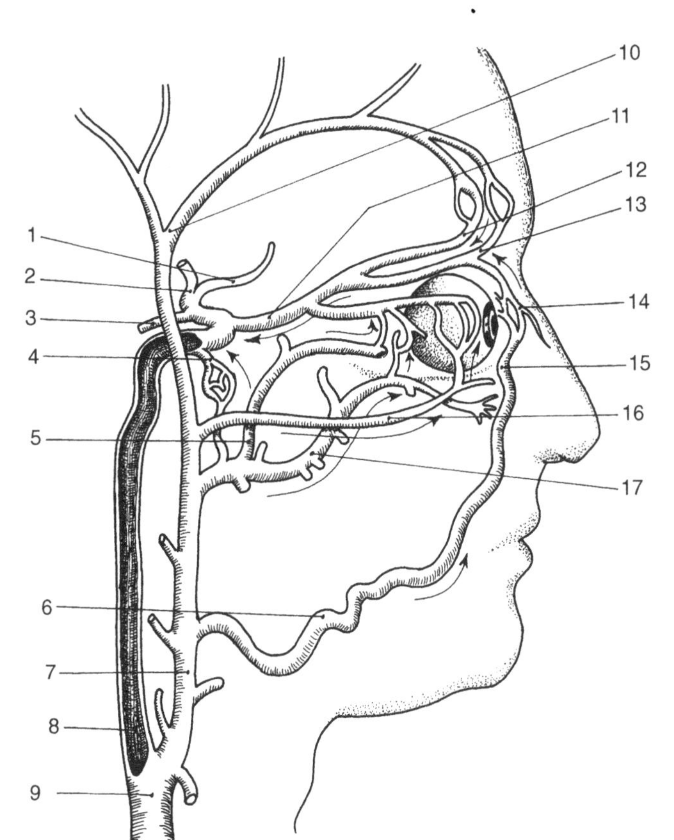

FIGURE 1–16. A patient with an occluded internal carotid artery with a reversal of flow through the ophthalmic artery via periorbital branches of the external carotid artery: (1) anterior cerebral artery, (2) middle cerebral artery, (3) posterior communicating artery, (4) caroticotympanic branch of the internal carotid artery, (5) middle meningeal artery, (6) fascial artery, (7) external carotid artery, (8) occluded internal carotid artery, (9) common carotid artery, (10) superficial temporal artery, (11) ophthalmic artery, (12) supraorbital artery, (13) supratrochlear artery, (14) dorsal nasal artery, (15) angular artery, (16) transverse fascial artery, (17) internal maxillary artery.

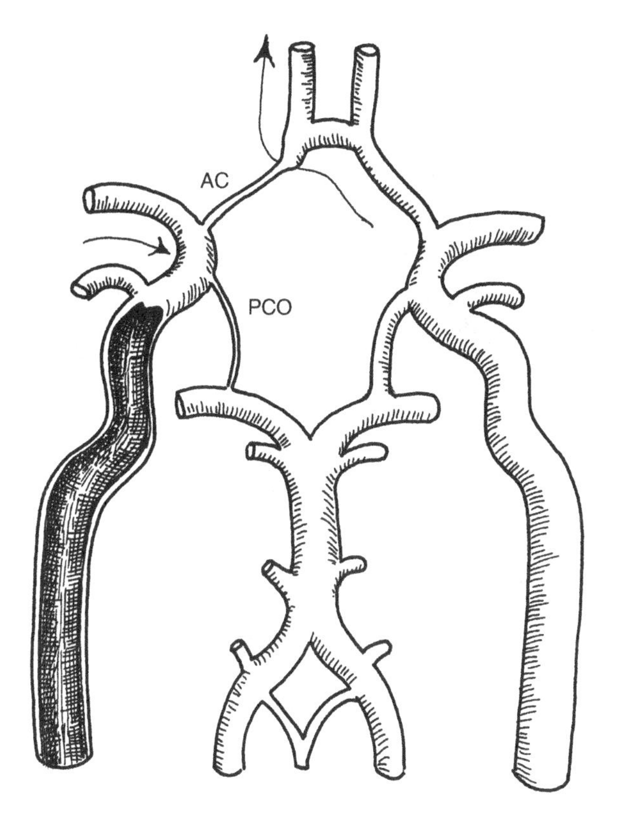

FIGURE 1–18. A patient with an internal carotid artery occlusion where the collateral flow may be reduced by the incomplete Circle of Willis [rudimentary right posterior communi-cating artery (PCO) and anterior cerebral artery (AC)].

arteries. Figures 1–16, 1–17, and 1–18 summarize the important collateral pathways in patients with an occluded internal carotid artery.

Pathology

Numerous theories exist as to the mechanism by which atherosclerosis develops in the carotid arteries, but whether you prescribe to the mechanical, sheer stress, chemical injury, or infectious theory,[18] the basic lesion is essentially the same. Atherosclerosis accounts for approximately 90% of extracranial cerebrovascular disease, with the remaining 10% being attributed to such disease processes as fibromuscular dysplasia, traumatic or spontaneous dissection, aneurysms, and arteritis, including Takayasu's arteritis.

The carotid plaque of atherosclerosis consists of cholesterol deposition in the arterial intima and an associated inflammatory reaction that results in fibroblast proliferation. These plaques occur preferentially at areas of vessel bifurcations and the process is similar to that seen with coronary artery disease. It can begin in the bulbous portion of the internal carotid artery on its posterior lateral wall. The atherosclerosis appears as a fatty strip subintimally with a collection of fat cells that progresses to a fibrous plaque in the subendothelial layer, causing gradually decreasing flow. These plaques can enlarge in several ways. They may just continue to slowly enlarge from an accumulation of cholesterol and fibroblasts, leading to a central necrosis and rupture of the intimal lining of the vessel. This will lead to discharge of athromatous debris into the lumen of the vessel, which can embolize. The exposed necrotic core of the lesion can then become a nidus for platelet deposition and further embolization to the brain. Progressive accumulation of the arteriosclerotic process, often with thrombotic debris, may result in stenosis or total occlusion in the carotid artery, with subsequent thrombosis of the internal carotid artery distal to the lesion (Figure 1–19). Another mechanism by which there may be sudden plaque enlargement is intraplaque hemorrhage.[19] Intraplaque hemorrhage may produce acute narrowing of the lumen. If the intima overlining the site of the plaque hemorrhage ulcerates, the necrotic contents of the atheromas escape into the lumen and cause cerebral embolization with transient

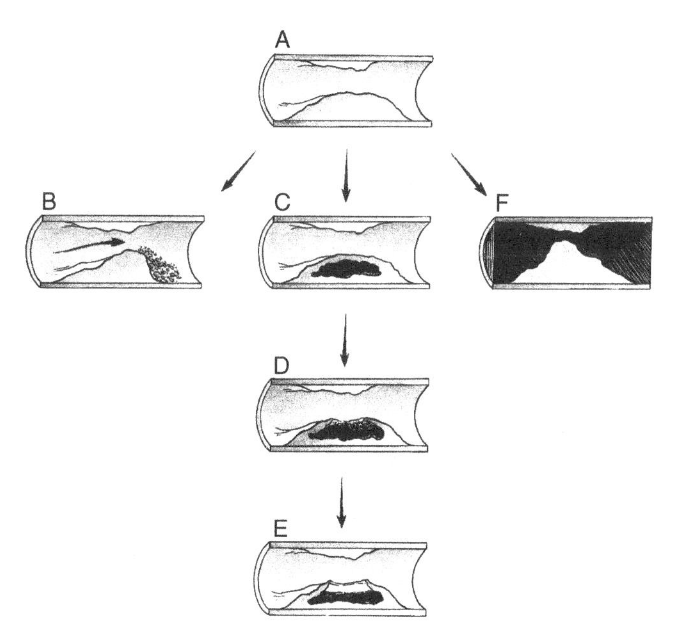

FIGURE 1–19. (A) Development of pathologic features in a plaque. (B) Partial obstruction created by a plaque may result in accumulation of a fibrin-platelet thrombus downstream from the obstruction. (C) The plaque may "soften" in its core. (D) This softening may break through to the surface, exposing the contents of the soft core to the bloodstream. (E) An ulceration may become covered by a fibrin deposit and even heal. (F) The increased size of the obstruction created by the plaque may result in thrombosis of the vessel lumen. (Courtesy of Springer-Verlag, *Surgery of the Arteries to the Head*, 1992, by Ramon Berguer and Edouard Kieffer, eds.)

ischemic attacks (TIAs) or cerebral infarcts. Nonulcerated lesions may alter flow and produce mural thrombi, which may fragment, causing embolization (Figure 1–20). The friability of these lesions is often not appreciated until seen by the vascular surgeon (Figure 1–21).

Blaisdell *et al.* and Hass *et al.*[20,21] studied the distribution of the atherosclerotic lesions involved in cerebrovascular disease and found that approximately one-third of responsible lesions occurred in the intracranial distribution that were surgically inaccessible. The remaining two-thirds of the lesions were in extracranial locations.

The common carotid bifurcation and the proximal internal carotid artery account for 50% of the lesions. Vertebral artery lesions account for 20%, left subclavian arterial lesions account for 10–15%, and lesions of the innominate and right subclavian arteries account for 15%. More than one lesion may be present (Figure 1–22).

Generally, the most common cause of cerebral ischemic events is embolic phenomena, primarily arterial in origin (carotid) and secondary to cardiac sources. The irregular plaque surface produces turbulence, which will act as a stimulus for platelet aggregation. If the platelet aggregates become large enough and embolize to an important vessel in the brain, symptoms will occur. If the platelet aggregates break up quickly from mechanical forces or from the effect of arterial prostacyclin, the symptoms will be transient, i.e., TIAs. If the embolic fragment persists, however, it can lead to focal infarction (Figure 1–23). As noted in Figure 1–24, the end result of the atherosclerotic plaque might be an internal carotid artery thrombosis. When an arteriosclerotic plaque expands to produce a critical reduction in blood flow, the vessel will ultimately undergo thrombosis. In the case of the internal carotid artery, this column of thrombus stops at the ophthalmic artery and remains stable, and if there is sufficient collateral circulation via the Circle of Willis, the thrombotic event may be entirely asymptomatic (Figure 1–24). However, if small thrombi rather than a thrombotic column form and are subsequently carried to the intracranaial vessels by continuous blood flow, then the patient will experience cerebral symptoms that can vary from transient amaurosis fugax or hemispheric events to a profound hemiplegia, depending upon the extent of the propagated thrombus or embolus (Figure 1–25). In addition, if the collateral circulation to the Circle of Willis is inadequate, the sudden loss of blood flow through a diseased internal carotid artery may induce a sudden drop in flow to the cerebral hemisphere, resulting in ischemic infarction as a consequence of inadequate proximal blood flow.

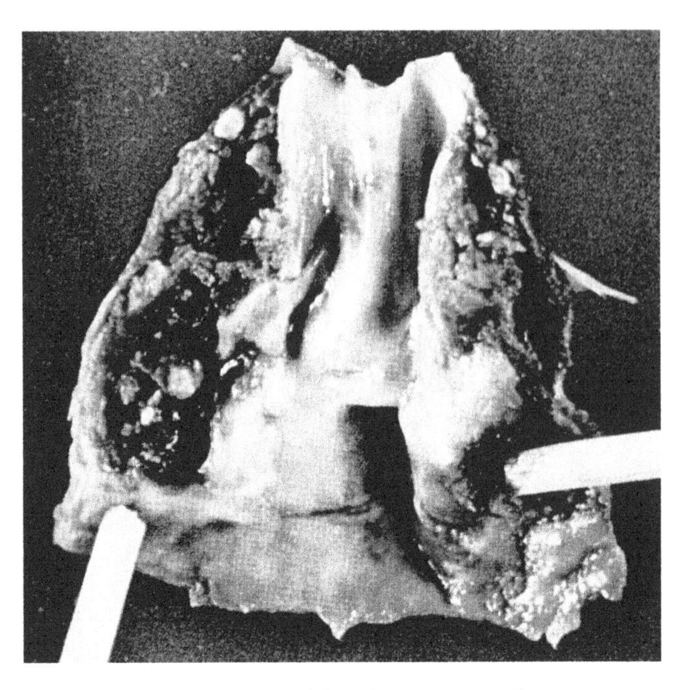

FIGURE 1–21. Carotid endarterectomy plaque.

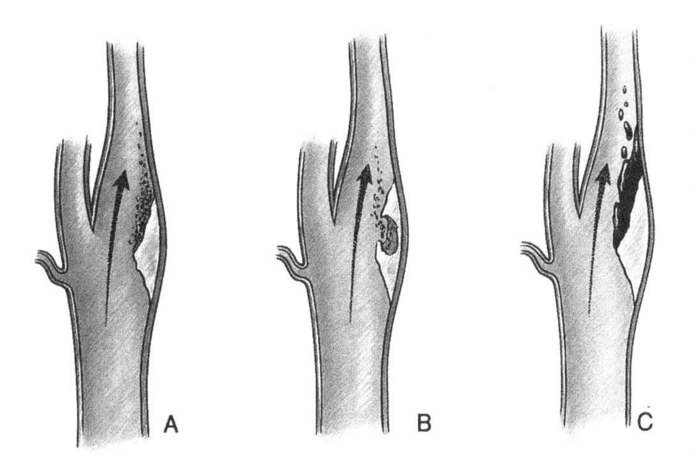

FIGURE 1–20. (A–C) Three mechanisms for thromboembolization from an internal carotid plaque. (A) Fibrin-platelet aggregates associated with an obstructing plaque. (B) Atheromatous contents. (C) Thrombus forming on the surface. (Courtesy of Springer-Verlag, *Surgery of the Arteries to the Head*, 1992, by Ramon Berguer and Edouard Kieffer, eds.)

A less common cause of cerebrovascular ischemia is fibromuscular dysplasia (FMD), which is usually more distally located in the internal carotid artery. The most common form of the disease is characterized by hyperplasia of the media producing alternating bands of thinned areas, leading to a beady appearance on angiography. Often the internal carotid artery is involved at long lengths. Always look for evidence of fibromuscular dysplasia elsewhere. It will involve both internal carotid arteries in 65% of patients.[22]

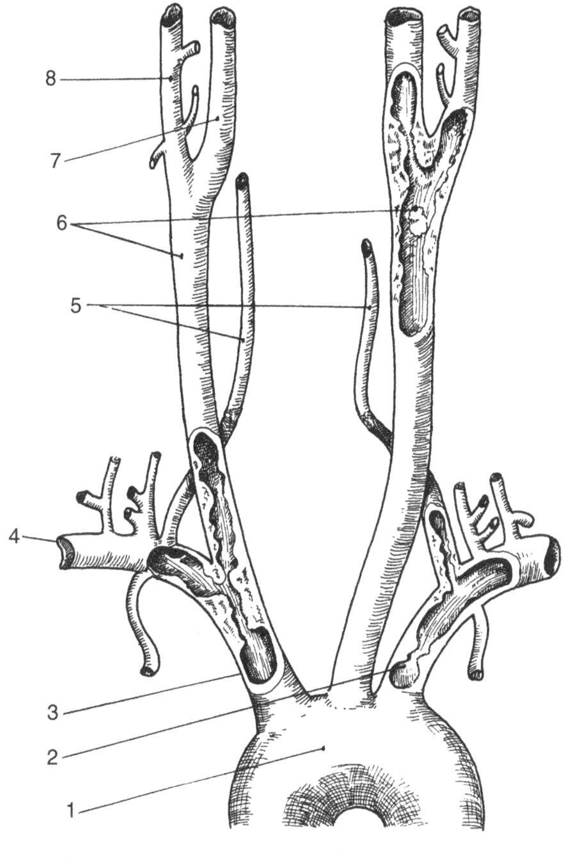

FIGURE 1–22. Sites of atheroclerosis of brachiocepahalic vessels: (1) aortic arch, (2) left subclavian artery, (3) innominate artery, (4) right subclavian artery, (5) right and left vertebral arteries, (6) right and left common carotid arteries, (7) right internal carotid artery, (8) right external carotid artery (note atherosclerosis at the left subclavian, left vertebral, innominate with proximal right common carotid and subclavian arteries, and left carotid bifurcation).

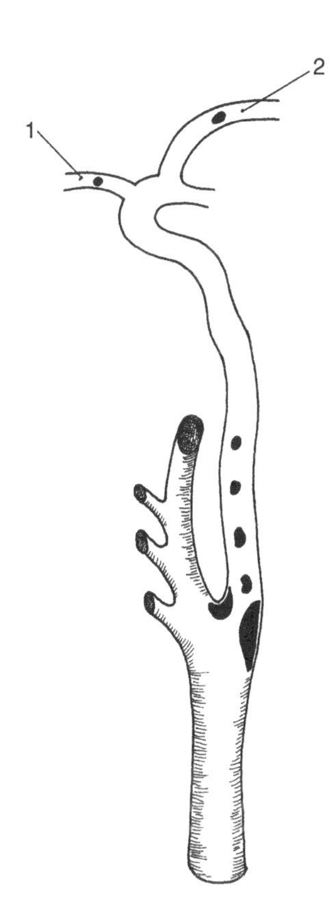

FIGURE 1–23. Embolization from an internal carotid artery stenotic lesion to the ophthalmic artery (1) and middle cerebral artery (2).

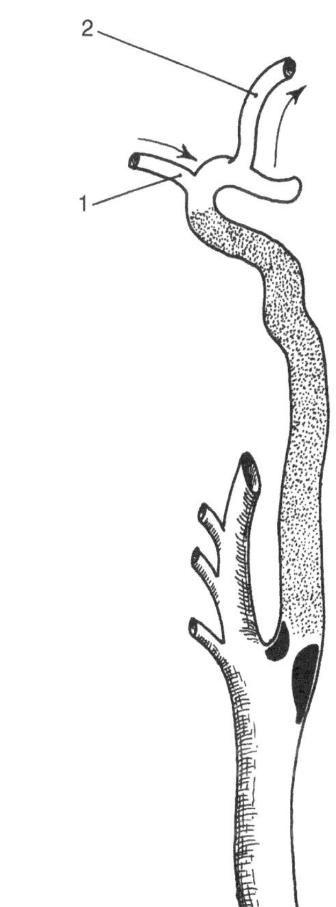

FIGURE 1–24. Internal carotid artery thrombosis with retrograde flow via the ophthalmic artery (1) to the terminal internal carotid artery and middle cerebral artery (2).

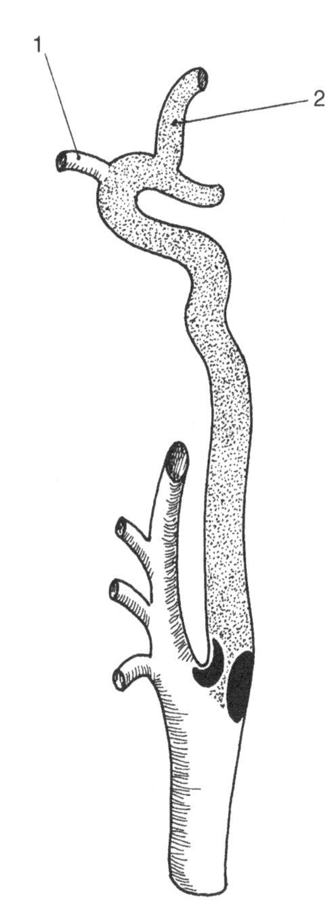

FIGURE 1–25. Internal carotid artery thrombosis that extends to the ophthalmic artery (1) and terminal internal carotid artery and middle cerebral artery (2).

Pathophysiology

It has been stated that a 70–80% reduction of the cross-sectional area of the arterial lumen must be present to produce a hemodynamically significant drop in the usual flow rate in the cerebrovascular system.[23] However, this may not always be the case. Important mechanisms of collateral flow and hemodynamic events that decrease cardiac output or systemic blood pressure, such as postural hypotension and cardiac arrhythmia, may produce transient episodes of ischemia. Embolization has been a documented cause of TIAs by proven ophthalmologic examination. Intraluminal particles of platelet fibrin aggregates, cholesterol fragments, and small clots have been noted. Most TIAs are probably caused by this mechanism. There is a permanent neurologic deficit as a result of permanently disrupted flow. A pale infarct occurs with focal cell necrosis and cerebral softening. The blood vessels lose integrity at the periphery of the infarct at a relatively ischemic spot. However, where neural death has not occurred, neurologic function may be altered and blood flow, while slow, may still be present.

Clinical Syndromes

The following well-defined syndromes of cerebrovascular ischemia have emerged:

1. TIAs are focal neurologic symptoms or deficits that usually clear completely within 2h. Some last for only a few moments, and others last for a few hours, but no longer than 24h.
2. Reversible ischemic neurologic deficits (RIND) are focal findings that clear over a period of days.
3. Minor stroke, which is defined as a neurologic deficit that clears completely in less than a week.
4. Major stroke, which is defined as a major neurologic deficit that lasts longer than a week.
5. Stroke in evolution or progressing stroke.
6. Complete stroke is a stroke with a significant return of function.
7. Diffuse cerebral ischemia or "low flow" syndrome.

Each of these syndromes requires a thorough history, physical, and neurologic evaluation with close attention to the severity of associated cardiovascular disease, hypertension, diabetes, neurologic aid, and diagnostic testing.

Over two-thirds of patients who have strokes have had prior TIAs. The mechanism by which TIAs occur is usually an embolic process. The source for these emboli can be from a number of sources—intracranial lesions, extracranial carotid, extracranial arch vessel lesions, primary cardiac thrombus, or even paradoxical emboli. The majority of TIAs will come from carotid bifurcation lesions, and this must be the site that is worked up first in these patients. When taking a history from patients who present with TIAs, it is important to obtain information as to previous episodes. Patients with a carotid source for their TIA will generally report having identical previous neurologic deficits, in contrast to cardiac TIAs that may vary; this is based on the principles of laminar flow within the carotid vessels that send the embolus to the same area each time.

The carotid TIA manifestations include transient ipsilateral blindness or visual impairment (amaurosis fugax) and contralateral sensory or motor deficit. There may be a degree of altered consciousness. Speech deficit may be present if the dominant hemisphere is affected.

The patient with amaurosis fugax will describe these episodes as someone pulling a shade over one of their eyes, which quickly resolves. A funduscopic inspection of these patients may reveal Hollenhorst plaques, bright yellow spots on the retina that represent cholesterol crystals. These may be present in asymptomatic patients with atherosclerotic disease as well.

Nonhemispheric TIAs present a dilemma to the vascular surgeon. These patients will present with symptoms of dizziness, ataxia, vertigo, bilateral neurologic or visual events, or even syncope. These symptoms may be related to an embolic event from primary atherosclerotic lesions involving the vertebrobasilar system, resulting in an ischemic event to the posterior brain or brain stem. Another mechanism for this may be a significantly diminished blood flow to the brain, or diffuse cerebral ischemia. To have this situation, the patient must have severe stenoses involving the majority of the extracranial vessels, incomplete Circle of Willis, or an altered flow state, i.e., subclavian steal syndrome.

Other clinical syndromes include reversible ischemic neurologic event (RIND). RIND is a focal neurologic deficit that takes several days to completely resolve. The mechanism by which RIND occurs is poorly understood. It is generally felt that these patients actually suffer focal cerebral infarctions, but these areas are very small and surrounding tissue compensates for the loss. Another syndrome is crescendo TIAs. These are hemispheric deficits that resolve within minutes, but occur with increasing frequency. Stroke in evolution is where initial neurologic symptoms may not completely resolve and subsequent neurologic events are progressive.

A completed stroke is a neurologic deficit that occurs and does not have a complete resolution of symptoms. This may be the result of a large embolus, a small embolus to an end vessel with surrounding vessel thrombosis, or thrombosis of the internal carotid artery.

Physical Examination

With a good history and thorough physical examination, it is possible to diagnose the nature and location of the vascular lesions with reasonable certainty, and the diagnosis can usually be confirmed by the noninvasive techniques to be described. The physical examination includes examining or checking the pulses of the superficial temporal artery, the carotid artery, both high and low in the neck, the subclavian artery above the mid-portion of the clavicle, and the radial artery. One side of the body should be compared with the other. The blood pressures in each arm should be compared. A 15–20 mm Hg difference in blood pressure may indicate a significant lesion of the subclavian or innominate arteries. Bruits in the neck, indicating turbulence in stenotic arteries, should be carefully evaluated. Listening for a bruit is also important. Remember that a near or total occlusion of the internal carotid artery has no bruit at all. A good pulsation may be felt under the mandible when a totally occluded internal carotid artery is present due to the palpation of the common carotid artery and the external carotid artery. These cannot be differentiated on a physical examination. It is sometimes difficult to palpate the subclavian arteries in obese or heavy-set individuals, and it is necessary to determine that cervical bruits are not really aortic ejection murmurs. A carotid bruit, heard louder at the level of the mandible than in the lower part of the neck, would probably indicate a stenosis of the internal carotid artery. This could also represent a stenosis of the innominate artery. Moderate stenosis may result in a systolic bruit, whereas more severe stenosis results in a systolic bruit that ends in diastole. A complete neurologic examination should be done.

Investigations

The work-up of patients presenting with asymptomatic carotid bruits or TIAs has changed over recent years. These changes have occurred because of recently published recommendations and improved noninvasive diagnostic tools. Initial screening in all of these patients must include carotid duplex scanning; and based on the findings of this study, the patient can take one of several routes. First, the patient may have no significant disease by duplex. These patients with classical hemispheric TIAs will require a cardiac work-up and, if negative, a systemic disease work-up, or possibly an arteriogram. Second, the patient may have a severe or tight stenosis or ulcerative plaque. In this situation, depending on the patient's operative risk, the surgeon's skill, the accuracy of the duplex, and the radiologist's complication rates, this patient could undergo magnetic resonance angiography or conventional arteriography, or surgery, without further work-up. Third, in patients with hemispheric TIAs and only mild to moderate disease by duplex, other sources should be explored, as well as carotid magnetic resonance angiography or arteriography. Again, many factors must be considered when working up patients for TIAs, and each patient must be individualized. A practical approach is described in Chapter 13.

Arteriography

Intraarterial injection is usually performed according to the Seldinger technique. The most commonly used artery is the common femoral artery, and to a lesser extent, the axillary or brachial arteries. Digital subtraction angiography (DSA) uses real-time digital video processing to detect the small amount of contrast medium that has been injected into the artery (Figures 1–26, 1–27, 1–28, and 1–29).

Interpretation of Stenosis

There are several methods of estimating stenoses. One of the most common methods described is the one

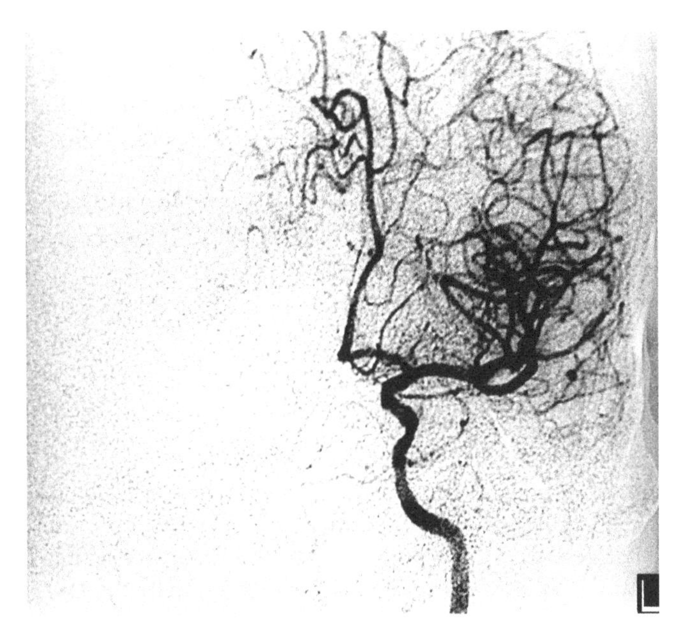

FIGURE 1–26. Carotid arteriogram showing a normal distal internal carotid artery and its two major branches: anterior and middle cerebral arteries.

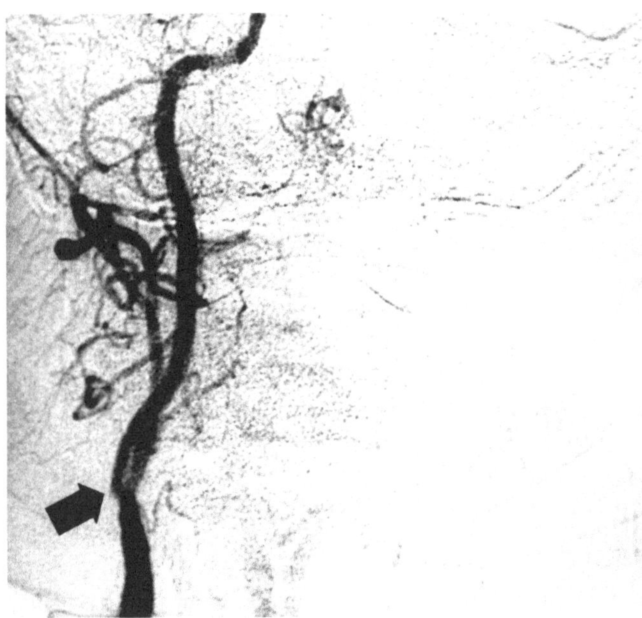

FIGURE 1–28. Carotid arteriogram showing severe stenosis of the carotid bifurcation and proximal internal carotid artery (arrow).

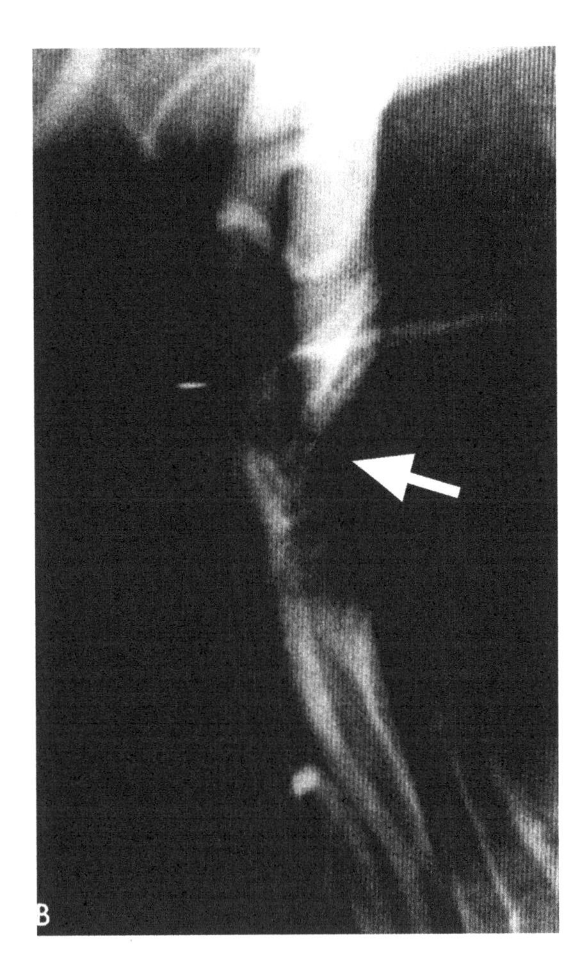

FIGURE 1–27. Carotid arteriogram showing tight stenosis of the proximal internal carotid artery (arrow).

used by the NASCET trial,[11] where the percentage of stenosis is calculated as a diameter reduction. The percentage of stenosis is determined by comparing the least transverse diameter at the stenosis to the diameter of the distal uninvolved internal carotid artery where the arterial walls become parallel (Figure 1–30). The percentage may then be expressed as the function of either the diameter or the cross-sectional area as follows.

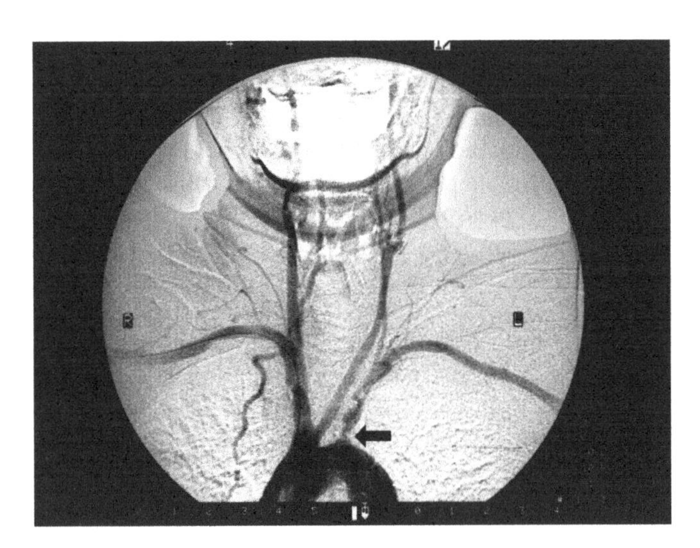

FIGURE 1–29. Four vessel arch aortogram showing severe stenosis of the proximal left subclavian artery (arrow).

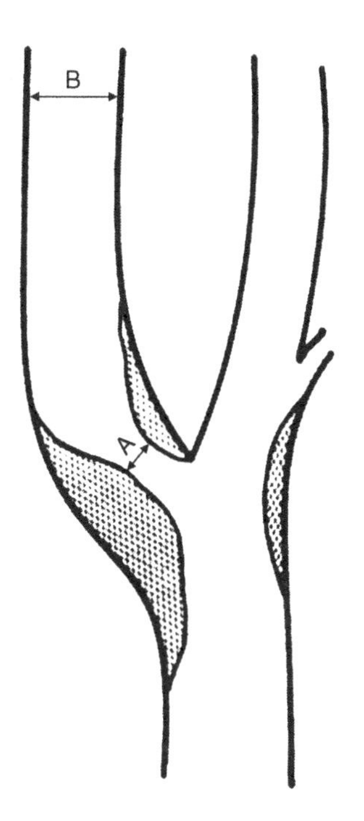

FIGURE 1–30. Information required for calculating the percentage of internal carotid artery stenosis. See text for details.

Percentage of Stenosis Calculation— Diameter Reduction

Percentage of stenosis equals 1 minus A divided by B multiplied by 100, i.e.

$$[1 - (A/B)] \times 100$$

Percentage of Stenosis Calculation— Area Reduction

To calculate the percentage of stenosis on the basis of the vessel cross-sectional area, and assuming the lesion is symmetrical, as seen in Figure 1–30, the percentage of stenosis (area reduction) will equal (1 minus A^2 divided by B^2) multiplied by 100, i.e.

$$[1 - (A^3/B^2)] \times 100$$

The third method of calculating the percentage of stenosis is to divide the area of residual lumen (A) by the area of the true lumen at the level of the stenosis (C), as adapted by the ECST, i.e.

$$\frac{C - A}{C} \times 100$$

This calculation will require a transverse view of the vessel in question.

Generally speaking, a stenosis that reduces the vessel diameter by 50% (which is equal to a 75% area reduction) is considered hemodynamically significant.

Treatment

Medical therapy generally includes control of risk factors, e.g., weight, a low-cholesterol diet that may enhance a normal endothelial cell metabolism, antihypertensive drugs for hypertensive patients to decrease shear forces on the endothelialized cells, and cessation of smoking. Specific medical therapy includes antiplatelet agents, such as aspirin, dipyridamole (Persantine, Boehringer), or combined aspirin and extended release dipyridamole (25 mg/200 mg capsule, Aggrenox, Boehringer), or clopidogrel (Plavix, Sanofi-Synthelabo).

Surgical intervention, a carotid endarterectomy, is indicated in patients with significant carotid artery stenosis (at least 50%) associated with TIA symptoms or strokes with a good recovery, as recommended by the NASCET study.[11] The NASCET study concluded, after analyzing 659 patients with TIAs or nondisabling strokes occurring within 6 months preceding presentations and with ipsilateral carotid stenosis of 70–99%, that the cumulative risk of an ipsilateral stroke occurring by the 18 month follow-up was 26% for 331 patients who were treated medically and 9% for 328 patients who were treated surgically. This yielded an absolute risk reduction of 17% ($p < 0.001$). The corresponding incidence of major or fatal ipsilateral stroke was 13% and 3% for medically and surgically treated groups, respectively. This translates into an absolute risk reduction of 11%, or a greater than 5 to 1 benefit in favor of operation ($p < 0.001$). The NASCET investigators concluded that carotid endarterectomy was highly beneficial for patients with recent hemispheric or retinal TIAs, or those with nondisabling stroke in the presence of ipsilateral high-grade carotid stenoses. The NASCET study also concluded that carotid endarterectomy was highly beneficial for symptomatic patients with 50% to <70% carotid artery stenosis.[24]

Patients with stenoses of >60% can be candidates for carotid endarterectomy if they are good risk patients.[7] The ACAS study also concluded that carotid endarterectomy was superior to medical therapy in good risk patients, and it reduced stroke by 55% over a 5-year period when surgical therapy was compared to medical therapy (5% versus 11%). Recently, the ACST Collaborative Group reported on the results of carotid endarterectomy in the prevention of stroke for ≥70% asymptomatic stenosis. Their conclusions were somewhat similar to the American study (the ACAS): in asymptomatic patients younger than 75 years of age with a carotid diameter reduction of 70%, immediate carotid endarterectomy decreased the net 5-year stroke risk by one-half, from 12% to 6% (including the 3% perioperative hazard). [9]

Recently, carotid angioplasty/stenting (CAS) has been recommended as an alternative to carotid endarterectomy. Several randomized and nonrandomized prospective trials have been conducted over the past few years to evaluate the efficacy of CAS in the prevention of strokes for both symptomatic and asymptomatic patients. Two of these studies are randomized prospective controlled trials. One of these, the SAPPHIRE study, just reported their early results comparing CAS to carotid endarterectomy in high-risk patients. The SAPPHIRE study was a randomized trial that compared carotid stenting using the angioguard emboli protection device to carotid endarterectomy in patients at increased risk for carotid surgery. Symptomatic patients with ≥50% stenosis and asymptomatic patients with ≥80% stenosis by ultrasound, who had one or more of the comorbidity criteria that placed them at increased risk for surgery, were included. The primary endpoints were death, stroke, and myocardial infarction at 30 days postprocedure, and ipsilateral stroke and death at 1 year. The composite endpoint of death, stroke, and myocardial infarction at 30 days was 5.8% for the stent group and 12.6% for the surgery group ($p = 0.047$). The trial concluded that carotid stenting in high-risk patients was comparable or somewhat favorable to carotid endarterectomy when combined death, stroke, and myocardial infarction were considered.[25]

The CREST (Carotid Revascularization Endarterectomy versus Stent trial), which compares the efficacy of carotid endarterectomy and carotid artery stenting in symptomatic patients in a randomized fashion, is presently being conducted. Recent data on the lead-in cases demonstrated a 30-day stroke and death rate of 3.6%. An update on 500 lead-in cases has demonstrated a 30-day stroke and death rate of 2.1% for asymptomatic patients and 5% for symptomatic patients with carotid artery stenting.[26]

References

1. Fields WS, North RR, Hass WK, *et al.* Joint study of extracranial arterial occlusion as a cause of stroke. I. Organization of study and survey of patient population. JAMA 1968;203:955–960.
2. Sherman DG, Dyken ML, Fisher M, *et al.* Antithrombotic therapy for cerebrovascular disorders. Chest 1989;95 (Suppl.):140S–155S.
3. Feldmann E. Intracerebral hemorrhage. In: Fisher M (ed). *Clinical Atlas of Cerebrovascular Disorders,* pp. 11.1–11.7. London: Mosby-Year Book Europe, 1994.
4. Eastcott HHG, Pickering GW, Robb CG. Reconstruction of internal carotid artery in a patient with intermittent attacks of hemiplegia. Lancet 1954;2:994–996.
5. DeBakey ME. Successful carotid endarterectomy for cerebrovascular insufficiency. Nineteen-year follow-up. JAMA 1975;233:1083–1085.
6. The CASSANOVA Study Group. Carotid surgery vs. medical therapy in asymptomatic carotid stenosis. Stroke 1991;22:1229–1235.
7. Asymptomatic Carotid Atherosclerosis Study Group. Study design for randomized prospective trial of carotid endarterectomy for asymptomatic atherosclerosis. Stroke 1989;20:844–849.
8. Hobson RW II. Management of symptomatic and asymptomatic carotid stenosis: Results of current randomized clinical trials. In: Bernstein EF (ed). *Vascular Diagnosis*, 4th ed., pp. 446–451. St. Louis, MO: Mosby, 1993.
9. MRC, Asymptomatic Carotid Surgery Trial (ACST) Collaborative Group. Prevention of disabling and fatal stroke by successful carotid endarterectomy in patients without recent neurological symptoms: Randomized controlled trial. Lancet 2004;363:1491–1500.
10. Mayberg MR, Wilson SE, Yatsu F. For the Veterans Affairs cooperative study program 309 trialist group. Carotid endarterectomy and prevention of cerebral ischemia in symptomatic carotid stenosis. JAMA 1991;266: 3289–3294.
11. North American Symptomatic Carotid Endarterectomy Trial Collaborators. Beneficial effect of carotid endarterectomy in symptomatic patients with high-grade carotid stenosis. N Engl J Med 1991;325:445–453.
12. European Carotid Surgery Trialists' Collaborative Group, MRC European Carotid Surgery Trial. Interim results for symptomatic patients with severe (70–99%) or with mild (0–29%) carotid stenosis. Lancet 1991;337:1235–1243.
13. Anson BJ, McVay CB. *Surgical Anatomy,* Vol. 1, pp. 3–6. Philadelphia, PA: WB Saunders Co., 1971.
14. Larson CP Jr. Anesthesia and control of the cerebral circulation. In: Wylie EJ, Ehrenfeld WK (eds). *Extracranial Cerebrovascular Disease: Diagnosis and Management,* pp. 152–183. Philadelphia, PA: WB Saunders Co., 1970.
15. Reivich M, Hooling HE, Roberts B, *et al.* Reversal of blood flow through the vertebral artery and its effect on cerebral circulation. N Engl J Med 1961;265:878–885.
16. Connolly JE, Stemmer EA. Endarterectomy of the external carotid artery: Its importance in the surgical management of extracranial cerebrovascular occlusive disease. Arch Surg 1973;106:799–802.
17. Ehrenfeld WK, Lord RSA. Transient monocular blindness through collateral pathways. Surgery 1969;65:911–915.
18. Cook PJ, Honeybourne D, LIP GY, *et al.* Chlamydia pneumoniae antibody titers are significantly associated with stroke and transient cerebral ischemia: The West Birmingham Stroke Project. Stroke 1998;29(2):404–410.
19. Sillesen H, Nielsen T. Clinical significance of intraplaque hemorrhage in carotid artery disease. J Neuroimaging 1998;8(1):15–19.
20. Blaisdell FW, Hall AD, Thomas AN, *et al.* Cerebrovascular occlusive disease. Experience with panarteriography in 300 consecutive cases. Calif Med 1965;103:321–329.
21. Hass WK, Fields WS, North RR, *et al.* Joint study of extracranial arterial occlusion. II. Arteriography, techniques, sites, and complications. JAMA 1968;203:961–968.
22. AbuRahma AF. Overview of Cerebrovascular disease. In: AbuRahma AF, Diethrich EB (eds). *Current Noninvasive*

Vascular Diagnosis, pp. 1–7. Littleton, MA: PSG Publishing, 1988.
23. Strandness DE Jr, Sumner DS. *Hemodynamics for Surgeons,* pp. 512–524. New York: Grune & Stratton, Inc., 1975.
24. Barnett HJM, Taylor DW, Eliasziw MA, *et al.* For the NASCET collaborators: Benefits of carotid endarterectomy in patients with symptomatic, moderate, or severe stenosis. N Engl J Med 1998;339:1415–1425.
25. Yadav JS, Wholey MH, Kuntz RE, *et al.* Protected carotid artery stenting versus endarterectomy in high-risk patients. N Engl J Med 2004;351:1493–1501.
26. Hobson RW II, Howard VJ, Roubin GS, Brott TG, Ferguson RD, Popma JJ, Graham DL, Howard G, CREST Investigators. Carotid artery stenting is associated with increased complications in octogenarians: 30-day stroke and death rates in the CREST lead-in phase. J Vasc Surg 2004;40:1106–1111.

2
Overview of Various Noninvasive Cerebrovascular Techniques

Ali F. AbuRahma

Contrast cerebrovascular arteriography has been the definitive diagnostic technique for evaluation of cerebrovascular disease; however, its limitations and complications played a great role in the drive to develop accurate, reliable noninvasive diagnostic procedures. Although arteriography serves to define anatomic lesions and is indispensable for most vascular surgery, it provides little objective data regarding physiologic disability, nor is it without risk.

Most complications of cerebral arteriography can be assigned to technical error, embolic events, or neurotoxic effects of the contrast material. Catheter-related injuries at the puncture site are near 0.2%, with mortality estimated at 0.02%.[1] Allergic reactions to the contrast medium occur in about 2% of cases, while the overall incidence of neurologic deficits is around 1% if the transfemoral approach is used (the figure is slightly higher with the transaxillary route). Both the North American Symptomatic Carotid Endarterectomy Trial Collaborators (NASCET) and the Asymptomatic Carotid Atherosclerosis Study Group (ACAS) reported stroke rates of around 1%.[2,3] Recent literature reported major complication rates of 5.9% and 9.1% for cerebral angiography.[4,5]

A technical shortcoming of cerebral arteriography is its failure to delineate shallow, superficially ulcerating lesions. Because of this, a potential source of cerebral emboli could be overlooked. If we add to these risks the disadvantages of patient discomfort, the need for hospitalization, and expense, there is little wonder that many physicians are reluctant to subject their patients to cerebral arteriography. This makes the noninvasive vascular diagnostic techniques highly desirable and cost-effective alternatives.

In the past 30 years extensive research has been done in the field of cerebrovascular diagnosis, resulting in the development of a broad range of noninvasive diagnostic tools, extending even to the use of radioactive isotope scanning. While these nuclear studies have been useful in detecting intracranial lesions, they have not been as effective as the noninvasive techniques in localizing extracranial disease, the main site of pathology in the carotid tree.

Ultrasound was first applied to the study of the carotid circulation as early as 1954,[6] but it was not until 1967 that its clinical application in velocity detection was reported.[7] Brockenbrough, in 1970, further refined the technique and popularized the flowmeter.[8]

In 1971, D. E. Hokanson, working in Eugene Strandness' laboratory at the University of Washington in Seattle, was able to piece together all the elements necessary to provide the first noninvasive visualization of an arterial segment using pulsed Doppler methods.[9] The concept was quite simple. If one knew the size and location of the Doppler transducer, the position of the pulsed Doppler sample volume, and could transfer this to a cathode ray tube, it should be possible to paint a picture containing all points within an arterial segment where flow was occurring. This led to the development of ultrasonic arteriography, which was successfully applied to the study of carotid artery disease. Although this method worked, there were significant limitations: (1) it was time-consuming, (2) an experienced technologist was required, (3) the image was distorted by the patient's movement, (4) arterial wall calcification blocked the transmission of ultrasound, and (5) the arterial wall and plaque were not visualized. Because of these limitations, Strandness and colleagues began exploring the use of B-mode ultrasound to visualize the arterial wall. Very early in their application of this method they studied a patient whose internal carotid artery appeared patent by ultrasonic imaging but was found to be occluded by arteriography. This led to the obvious conclusion that thrombus may have acoustic properties similar to flowing blood and, thus, would be missed by imaging alone. The solution appeared to be the addition of a Doppler probe to the ultrasonic imaging to permit assessment of the presence or absence of flow. It was this combination of imaging plus Doppler that led to the term ultrasonic duplex scanner.[10] When real-time fast

A.F. Aburahma, J.J. Bergan (eds.), *Noninvasive Cerebrovascular Diagnosis*, DOI 10.1007/978-1-84882-957-2_2,

Fourier transform (FFT) spectrum analysis was added, the basic components of the systems that are in widespread use today became available.

Another breakthrough came in 1974, when Gee *et al.*[11] introduced the use of the oculopneumoplethysmograph for carotid disease screening.

Due to the propensity for atherosclerotic disease to attack the extracranial (vs. intracranial) carotid network, noninvasive testing has concentrated on this area.

Generally speaking, there are two types of noninvasive approaches to extracranial circulation: direct, which examines flow changes in the cervical portion of the carotid artery near the bifurcation (site of the majority of lesions); and indirect, which detects significant stenotic lesions by assessing flow changes at locations distal to the bifurcation.

Duplex with color flow imaging systems using pulsed wave Doppler signals are now the most common direct methods for carotid evaluation; indirect methods such as continuous wave Doppler technique, periorbital Doppler,[8,12] and oculopneumoplethysmography[11,13,14] are outdated and are no longer used in the modern vascular laboratory for the diagnosis of carotid artery disease.

Indirect Methods

From a historical perspective, oculopneumoplethysmography (OPG/Gee) detects the ophthalmic artery pressure by suction ophthalmodynamometry. The main indication for OPG/Gee is the identification of carotid artery stenosis,[11,13,14] however, it can also be used in measuring ophthalmic artery pressure during external compression of the common carotid artery, reflecting the collateral pressure of the ipsilateral internal carotid artery. It may also be helpful in determining the safety of ligating or resecting the carotid artery.

This procedure has some limitations in common with all other types of oculoplethysmography, such as it cannot be used with certain types of eye disease and cannot be applied to some patients with severe hypertension if the systolic endpoint cannot be measured (fewer than 2% of patients). Also, it cannot distinguish between total occlusion and severe stenoses cannot detect subcritical stenoses or locate the exact site of the stenoses, and is not useful in documenting the progression of disease.

OPG/Gee measures the ophthalmic arterial systolic pressure by applying a vacuum to the eye. As the vacuum distorts the shape of the globe, intraocular pressure increases to the point at which it obliterates the arterial inflow. Strip chart recordings are then made as the vacuum is slowly decreased. The pulse wave reappears when the ophthalmic arterial pressure exceeds the intraocular pressure. A vacuum of 300 or 500 mm Hg is applied according to the patient's baseline blood pressure. Since the pressure in the ophthalmic artery reflects the pressure in the distal internal carotid artery, the measurement of ophthalmic arterial pressure using this test can be useful in detecting hemodynamically significant carotid stenoses.

Abnormal findings are ophthalmic systolic pressures that differ by equal to or more than 5 mm Hg and/or an abnormal ratio of ophthalmic-to-systolic pressure.

Another indirect test that was used in the past is the periorbital Doppler examination (ophthalmosonometry), the principle of which is based on evaluating the Doppler velocity flow pattern in the accessible branches of the ophthalmic artery and assessing the response to compression of the branches of the external carotid. The identification of advanced internal carotid stenosis by examination of the periorbital flow patterns with the Doppler detector was first described by Brockenbrough in 1969.[8] The original technique described by Brockenbrough used a nondirectional velocity detector to examine the signal obtained from the supraorbital artery and the response to the compression of the superficial temporal artery.[8] Further refinement became possible with the development of the directional Doppler detector, which permitted the documentation of reverse flow in the branches of the ophthalmic artery.[15,16]

Direct Methods

Several direct methods that were used in the past are now outdated, including pulsed Doppler arteriography,[17] carotid phonoangiography,[18] color-coded echoflow,[19] radionuclide arteriography, and carotid scanning.[20,21]

Real-Time B-Mode Carotid Imaging

B-mode ultrasound imaging has been used extensively for visualizing soft tissue structures. Carotid arteries, however, could not be seen properly until the advent of real-time techniques that have overcome the problem of visualization. With B-mode imaging alone, variations in the acoustic properties of different tissues reflect ultrasound waves and generate an image of the tissues being examined. These variations in acoustic reflectance are represented visually by shades of gray on the image, which facilitates identification of different tissues. The vessel wall, because of its high reflectively, may thus be visualized. Yet it is this tissue interaction with ultrasound that has imposed severe limitations on techniques that use this method for visualizing atherosclerotic plaques and occluded arteries.

Unfortunately, methods currently used for processing the reflected ultrasound waves are often incapable of differentiating flowing blood, thrombus, and noncalcified

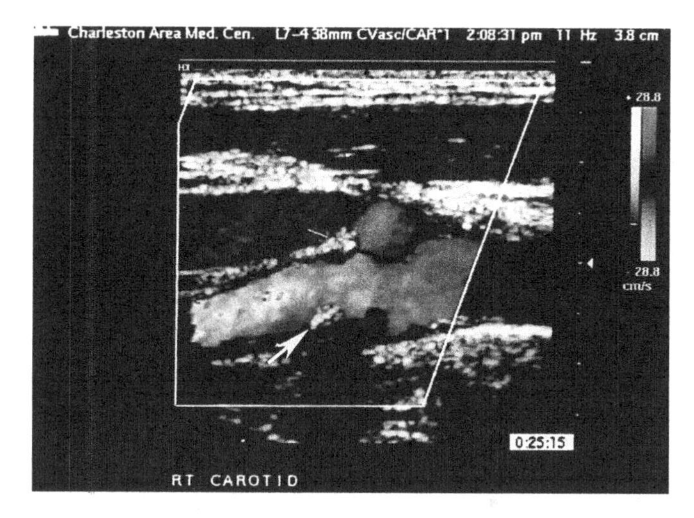

FIGURE 2–1. Color duplex ultrasound image of an internal carotid artery showing calcified plaque where a very dense acoustic signal is registered (arrow) with acoustic shadowing (underneath the arrow).

plaques. Thus, vessels that are completely occluded may appear patent. Likewise, noncalcified plaques may be entirely missed or, at best, only partly visualized. In addition, when atherosclerotic disease at the carotid bifurcation exists, calcium is a common component of the plaque and prevents the passage of ultrasound waves through this area. Thus, if there is a calcified plaque on the anterior wall of the vessel a very dense acoustic signal will be registered, but there will be no information concerning the lumen beneath the calcified segment. This is commonly referred to as acoustic shadowing (Figure 2–1). These limitations are largely overcome by combining B-mode imaging with flow detection techniques using Doppler, such as spectral waveform analysis and color flow imaging. Experience with B-mode imaging techniques for the classification of carotid artery disease has generally shown that interpretation of the image is most accurate for lesions of a minimal to moderate degree of stenosis, and least accurate for high-grade stenoses or occlusions. It is often difficult to estimate the size of the arterial lumen from a B-mode image because the interface between the arterial wall and flowing blood is not clearly seen. Calcified atherosclerotic plaque, which is extremely echogenic, results in bright echoes with acoustic shadows (Figure 2–1).

Continuous Wave and Pulse Doppler Wave Analysis

Nonimaging Doppler techniques can directly interrogate the common carotid, the internal carotid, and the external carotid arteries to detect a hemodynamically significant stenosis. Since these are nonimaging techniques, they provide only physiologic information and cannot differentiate a tight stenosis from occlusion. Information from more than one vessel along the path of the beam may also be included. A collateralized external carotid artery may be mistaken for an internal carotid artery when the internal carotid artery is actually occluded. These techniques require an experienced technologist.

Principles and Instrumentation

Either continuous wave Doppler or pulse Doppler can be used. Continuous wave Doppler emits ultrasound continuously and receives reflected wave continuously. The difference between the transmitted and received signals falls within the hearing range. The received signals can then be distinguished by their auditory characteristics. In addition, the signal can be evaluated visually on a strip chart recorder or with a spectral analysis. In pulse Doppler the beam of pulse Doppler ultrasound is not continuously transmitted and received. Range-gating allows signals only from specific depths to be processed, thereby controlling sample size and range resolution. Two vessels located directly above one another can be evaluated separately, and vessels can also be followed as their course changes.

Doppler Signal Displays

The display can be done using the following methods. (1) auditory—achieved by simply displaying the Doppler-shifted frequencies as an audible sound. (2) Analog recording—Doppler-shifted frequencies can be displayed on a strip chart recorder that incorporates a zero-crossing detector. The circuitry counts every time the input signal crosses the 0 baseline within a specific time span. Because the number of times the sound waves oscillate each second varies, for example, high-frequency waves have many oscillations while low-frequency waves have few, and because the direction of flow varies during the cardiac cycle, the machine estimates the frequency of the reflected signal and displays it.

The vertical access represents the amplitude of the Doppler-shifted frequencies while the horizontal axis represents time. Analog recording has the following limitations: it works poorly in the presence of background noise, it is amplitude dependent, it does not display two peak frequencies, and its poor directional resolution may cause a venous and arterial signal to be added together. (3) Spectrum analysis—the FFT method makes it possible to display the individual frequencies that make up the return signal. Information related to the intensity of the spectrum is also possible: for example, a narrow well-defined spectrum is displayed when a limited number of frequencies is evident in a laminar flow. Spectral broadening represents a variety of frequencies and is often associated with turbulent flow. The velocity profile shows various frequency shifts on the vertical axis and time on the horizontal axis.

Technique

The patient is positioned supine with the head on a pillow. Optimal signals are usually obtained with the neck slightly hyperextended and the head slightly rotated away from the side being examined. Acoustic coupling gel is applied to the area to be examined. Pointing cephalad and maintaining a 45° to 60° angle of insonation, the continuous wave Doppler probe is placed on one side of the trachea and just above the clavicle to investigate the common carotid artery. As the examiner moves the probe cephalad, a change in the Doppler arterial signal signifies the bifurcation of the common carotid artery into the external carotid artery, which usually courses medially, and the internal carotid artery, which usually courses laterally.

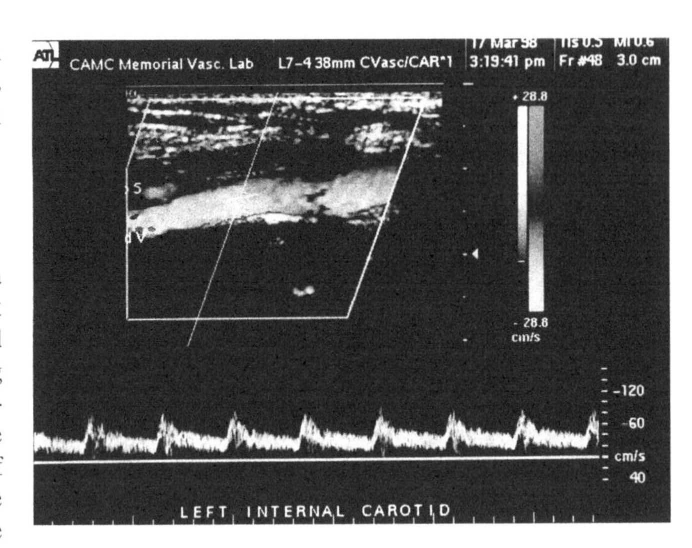

FIGURE 2–3. Color duplex ultrasound image of the internal carotid artery. Note that the waveform of the internal carotid artery has a rapid upstroke and downstroke with a high diastolic component. The diastolic notch may not be evident.

Interpretation

Normal Findings

The external carotid artery supplies blood to the vascular bed that has high peripheral resistance. Therefore, its signal is more pulsatile and very similar to the signal from peripheral arteries, such as the common femoral artery. As shown in Figure 2–2 the external carotid artery has a rapid upstroke and downstroke with a very low diastolic component. The diastolic notch is clearly seen and tapping the superficial temporal artery causes oscillations in the waveform (Figure 2–2).

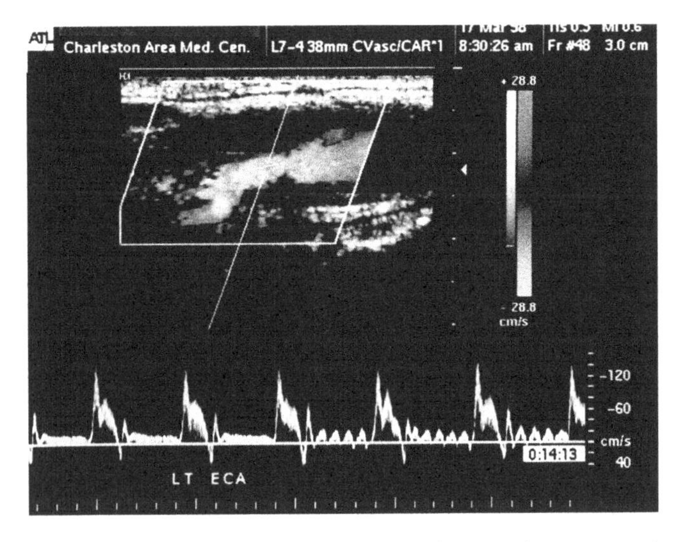

FIGURE 2–2. Color duplex ultrasound image of an external carotid artery. Note that the external carotid artery has a rapid upstroke and downstroke with a very low diastolic component. The diastolic notch is clearly seen and tapping of the superficial temporal artery causes oscillations in the waveform (bottom right).

The internal carotid artery signal is slightly more high-pitched and continuous than the signal from the external carotid artery. The blood flow in the internal carotid artery is less pulsatile since the brain is a low-resistance vascular bed, with increased flow during diastole. As shown in Figure 2–3, the waveform of the internal carotid artery has a rapid upstroke and downstroke with a high diastolic component. A diastolic notch may not be evident. The common carotid artery, meanwhile, has a flow characteristic of both the internal and external carotid arteries (Figure 2–4).

In a pulsed Doppler tracing, and because the sample volume would be more precisely placed in a center stream, the signals will have a narrow band of frequencies in systole with a blank area under that narrow band. The narrow band is called the spectral envelope; the blank area is called the frequency window or spectral window. The presence of these features is generally seen in laminar flow (Figure 2–5). In contrast, in continuous wave Doppler, because of the inability to regulate sample size or depth, a frequency window is not clear (Figure 2–6).

Abnormal Findings

The auditory signal from a stenotic vessel is characterized by a higher than normal pitch, with a very high-pitched hissing or squealing type of signal evident at significant stenosis. The waveform from a stenotic vessel has a higher than normal amplitude because of the accelerated flow through

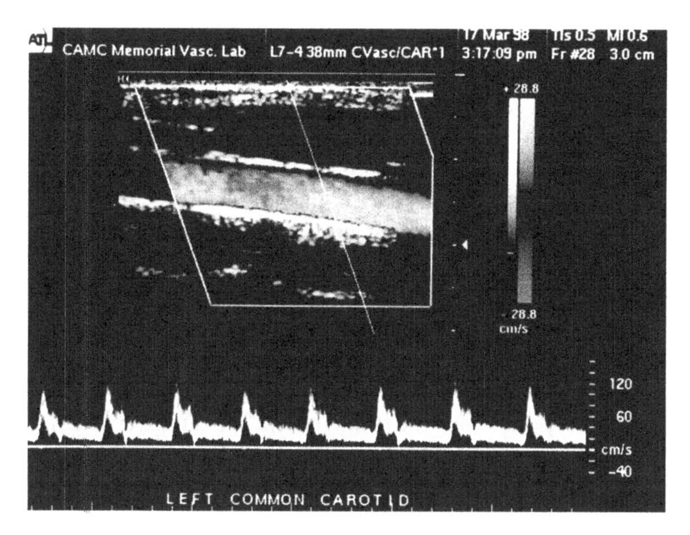

FIGURE 2–4. A color duplex ultrasound image of the common carotid artery. The common carotid artery signal has a flow characteristic of both the internal and external carotid arteries.

the stenosis (Figure 2–7). The very high-pitched hissing signal that is evident at a significant stenosis has a higher than normal amplitude in systole and diastole. In a spectral analysis, the band evident along the top of the waveform during systole may fill in the spectral window to create the spectral broadening that is consistent with turbulent flow (Figure 2–7). As seen in Figure 2–7, the more significant the stenosis, the greater the increase in systolic and diastolic frequencies. In severe stenoses there will be complete loss of the window. Distal to a stenosis, disturbed flow patterns are evident, i.e., damped monophasic flow (turbulence). It should be noted that an absent signal may suggest occlusion; however, a tight stenosis cannot be ruled out since blood flow may be difficult to detect with velocities of less than 6 cm/s.

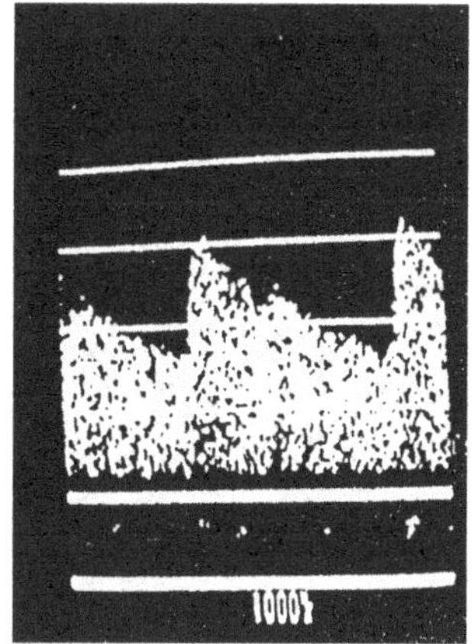

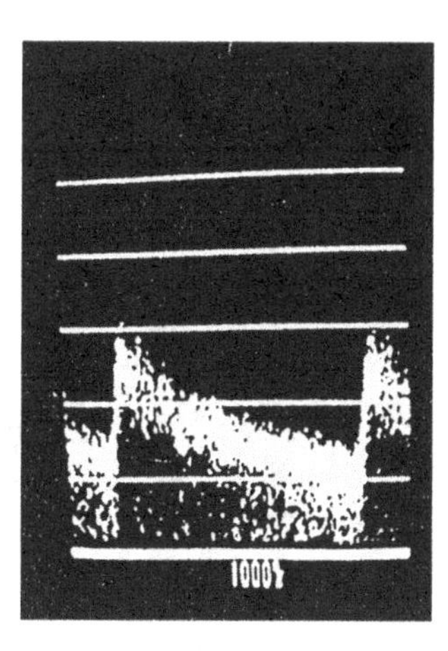

FIGURE 2–6. Left: continuous wave Doppler signal. Note the absence of a frequency window. Right: in contrast the pulse wave Doppler signal has a frequency window.

Occlusion of the internal carotid artery (Figure 2–8) is usually associated with a loss of the diastolic component in the ipsilateral common carotid artery. If the contralateral common carotid and internal carotid arteries are serving as collateral pathways, increased systolic and diastolic velocities may be evident in these arteries. If a carotid siphon stenosis is present, high resistance flow patterns may be evident in the extracranial internal carotid artery. Flow characteristics from one side must be compared with those on the other, as well as those in proximal to distal segments of the ipsilateral carotid system. Generally, this test is somewhat limited in patients with poor cardiac output or stroke volume, which may result in bilaterally diminished common carotid artery velocities. Unilateral reduction of velocities may

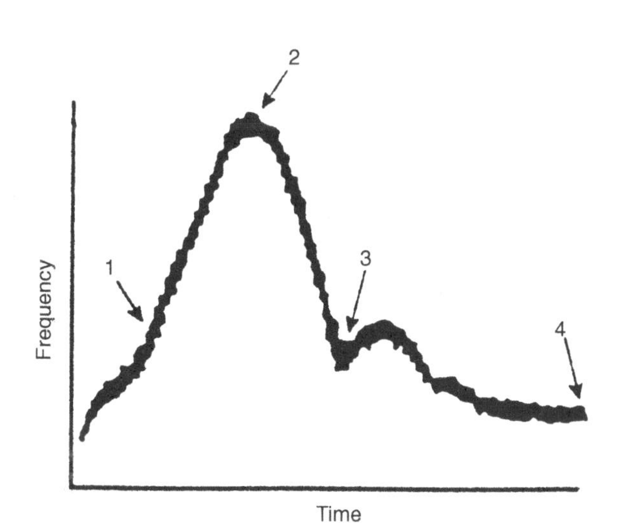

FIGURE 2–5. Spectral analysis of pulse Doppler waveform: 1, spectral envelope; 2, peak systole; 3, frequency window; 4, dicrotic notch; 5, diastole.

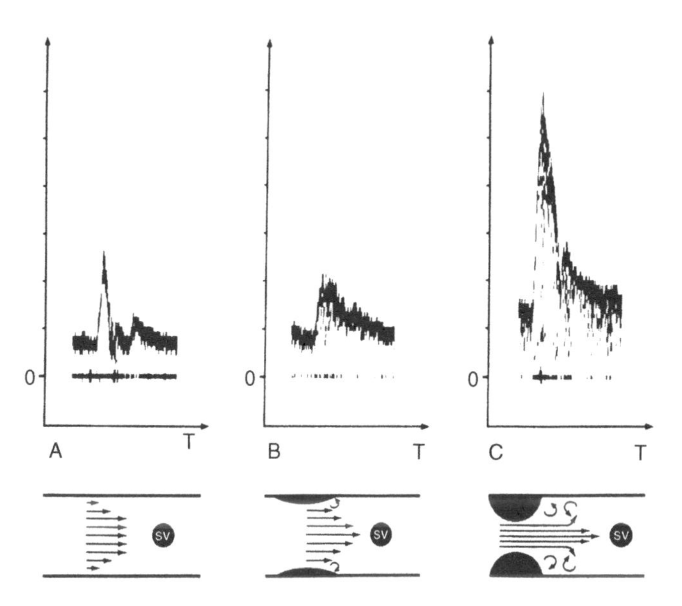

FIGURE 2–7. Waveforms from a normal vessel (A) in contrast to a mildly stenotic vessel (B) and a severely stenotic vessel (C). See text for a more detailed description.

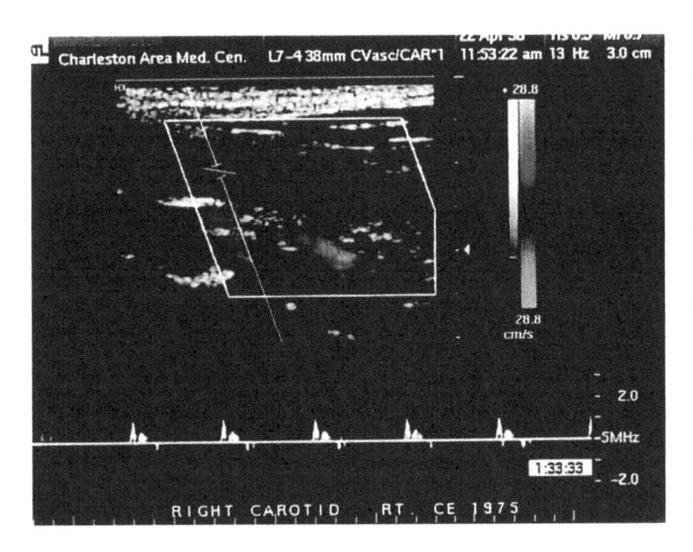

FIGURE 2–8. A color duplex ultrasound image of a patient with occlusion of the internal carotid artery, which is usually associated with a loss of the diastolic component in the ipsilateral common carotid artery (bottom).

suggest proximal disease, such as innominate or common carotid artery stenoses.

Duplex Carotid Scanning

Duplex carotid scanning, originally developed at the University of Washington, combines real-time, B-mode ultrasound imaging with a pulsed Doppler detector. As mentioned previously, although calcified plaques can readily be identified on a B-mode scan due to the high acoustic reflectivity, noncalcified plaques and thrombi have approximately the same acoustic impedance as flowing blood. Therefore, a completely thrombosed vessel may not be distinguished from a patent one based on the B-mode image alone. By using Doppler flow investigation of the vessels that can be imaged, this difficulty can be overcome.

In the initial model of the duplex scanner, the same transducer housed both pulsed echo and pulsed Doppler functions, as well as the multigated pulsed Doppler flow detector. However, after clinical trials it was apparent that separate transducers would be advisable due to the conflicting transducer alignment requirements for the pulsed echo and the pulsed Doppler functions.

The next generation of duplex scanners utilized separate echo and Doppler transducers that alternated pulse transmission in a time-sharing fashion. The scanner also contained a movable, single-gated pulsed Doppler detector. By using the B-mode image as a guide for precise placement of the pulsed Doppler range gate, the characteristics of flow at various points in the carotid arteries could be determined. This duplex scan also had the capability of spectral sound analysis of the Doppler signals. This helped to differentiate high-grade stenosis from occlusion in the carotid arteries accurately, as well as aiding in the detection of many lesions that were not severe enough to reduce pressure or flow. The strength of an echo is indicated by its brightness on an oscilloscope screen, a double display term brightness modulation, or B-mode. B-scan refers to the imaging technique that utilizes brightness modulation and a moving transducer. A primary difference between the pulsed Doppler and pulsed echo systems is the type of electronic signal processing used to detect the Doppler shift. In the conventional continuous wave Doppler instrument, separate transmitting and receiving transducers are used that operate constantly to detect flow at any point along the sound beam. The duplex scan generally employs a 5-MHz pulsed Doppler instrument with a single transducer that acts as both transmitter and receiver. The transducer emits short pulses of ultrasound, and then by varying the time interval before it operates as a receiver, flow at different depths in tissue can be detected. This technique is referred to as a range-gating.

In the past two decades a number of commercial versions have become available. Blackshear *et al.*[22] reported 92% correct diagnosis of high-grade stenosis or occlusion in a series of 120 patients. A follow-up study from the University of Washington showed an overall accuracy of 96%. Duplex scanning of the carotid bifurcation provides a highly accurate method of identifying significant lesions of the internal carotid artery, as well as of separating lesions into general pathologic categories. It also has the advantage of real-time visualization, so that a satisfactory scan does not depend on the patient. This system and its clinical applications are described in detail in Chapter 3. Its major disadvantages are the high cost of the equipment and the extensive operator training required.

Duplex scanning of the carotid arteries has become the method of choice for noninvasive assessment of extracranial carotid artery disease. The addition of color-coded flow mapping facilitates the examination and allows more accurate frequency and/or velocity measurement. Accuracies of equal to or more than 90% have been reported by several investigators in the past several years.[23–36]

Color Duplex Carotid Scanning

In addition to the technology described for duplex ultrasound, the color duplex carotid scanner utilizes a large number of sampling sites to determine the backscattered frequency and visually depicts this information as a real-time flow image. This development has occurred because of advances in computer technology that enable the rapid processing of large amounts of information. The instrument simultaneously analyzes Doppler information obtained from over 300 small sampling sites in the zone of insonation. This frequency information is subprocessed and displayed in a color-coded format rather than a gray-scale format. The color depiction of the frequencies facilitates identification of focal areas of abnormal flow patterns. This technique is performed in a manner similar to that described for duplex ultrasound with the addition of a hard copy of the real-time color flow image.

Color flow imaging is an alternative to spectral waveform analysis for displaying the pulsed Doppler information obtained by duplex scanning. In contrast to spectral analysis, which evaluates the entire frequency and amplitude content of the signal at a single sample site, color flow imaging provides an estimate of Doppler-shifted frequency or flow velocity for each site within the B-mode image. The color assignments are based on flow direction and a single mean or average frequency estimate for each site in the B-mode image plane. Accordingly, the peak Doppler frequency shifts or velocities shown by spectral waveforms are generally higher than the frequencies or velocities indicated by color flow imaging. In color flow imaging, shades of two or more distinct colors, usually red and blue, indicate the directional flow relative to the ultrasound scan lines. Variations in the Doppler-shifted frequency or flow velocity are then indicated by changes in color, with lighter shades typically representing high-flow velocities. A single sample volume-pulsed Doppler and spectrum analyzer are always available for a detailed evaluation of the flow patterns at specific arterial locations. One of the main advantages of color flow imaging is that it presents simultaneous flow information on the entire image. Although color flow imaging may be helpful in identifying flow disturbances, some high-velocity jets may not be clear on the color flow imaging because the colors are based on mean Doppler frequency estimates rather than peak systolic frequency. Color flow imaging has been especially helpful in identifying unusual anatomic features such as kinking or tortuosity, which can be difficult to recognize with conventional duplex scanning. Color flow imaging is also valuable for documenting internal carotid artery occlusion.[28]

This technology generally is user-friendly because it provides a real-time anatomic and flow imaging of the vessels being examined. Although this information can be obtained fairly rapidly initially, additional time is required for determining the optimal location of the sample volume for discrete spectra. The major drawback of this technique currently is its high cost and the fact that a detailed knowledge of Doppler technology is essential for meaningful interpretation of the color images.[37] This technology will be described in more detail in Chapter 3.

Transcranial Doppler

Transcranial Doppler (TCD) is capable of detecting intracranial stenoses and occlusions. It can also evaluate the collateral circulation in patients with severe carotid artery stenosis or occlusion. One of the most important applications of TCD is its ability to evaluate the onset, severity, and time course of vasoconstriction caused by subarachnoid hemorrhage. Other applications include evaluation of intracranial arteriovenous malformations and assessment of patients with suspected brain death. TCD also allows for the identification of flow abnormalities during many cerebrovascular and cardiovascular procedures, such as carotid endarterectomy and cardiopulmonary bypass. A significant decrease in the middle cerebral artery flow velocities during the cross-clamping of carotid endarterectomy may signal the need for carotid shunting.[38] Auditory signals related to microemboli may also lead the surgeon to alter the operative technique. TCD is usually done using 2-MHz pulse Doppler with a spectrum analyzer with an assumed angle of insonation of 0°. Three acoustic windows provide access to the intracranial circulation: transtemporal, transorbital, and transforaminal. The transtemporal approach allows for three windows: anterior, middle, and posterior. Accurate vessel identification requires appropriate sample volume size and depth, knowledge of the direction and velocity of the blood flow, the relationship of the various flow patterns to one another, and common carotid artery compression and oscillation maneuvers. This technology will be described in detail in Chapter 6.

Conclusions

As noted, various noninvasive vascular tests have been utilized for the diagnosis of extracranial carotid artery disease with varying degrees of overall accuracy. A review of these conflicting results reveals problems in study design and analysis: for example, lack of a prospective blinded approach; differences in criteria or standards indicative of carotid stenosis; failure to compare carotid noninvasive tests against standards; an assumption that the percentage of carotid stenosis on angiography correlates with hemodynamic alterations produced by the lesion; differences in the prevalence of carotid stenosis in the particular population examined; incomplete angiography; and lack of criteria for abnormal test results, skill of technicians, and the inherent accuracy of the test. Although angiography has been the standard against which most noninvasive tests have been measured, it is far from ideal for comparison with physiologic tests designed to detect altered hemodynamics. Furthermore, any significant stenosis in the carotid artery from its origin at the aorta up to and including the ophthalmic artery can result in abnormal test results in the indirect methods of testing. In addition, long-standing collateral pathways that compensate effectively for the hemody-

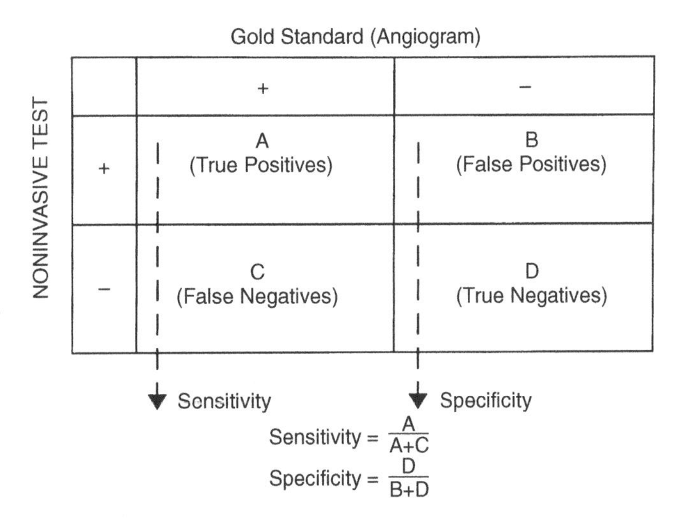

FIGURE 2–9. Method for calculating sensitivity and specificity.

namic effects of the stenotic lesion can produce a normal result in an indirect carotid test.

Direct methods do not detect lesions in the upper part of the internal carotid artery, where such lesions can also produce an abnormal result with an indirect test.

In an unbranched artery, blood flow is determined by the cross-sectional area of its narrowest portion and by the pressure gradient across it. Accordingly, the extent of stenosis caused by a carotid bifurcation plaque should be calculated by comparing the narrowest diameter of its diseased lumen with the diameter of the undiseased distal internal carotid artery. Although the term "critical stenosis" is generally used to compare the results of noninvasive testing, the exact value necessary to cause a measurable decrease in pressure or alteration in arterial blood flow remains controversial. DeWeese *et al.*[39] reported that lesions that narrowed the lumen less than 47% and left a residual lumen larger than 3 mm in diameter never caused measurable pressure drops, whereas stenoses greater than 63% of the luminal diameter with residual lumens smaller than 1 mm in diameter always did. Therefore, if systolic pressure distal to an arterial stenosis is measured, lesions that reduce the diameter 50% or more, thus reducing the cross-sectional area by 75% or more, are generally detected. However, if alterations in blood flow are measured, diameter reductions in excess of 67% (more than 90% of the cross-sectional area) are necessary for abnormal test results.[40] Clinically, a stenosis greater than 75% of the diameter or 94% of the area is necessary to cause symptomatic reduction of cerebral blood flow.[41] Since various reports have used diameter reductions from 40% to 75% as their standard of comparison, some variations in the reported results can be explained on this basis.

In addition to problems in study design, many of the carotid noninvasive studies report their results in terms of diagnostic accuracy. Since diagnostic accuracy may vary with the prevalence of disease in the population, it is impossible to compare different series if this term is used. By contrast, if results of carotid noninvasive studies are expressed in terms of sensitivity, i.e., the ability to detect the presence of the disease (true-positive rate) and specificity, i.e., the ability to detect the absence of disease (true-negative rate), these terms should be independent of disease prevalence and allow comparison of one series with another.

The following terms are generally used in comparing the accuracy of various noninvasive vascular tests. (1) Sensitivity is calculated by dividing the number of true-positive tests detected noninvasively by the total number of true-positive tests detected by angiography. (2) Specificity is calculated by dividing the true-negative tests detected noninvasively by the total true-negative tests detected by angiography. (3) The false-positive rate is calculated by dividing the number of false-positive tests detected noninvasively by the total number of noninvasive positive tests. (4) The false-negative rate is calculated by dividing the number of false-negative tests detected noninvasively by the total number of negative noninvasive tests. (5) The positive predictive value is the percentage of noninvasive test results that accurately predicts abnormality, in other words, the percentage of positive noninvasive tests that correctly predicted disease as supported by "gold standard" arteriography. It is calculated by the number of true-positive noninvasive testing divided by the number of all positive noninvasive studies (i.e., true plus false-positives). (6) Negative predictive value is defined as the percentage of noninvasive test results that accurately predicts normality. In other words, the percentage of negative noninvasive studies that correctly predicted the absence of disease as supported by "gold standard" arteriography. It is calculated by dividing the number of true-negative noninvasive tests by the number of all negative noninvasive studies (i.e., true plus false-negatives). (7) The overall accuracy is defined as the sum of the true-positive and the true-negative values compared with the total number of tests performed. Figures 2–9, 2–10, and 2–11 are simplified

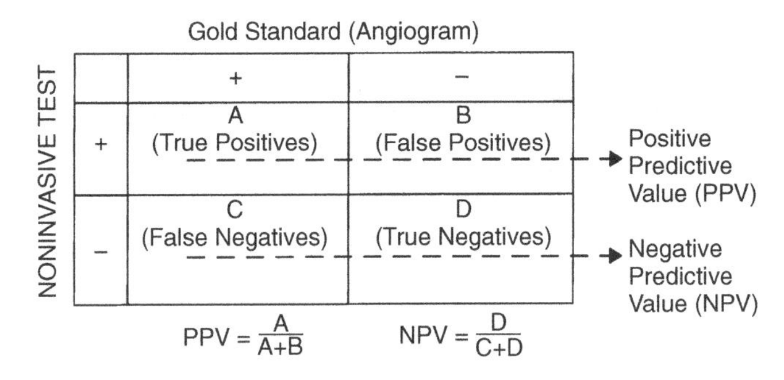

FIGURE 2–10. Method for calculating positive predictive values and negative predictive values.

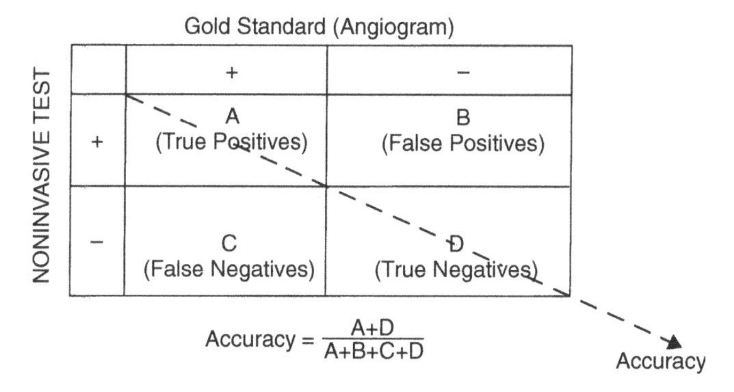

FIGURE 2–11. Method for calculating overall accuracy.

methods of calculating sensitivity, specificity, positive predictive values, negative predictive values, and overall accuracy.

Although specificity and sensitivity possess certain advantages, they are limited to fixed threshold criteria that are taken as positive for the noninvasive carotid screening test. Expressing the result of a screening test as a receiver operator-characteristic curve avoids the limitations of fixed threshold criteria.[41] This curve plots the dynamic relationship between sensitivity and specificity and allows the examiner to increase or decrease the sensitivity of the tests by varying the threshold criterion for a positive result of that particular test.

References

1. Hessel SJ, Adams DF, Abrams HL. Complications of angiography. Radiology 1981;138:273–281.
2. North American Symptomatic Carotid Endarterectomy Trial Collaborators. Beneficial effect of carotid endarterectomy in symptomatic patients with high-grade carotid stenosis. N Engl J Med 1991;325:445–453.
3. The Asymptomatic Carotid Atherosclerosis Study Group. Study design for randomized prospective trial of carotid endarterectomy for asymptomatic atherosclerosis. Stroke 1989;20:844–849.
4. Balduf LM, Langsfeld M, Marek JM, *et al.* Complication rates of diagnostic angiography performed by vascular surgeons. Vasc Endovasc Surg 2002;36:439–445.
5. Egglin TK, Moore PV, Feinstein AR, *et al.* Complications of peripheral arteriography: A new system to identify patients at increased risk. J Vasc Surg 2000;22:787–794.
6. Miyazaki M, Kato K. Measurement of cerebral blood flow by ultrasonic Doppler technique: Hemodynamic comparison of right and left carotid artery in patients with hemiplegia. Jpn Circ J 1954;29:383.
7. Goldberg RD. Doppler physics and preliminary report for a test for carotid insufficiency. In: Goldberg, RD, Saris LV (eds). *Ultrasonics in Ophthalmology: Diagnostic and Therapeutic Applications,* p. 199. Philadelphia, PA: WB Saunders, 1967.
8. Brockenbrough EC. Screening for prevention of stroke: Use of a Doppler flow meter. Seattle: Seattle Parks Electronics, 1970.
9. Mozersky BJ, Hokanson DE, Sumner DS, *et al.* Ultrasonic visualization of the arterial lumen. Surgery 1972;72: 253–259.
10. Barber FE, Baker DW, Strandness DE Jr, *et al.* Duplex scanner. II. For simultaneous imaging of artery tissues and flow. Ultrasonic symposium. Proc IEEE 1974;74:CHO 8961SU.
11. Gee W, Smith CA, Hinson CE, *et al.* Ocular pneumoplethysmography and carotid artery disease. Med Instrum 1974;8:244–248.
12. Barnes RW, Russell HE, Bone GE, *et al.* Doppler cerebrovascular examination: Improved results with refinements in technique. Stroke 1977;8:468–471.
13. AbuRahma AF, Diethrich EB. Diagnosis of carotid arterial occlusive disease. Vasc Surg 1980;14:23–29.
14. AbuRahma AF, Osborne L. Comparison of the pneumoculoplethysmography (Gee) and the digitalized pulse timing oculoplethysmography (Zira). Am Surg 1983;49:548–550.
15. Muller HR. The diagnosis of internal carotid artery occlusion by the directional Doppler sonography of the ophthalmic artery. Neurology 1972;22:816–832.
16. Burger R, Barnes RW. Choice of ophthalmic artery branch for Doppler cerebrovascular examination: Advantages of the frontal artery. Angiology 1977;28:421–426.
17. Sumner DS, Russell JR, Ramsey DE, *et al.* Noninvasive diagnosis of extracranial carotid artery disease. Arch Surg 1979;114:1222–1229.
18. Kartchner MM, McRae LP, Morrison FD. Noninvasive detection and evaluation of carotid occlusive disease. Arch Surg 1973;106:528–535.
19. White DN. Color-coded Doppler carotid imaging. In: Bernstein EF (ed). *Noninvasive Diagnostic Techniques in Vascular Disease,* pp. 258–264. St Louis, MO: CV Mosby, 1982.
20. Foo D, Henriskson L. Radionuclide cerebral blood flow and carotid angiogram: Correlation in internal carotid artery disease. Stroke 1977;8:39–43.
21. Mettinger KL, Larsson S, Ericson K, *et al.* Detection of atherosclerotic plaques in carotid arteries by the use of ^{123}I-fibrinogen. Lancet 1978;I:242–244.
22. Blackshear WM, Phillips DJ, Thiele BL, *et al.* Detection of carotid occlusive disease by ultrasonic imaging and pulse Doppler spectrum analysis. Surgery 1979;86:698–706.
23. Polak JF, Dobkin GR, O'Leary DH, *et al.* Internal carotid artery stenosis: Accuracy and reproducibility of color Doppler assisted duplex imaging. Radiology 1989;173: 793–798.
24. Spadone DP, Barkmeier LD, Hodgson KJ, *et al.* Contralateral internal carotid artery stenosis or occlusion: Pitfall of correct ipsilateral classification. A study performed with color-flow imaging. J Vasc Surg 1990;11:642–649.
25. Londrey GL, Spadone DP, Hodgson KJ, *et al.* Does color-flow imaging improve the accuracy of duplex carotid evaluation? J Vasc Surg 1991;13:359–363.
26. Mattos MA, Hodgson KJ, Ramsey DE, *et al.* Identifying total carotid occlusion with color-flow duplex scanning. Eur J Vasc Surg 1992;6:204–210.

27. AbuRahma AF, Robinson PA, Khan S, *et al.* Effect of contralateral severe stenosis or carotid occlusion on duplex criteria of ipsilateral stenoses: Comparative study of various duplex parameters. J Vasc Surg 1995;22:751–762.
28. AbuRahma AF, Pollack JA, Robinson PA, *et al.* The reliability of color duplex ultrasound in diagnosing total carotid artery occlusion. Am J Surg 1997;174:185–187.
29. AbuRahma AF, Robinson PA, Stickler DL, *et al.* Proposed new duplex classification for threshold stenoses used in various symptomatic and asymptomatic carotid endarterectomy trials. Ann Vasc Surg 1998;12:349–358.
30. Lovelace TD, Moneta GL, Abou-Zamzam AH, Edwards JM, Yeager RA, Landry GJ, Taylor LM, Porter JM. Optimizing duplex follow-up in patients with an asymptomatic internal carotid artery stenosis of less than 60%. J Vasc Surg 2001;33:56–61.
31. Nederkoorn PJ, Mali WPTM, Eikelboom BC, Elgersma OEH, Buskens E, Hunink MGM, Kappell LJ, Buijs PC, Wust AFJ, van der Lugt A, van der Graaf Y. Preoperative diagnosis of carotid artery stenosis: Accuracy of noninvasive testing. Stroke 2002;33:2003–2008.
32. Ricco JB, Camiade C, Roumy J, Neau JP. Modalities of surveillance after carotid endarterectomy: Impact of surgical technique. Ann Vasc Surg 2003;17:386–392.
33. Moore WS. For severe carotid stenosis found on ultrasound, further arterial evaluation is unnecessary. Stroke 2003;34:1816–1817.
34. Rothwell PM. For severe carotid stenosis found on ultrasound, further arterial evaluation prior to carotid endarterectomy is unnecessary: The argument against. Stroke 2003;34:1817–1819.
35. Nederkoorn PJ, van der Graaf Y, Hunink Y. Duplex ultrasound and magnetic resonance angiography compares with digital subtraction angiography in carotid artery stenosis. Stroke 2003;34:1324–1332.
36. Kern R, Szabo K, Hennerici M, Meairs S. Characterization of carotid artery plaques using real-time compound B-mode ultrasound. Stroke 2004;35:870–875.
37. Sumner DS. Use of color-flow imaging technique in carotid artery disease. Surg Clin North Am 1990;70:201–211.
38. Ackerstaff RGA, Moons KGM, van de Vlasakker CJW, Moll FL, Vermeulen FEE, Algra A, Spencer MP. Association of intraoperative transcranial Doppler monitoring variables with stroke from carotid endarterectomy. Stroke 2000;31:1817–1823.
39. DeWeese JA, May AG, Lipchik EO, *et al.* Anatomic and hemodynamic correlations in carotid artery stenosis. Stroke 1970;1:149–157.
40. Gee W. Discussion following: Archie JP, Feldtman RW. Critical stenosis of the internal carotid artery. Surgery 1981;89:67–72.
41. O'Donnell TF, Pauker SG, Callow AD, *et al.* The relative value of carotid noninvasive testing as determined by receiver operator characteristic curves. Surgery 1980;87:9–19.

3 Duplex Scanning of the Carotid Arteries

Ali F. AbuRahma and Kimberly S. Jarrett

Historical Perspectives and the Duplex Concept

The past 30 years have seen a significant evolution in the application of noninvasive technology for the diagnosis of extracranial vascular disease with more widespread utilization of direct methods of diagnosis. Of these, duplex scanning has achieved major prominence. In this time, a technology that was initially highly experimental has achieved clinical maturity with validation of its application by many comparative studies. An appreciation of why this technology has enjoyed such acceptance is best obtained by understanding the evolution of the concept of using combined imaging and velocity detection techniques.

When Kosoff [1] applied gray scale techniques to imaging, he paved the way for identifying vessels with ultrasound. In 1969, Olinger[2] reported on the use of ultrasound echo techniques to identify the carotid arteries and was active in the development of high-resolution imaging technology. In these studies, the walls of vessels were identified as echo-dense parallel structures, while the lumen was an echo-free zone contained between the walls. Atherosclerotic lesions would theoretically be identified as projections into the lumen and, thus, it appeared that this technique alone would be suitable for identifying all degrees of occlusive disease. Early experimental application, however, encountered three major problems, which in retrospect, seem obvious.

The first of these related to the complex acoustic density of atherosclerotic plaques, particularly as the lesions became more severe with zones of hemorrhage and calcification. The areas of hemorrhage were relatively echo free and appeared as defects within the substance of the plaque, rendering accurate delineation of the plaque surface difficult. The presence of calcification served as an acoustic barrier to deeper penetration of the ultrasound beam, resulting in the production of an acoustic window with subsequent loss of resolution of deeper structures.[3] While a pure imaging technique might accurately identify the surface characteristics if a plaque is homogeneous, the presence of so-called "complicated plaques" introduced a source of significant error. Finally, because thrombus and flowing blood had similar acoustic densities, it was difficult to differentiate between occluded and nonoccluded arteries.

To overcome this problem, a Doppler device was added to the imaging system, and its initial application was reported by Barber *et al.* in 1974.[4] It soon became apparent that changes in the flow patterns detected by the Doppler velocity apparatus correlated closely with the severity of stenosis as judged by arteriography.[5] The emphasis in instrument development, therefore, shifted from imaging to Doppler detection of velocity changes.

Thus, the duplex concept of combining B-mode imaging and pulsed Doppler flow detection for direct evaluation of arterial disease led to the creation of the first duplex scanning instruments. Using duplex ultrasonography, anatomical and physiological information can be obtained directly from the sites of vascular disease. This is based on the concept that arterial lesions produce disturbances in blood flow patterns that can be characterized by Doppler flow signal analyses. B-mode imaging is used as a guide for placement of a pulsed Doppler sample volume within the artery of interest, and the local flow pattern is evaluated by spectral wave analysis. Duplex scanning permits evaluation of the arterial flow pattern at a discrete site within the B-mode image, using pulsed Doppler. The sample volume of the pulsed Doppler is the region in which flow is actually detected. Adjusting the position and size of the sample volume aids in allowing the center stream pattern to be evaluated without interference from flow disturbances near the arterial wall or in adjacent blood vessels. B-mode imaging is useful in identifying anatomical variants and arterial wall pathology, including thickening or calcifications, however, the classification of arterial disease severity is

A.F. Aburahma, J.J. Bergan (eds.), *Noninvasive Cerebrovascular Diagnosis*, DOI 10.1007/978-1-84882-957-2_3,

based primarily on an analysis of the pulsed Doppler spectral waveforms.

Duplex Ultrasound Components

B-Mode Imaging

B-mode imaging has been used with varying degrees of success to evaluate carotid plaque morphology at the level of the carotid bifurcations, and to assess the histologic features of the plaques. Calcified atherosclerotic plaque, which is very echogenic, results in bright echoes and acoustic shadows (Figure 3–1). The ultrasonic carotid plaque morphology may correlate qualitatively with its histological composition, however, the clinical relevance of this information is somewhat controversial.[6–9] The B-mode characteristic of the carotid plaque that appears to correlate most closely with the clinical outcome is heterogeneity. This is generally defined as a plaque that has a mixture of hyperechoic, hypoechoic, and isoechoic plaques, a feature that may be attributed to the presence of intraplaque hemorrhage. This feature has been noted more frequently in patients with neurological events than in asymptomatic carotid stenoses. The size of the arterial lumen or the degree of stenosis may be difficult to evaluate using B-mode ultrasound only, because the interface between the arterial wall and the flow in blood is not always clearly seen. Acoustic shadowing from calcified plaques may also prevent thorough visualization of the arterial wall and lumen. These limitations are largely overcome by adding Doppler flow sampling, i.e., duplex technology. Generally speaking, B-mode imaging has been helpful in determining lesions of minimal to moderate severity, but least accurate for high-grade stenoses or occlusion.

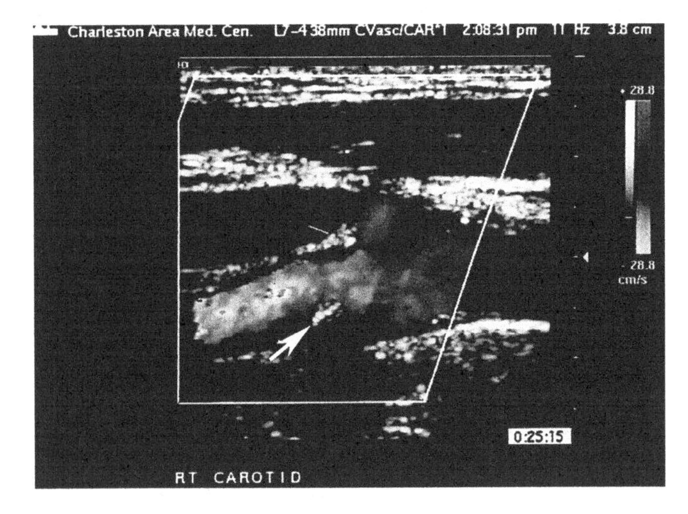

FIGURE 3–1. A color duplex ultrasound image of the carotid artery showing a calcified plaque (arrow) with acoustic shadowing underneath (under the arrow).

Doppler Spectral Waveform Analysis

A valuable adjunct to B-mode imaging is the use of spectral analysis to analyze the backscattered Doppler signal. Spectral analysis, as applied to Doppler ultrasound, is merely a method of determining the frequency content of the backscattered signal and the relative strengths or amplitude of these component frequencies. The original technique was utilized off line and employed a Kay sonograph, which although providing more information than was previously available with analog displays, was time-consuming and did not depict forward and reverse flow. Real-time spectral analysis was introduced using fast Fourier transform analysis. This has the advantages of saving time and detecting both forward and reverse flow. This method of signal processing was particularly suitable because pulsed Doppler beams were being utilized in the echo component. Other techniques of spectral analysis, including multiple bandpass filter analysis and time compression analysis, have been used, but have not achieved widespread acceptance.

The availability of the pulsed Doppler technique made it possible to obtain velocity information from a known location and, depending on the sample volume size, from a finite volume of the flow stream. The continuous-wave (CW) instruments utilized widely at that time for the detection of disease in the lower extremity were known to have a large sample volume that traversed the whole width of the vessel being insonated, and were really most suitable for determining the mean velocity in the forward or reverse direction. Also, the data analyzed by CW instruments were obtained not only from the vessel of interest, but also from other vessels in close proximity. With the pulsed instrument, the examiner could be certain that the data were being obtained from the vessel of interest. It was also possible, because of the finite sample volume, to interrogate a segment of the velocity profile and, perhaps, to detect changes that would not otherwise be apparent with a CW device.

A series of animal studies were conducted to determine the relationship between varying degrees of stenosis and spectral changes as identified by pulsed Doppler and fast Fourier spectrum analysis.[10] In these studies, artificial stenoses in the canine thoracic aorta were constructed using a snare loop technique, and the severity of stenosis was confirmed by arteriography. Validation that concentric stenoses were constructed was obtained by endoscopy under experimental perfusion pressures. A high-frequency (20-mHz) pulsed Doppler instrument was used to obtain center stream velocity samples at one, two, and three diameters distal to the areas of artificially created stenosis. The signals were subsequently analyzed

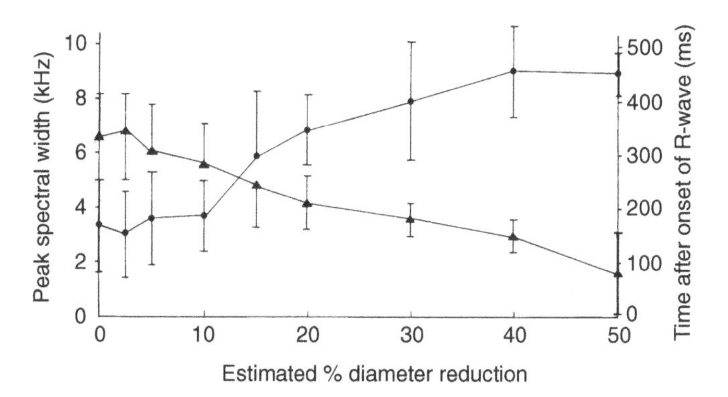

FIGURE 3–2. Results of an experimental study in canine thoracic aorta depicting the relationship between peak spectral width and percent diameter stenosis. The two graphs represent the maximum spectral width values obtained during the study as depicted by values on the left side and time after the onset of the R wave at which these values occurred as depicted on the right. Maximum spectral width increased gradually from a 15% diameter reducing stenosis to a 50% diameter reducing stenosis, while the time at which the maximum spectral width occurred appeared earlier in the cycle as this value increased.

by spectral analysis and a computer program that measured peak spectral width as defined by the upper and lower frequency plots 8 dB on either side of the mode frequency. The time in the cycle at which maximum spectral broadening occurred could be determined, as an ECG timing device was utilized during the studies. The relationship between maximum spectral width and percent stenosis, and the time of maximum spectral width were determined and are depicted in Figure 3–2.

As noted, spectral broadening was present in normal vessels, and those with minimal degrees of stenosis up to a 15% diameter reduction, at which point this parameter gradually increased reaching a maximum value at 50% diameter-reducing stenosis. Statistical analysis of these results confirmed that this parameter could be utilized to differentiate between stenoses of 15% diameter and increments between 15% and 50% diameter reducing stenosis. In addition, it should be noted that maximum spectral width in normal or minimally stenotic arteries occurred late in the pulse cycle and, as the stenosis became more severe, occurred earlier in the cycle. While the velocity profile in the canine thoracic aorta differs from that seen in the human internal carotid artery, this study provided validation of the relationship between spectral broadening and nonhemodynamically significant stenoses.

The Doppler spectral waveform analysis is a signal processing technique that displays the complete frequency and amplitude content of the Doppler signal. This Doppler-shifted frequency is directly proportional to blood cell velocity, and the amplitude of the Doppler signal depends on the number of cells moving through the pulsed Doppler sample volume. The signal amplitude becomes stronger as the number of cells producing

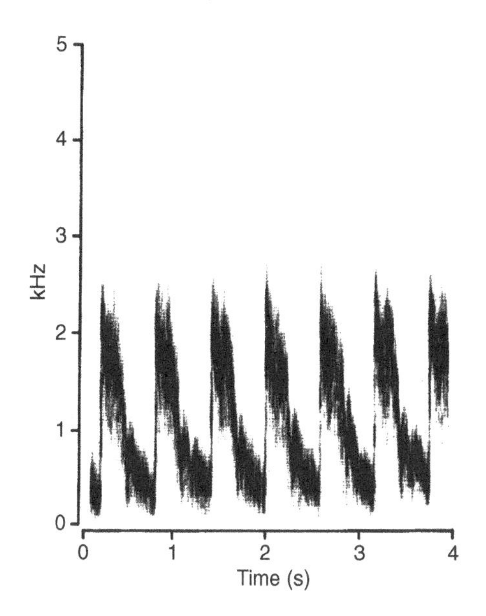

FIGURE 3–3. A normal internal carotid artery Doppler spectra.

Doppler frequency shift increases. This spectral information is usually presented graphically with time on the horizontal axis and frequency or velocity on the vertical axis; and amplitude is indicated by shades of gray (Figure 3–3).

The following is an explanation of these findings as it applies to the flow patterns within vessels. The center stream flow pattern in a normal artery is uniform or laminar, and a spectral waveform taken with the pulsed Doppler sample volume in the center of the lumen shows a relatively narrow band of frequency. It appears that even relatively mild degrees of stenosis are capable of producing deviations from laminar flow (as zones of vorticeal shedding) in the area distal to the stenosis (Figure 3–4), with the magnitude of these disturbances being

FIGURE 3–4. Schematic representation of a minor flow disturbance generated by nonhemodynamically significant stenosis with production of vorticeal shedding immediately beyond the area of the stenosis with resumption of a normal laminar flow pattern further downstream.

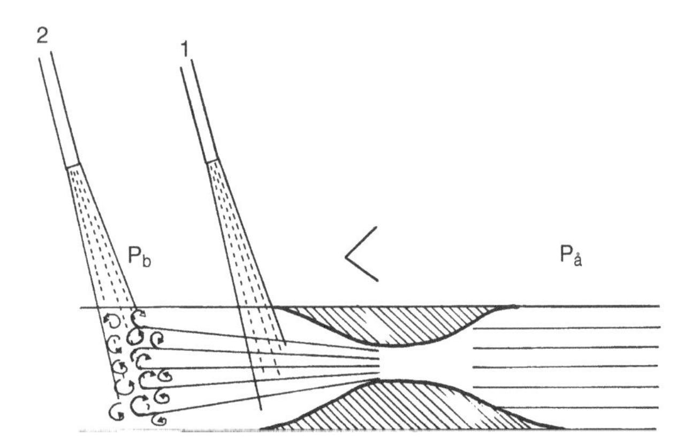

FIGURE 3–5. Schematic representation of major flow disturbance produced by hemodynamically significant stenosis with both increases in peak velocity in and immediately beyond the stenosis with decay of laminar flow to turbulent flow occurring at a maximum two diameters distal to the stenosis.

depicted by the magnitude of change in spectral width (spectral broadening). With hemodynamically significant stenoses, not only is spectral broadening present, which is produced by a major decay in the laminar flow pattern, but there is also a marked elevation in peak frequency or peak velocity at systole as a result of the high-speed jet of blood passing through and immediately beyond the stenosis (Figure 3–5). High-grade stenoses can, therefore, be recognized by the presence of both elevations in peak frequency at systole and diffuse spectral broadening.[5]

The end diastolic frequency or velocity is also increased in very severe stenoses. The Doppler spectral waveform criteria for classifying severity of carotid artery stenosis will be described in detail later.

The current application of duplex scanning in the detection of carotid artery disease utilizes this principle of identification of flow disturbance patterns by Doppler velocity detection instrumentation, with the emphasis in later years being on technical improvements in instrument design. A variety of duplex scanning instruments are available, the major differences among them being in the Doppler component. These are of two types: those utilizing CW Doppler and those utilizing pulsed Doppler beams. The outline below applies to the instrumentation available that currently uses pulsed Doppler beams for velocity detection and image generation.

Instrumentation

Originally, three fixed-focus 5-mHz transducers, mounted in a rotating wheel, generated a two-dimensional soft tissue image with 16 levels of gray, for characterization at a rate of 30 frames per second. The image information is digitized, as a result of which the image can be frozen, and one of the transducers is used solely as a pulsed Doppler source. The axis of the Doppler beam is superimposed on the image with the location of the sample volume depicted by a prominent white dot (Figure 3–6). The backscattered Doppler signal is processed using fast Fourier transform spectral analysis with display of the spectra on an oscilloscope screen. Hard copy reproduction is obtained using either a Polaroid camera or light-sensitive paper.

The most significant changes in instrumentation have occurred in scan head design. The shape of the pulsed Doppler beam, and therefore its sample volume, has been modified using either medium-focus or short-focus scan heads. The medium-focus scan head, operating at 5 mHz, has a 40-mm focal point, while the short-focus scan head, at a transmitting frequency of 5 mHz, has a 20-mm focal point. The beam width of the medium-focus scan head is most narrow at 35–45 mm depth, whereas that of the short-focus scan head is most narrow at 20–30 mm. The medium-focus scan head is, therefore, more appropriate for evaluating blood flow in vessels deeper than 30 mm, while the short-focus scan head is ideal for evaluating flow in vessels located close to the surface, 2–3 cm from the skin. Because the carotid arteries lie within 30 mm of the skin surface in the majority of human subjects, the short-focus scan head, at least theoretically, is ideal for evaluating these vessels.

These features are not only important in a consideration of the depths of the vessels studied, but also in understanding the effects of the sample volume size on the velocity profile being evaluated. If a large sample volume

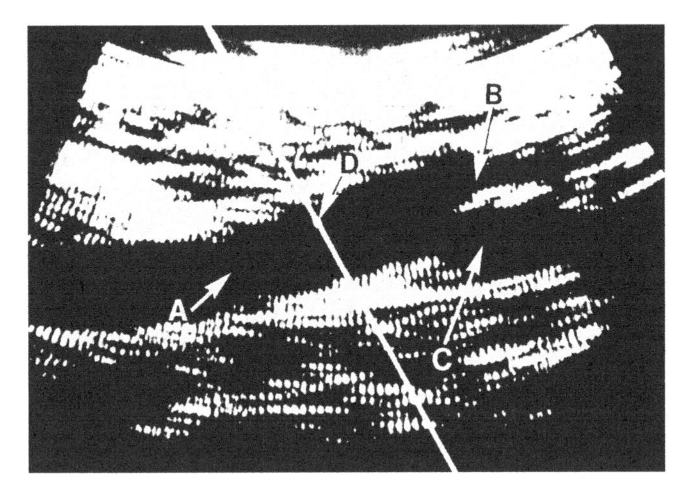

FIGURE 3–6. Oscilloscope screen depiction of the pulsed echo image generated by the duplex scanner with the Doppler beam axis depicted by the continuous white line and the location of the sample volume depicted by the bright white dot(D).

size is used in the evaluation of small-diameter vessels, a wide range of velocities will be detected under normal circumstances, which on spectral analysis will appear as spectral broadening. In these circumstances, this finding is normal and is similar to the spectra generated by CW instruments. Conversely, if a small sample volume is used in a large vessel, particularly if flow is axisymmetric, the velocities in the sample volume are likely to be similar, and on spectral analysis, will not display spectral broadening. At a range of 25 mm, the beam widths for the medium- and short-focus scan heads are 5.5 mm and 2 mm, respectively, at the 20 dB level. At this range, the sample volumes have been calculated at $3 mm^3$ and $24 mm^3$ for the short- and medium-focus scan heads, respectively. If spectral broadening, therefore, is an important feature in the evaluation, it is apparent that a short-focus scan head should be more sensitive than a medium-focus scan head.

An additional feature of the current instruments is the dedicated use of the pulsed signal to the Doppler component, which avoids the problem of aliasing encountered in the original prototypes. In the latter, the signal was shared between the echo and Doppler components and resulted in a limited peak frequency detection capability that could be exceeded when severe disease was present. With the pulsed echo component nonoperative, the usual pulse repetition frequency available to the Doppler component is doubled, increasing the frequency response of the 5-mHz instrument at 60° to 9.5 kHz, which is more than adequate to detect the frequencies associated with severe disease.

The quadrature outputs of the pulsed Doppler signal are then analyzed using an on-line fast Fourier transform spectral analyzer, providing a full-scale frequency display of 10 kHz, with 7 kHz usually being used for forward frequencies and 3 kHz for reverse frequencies. The amplitude of the component frequencies in the signal is depicted in gray-scale format on the oscilloscope screen.

To improve the signal-to-noise ratio on the spectral display, the signal in many instruments is "normalized," a principle that increases the highest amplitude of each analysis in the spectrum to a particular reference level with the subsequent same scaling factor being applied to all other amplitudes. Following this normalizing process, a variable amount of signal is then displayed depending on the dynamic range used with the Doppler signal. The use of a wide dynamic range enhances the likelihood that in addition to the Doppler backscattered signal, noise will also be displayed. Narrow dynamic range is ideal for evaluating the Doppler signal only.

The addition of high definition imaging (HDI) technology revolutionized the front end of the ultrasound image formation process. The extended signal processing, or ESP technology (Advanced Technology Laboratories/Phillips System), extends the momentum into the area of signal processing. The result is a substantial reduction in speckle noise, allowing a higher level of clarity and detail than has ever been seen in ultrasound images. Tissue differentiation and resolution of fine anatomical detail, already hallmarks of HDI images, are enhanced even further through the addition of ESP technology.

The technology developments that make high HDI and extended signal processing possible are many and complex. Perhaps the most appropriate place to begin is with the acoustic information that is returned to the ultrasound system from the body.

Each tissue within the body responds to ultrasound energy of different frequencies in a characteristic way, which is often referred to as the tissue signature. The tissue signature information is carried within the spectrum of ultrasound frequencies returning from the tissue. This band of frequencies is referred to as the frequency spectrum bandwidth, or simply, bandwidth.

HDI preserves the quantity and quality of tissue signature through the capture and preservation of the entire bandwidth. This results in more sonographic information with better detail and definition.

The ultrasound beamformer, together with the scanhead, determines the ultimate contrast resolution, spatial resolution, penetration, and consistency of the image. If the acoustic information containing the tissue signature is reduced in quantity, or distorted in the beamformer, there is no way of recovering it.

Beam formation is accomplished by pulsing the transducer elements in the scanhead to insonify the target. Sound waves reflected by the target return to the elements of the transducer, generating signals that are essentially separated in time. The beamformer delays these signals so when all the channels are summed together, the time variations in the signals are compensated for and the exact tissue definition is obtained.

The critical design requirements of the beamformer are to preserve the entire bandwidth, which contains all of the acoustic information and to prevent distortion of the signal during delay.

More recently, SonoCT real-time compound imaging was incorporated into duplex technology. Using up to nine "lines of sight," SonoCT imaging dramatically enhances image quality by providing up to nine times more information than conventional two-dimensional imaging. The resulting real-time image is a more realistic representation of actual tissue.

The clinical benefits of SonoCT real-time compound imaging include improved visualization of plaque border delineation, allows better assessment of plaque morphology, reduction of clutter artifacts seen in difficult-to-image patients, and reduction of posterior plaque shadowing to reveal the full extent of vascular disease.

The new HDI 5000 SonoCT systems (Advanced Technology Laboratories, Phillips) have a breakthrough pro-

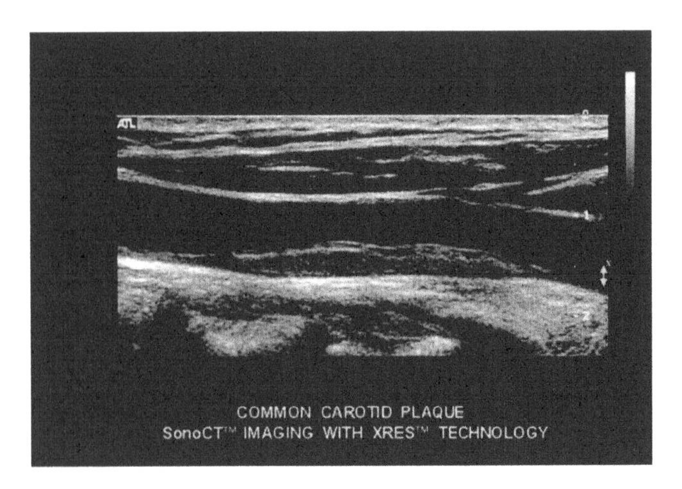

FIGURE 3–7. A SonoCT image showing tissue texture, borders, and margins.

cessing technology that optimizes image quality down to the pixel level. It displays a SonoCT image with unprecedented visualization of tissue texture, borders, and margins, almost free of image-degrading artifacts (Figure 3–7).

Carotid Examination Technique

The examination is conducted with the patient supine and the head slightly extended and turned slightly away from the side being examined and supported to eliminate lateral movement. Copious quantities of water-soluble acoustic gel are applied along the anterior border of the sternomastoid muscle and the scan head is applied to the skin surface. A 7.5- or 5-mHz transducer is usually used. Presently, we are using the HDI 5000 system, Advanced Technology Laboratory, Bothell, WA (Figure 3–8). If color flow imaging is used, Doppler information is displayed on the image after it is evaluated for its phase (i.e., direction toward or away from the transducer) and its frequency content (i.e., a hue or shade of color). The sample volume of the pulsed Doppler should be kept as small as possible and placed in the center of the vessel or the flow channel. A Doppler angle of 45–60° should be maintained to obtain consistent results in velocity measurements. The vessels are examined both in longitudinal (Figure 3–9) and transverse views (Figure 3–10), and followed from the clavicle to the mandible with anterior oblique, lateral, and posterior oblique projections to identify and evaluate any carotid plaques or pathology.

The scan head is then moved cephalad with the B-mode imaging display activated, and with frequent sampling of the center stream velocity signal. Audible interpretation alone is usually used during this phase of the examination. The region of the carotid bifurcation is identified by the presence of two vessels and visualization of the superior thyroid artery branch of the external carotid artery. This may be confirmed by sampling in the center stream just distal to the origin of these vessels and identifying the characteristic differences between the two arteries.

It is recommended that the dynamic range be set to 40–50 dB to optimize the gray-scale image and the time gain compensation (TGC) as needed, in regards to the depth of the carotid and vertebral arteries examined.

The external carotid signal is recognized by the presence of flow reversal, while the internal carotid signal is identified by the absence of flow reversal and the presence of forward flow during diastole. The scan head is moved further cephalad to insonate the proximal few centimeters of the internal carotid artery, which is the common site of disease. Abnormalities in the velocity spectra displayed on the screen are noted for subsequent reference. Once the general anatomy has been outlined, a detailed examination is performed. The initial quick scanning of the vessels provides a reference for deter-

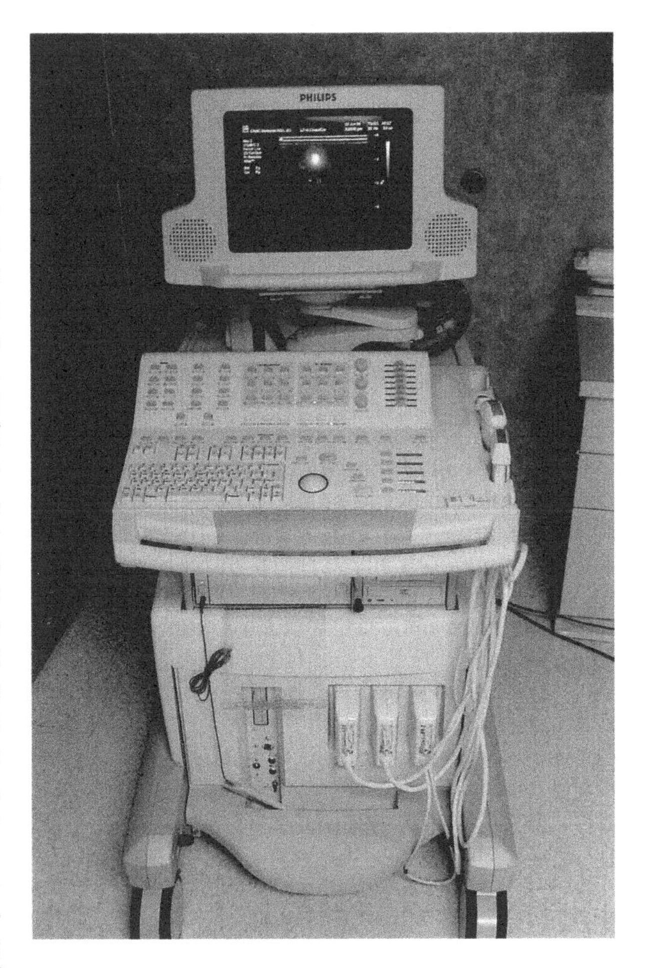

FIGURE 3–8. A duplex ultrasound machine, HDI 5000 system, Advanced Technology Laboratory/Phillips, Bothell, WA.

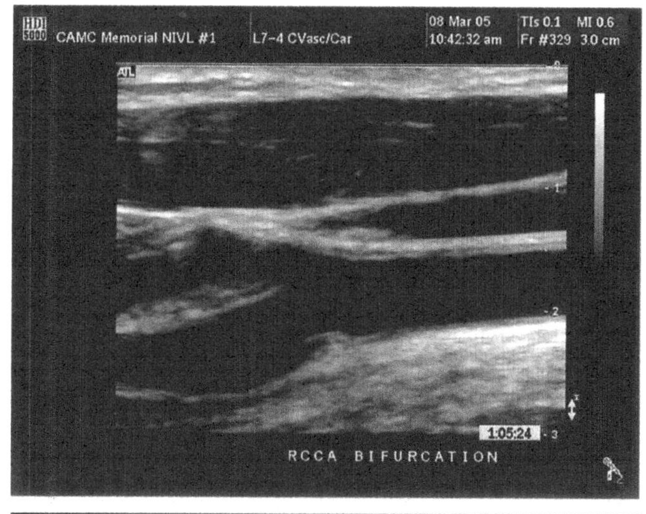

A

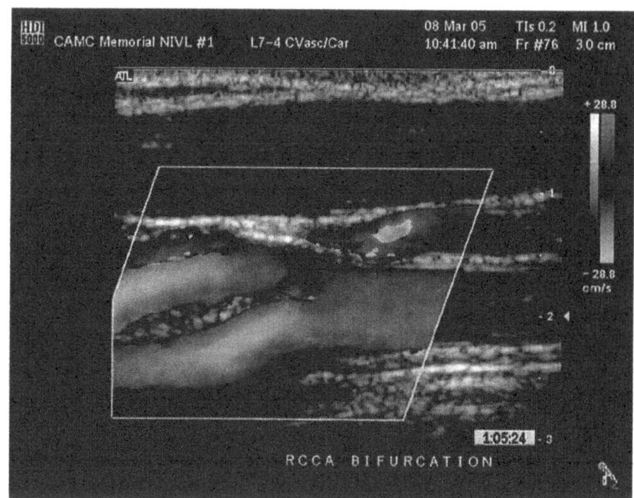

B

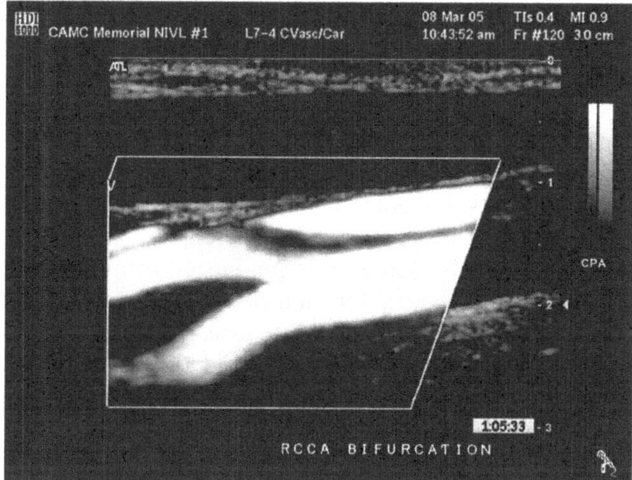

C

FIGURE 3–9. (A) Gray scale of right common carotid artery bifurcation in longitudinal view. (B) Color duplex ultrasound of right common carotid artery bifurcation in longitudinal view. (C) Power Doppler image of right common carotid artery bifurcation in longitudinal view.

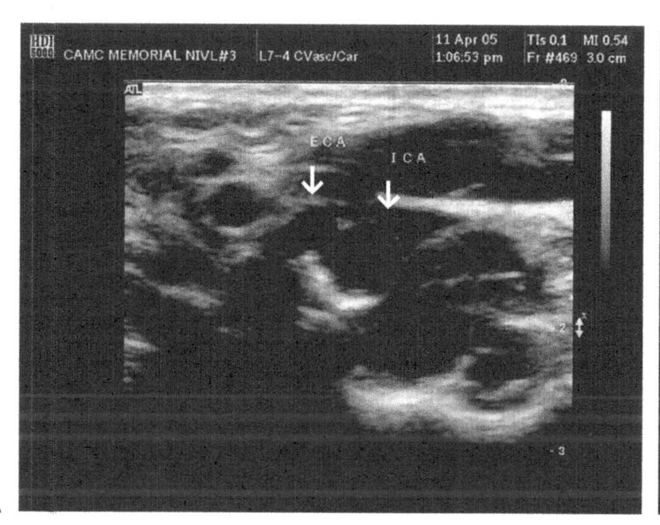

A

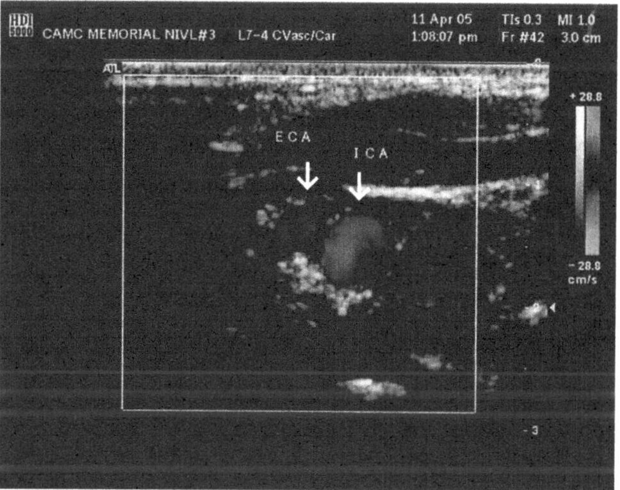

B

FIGURE 3–10. (A) Common carotid artery bifurcation in transverse view (grayscale). (B) Common carotid artery bifurcation in transverse view (color flow).

mining whether disease is present and, if so, its severity. It is likely that these areas will require more detailed interrogation than areas that are normal.

Following the preliminary scan, the scan head is returned to the base of the neck over the anterior border of the sternomastoid muscle, and the common carotid artery is again visualized. Note is taken of the presence or absence of calcification in the wall represented by dense acoustic shadows and a deeper acoustic window. Representative spectra are then obtained from the center stream with the Doppler beam axis at 60° and the signals recorded on videotape for subsequent analysis. During this part of the examination, the peak frequency or velocity should be noted and whether the velocity is always in the forward direction throughout the whole of the cycle.

Low peak systolic frequencies or velocities suggest occlusions of the internal or external carotid arteries, while frequencies approaching zero are suggestive of either high-grade stenosis or occlusion of the internal carotid artery. Other variations in the waveform may occur as a result of significant aortic disease.

The scan head is again moved cephalad with a second center stream sample being obtained just proximal to the region of the bulb. With rapid shifting from B-mode to Doppler mode imaging, the evaluation is continued through and into the proximal internal carotid artery, looking for abnormal spectral displays. Care must always be taken during sampling to ensure that the sample volume cursor is located in the center stream of the vessel, and the incident angle of the Doppler beam to the long axis of the vessel is as close as possible to 60°. The presence of disease is suspected by echogenic shadows impinging on the lumen of the vessel associated with either changes in spectral broadening or fluctuations in peak systolic and diastolic frequencies or velocities. It is frequently necessary to obtain multiple spectra along the center stream axis of the internal carotid artery to determine the location at which the most abnormal spectra occur. These should be recorded on videotape for future reference.

Attention is then directed to the subclavian artery in the posterior triangle of the neck and the vessel is visualized. Scanning proceeds proximally with identification of the origin of the vertebral artery and subsequent sampling with the Doppler component of the orifice in the proximal centimeter of the first portion of this vessel, as this is the usual site of stenotic disease.

With a clear view of the common carotid artery, the probe is slowly angled more posterior-laterally to identify the vertebral artery. This artery will have vertical shadows running through it from the spinous processes of the vertebrae, giving it the appearance of a series of Hs (Figure 3–11). Vertebral flow is documented, either antegrade or retrograde flow. Major elevations in peak frequency are characteristic of high-grade orifice stenosis. The contralateral side of the neck is then evaluated in a similar manner and representative recordings from the common carotid, external, and internal carotid arteries are obtained.

The following considerations are generally helpful in optimizing color flow setup and value. The appropriate color pulse repetition frequency (PRF) must be chosen by setting the color velocity scale for the expected velocities in the examined vessel. The scale should be adjusted to avoid systolic aliasing (low PRF) or diastolic flow gaps (high PRF) in normal vessels. Every effort should be made to avoid using large wider color boxes, which may slow down frame rates and resolution of the imaged vessel. It is recommended that color boxes that cover the entire vessel diameter and are approximately 1–2 cm of its length be used. The color, power, and gain should be optimized so that flow signals are recorded throughout the lumen of the examined vessel with no bleeding of color into the adjacent tissues.

The zero baseline of color bar (BRF) is set at approximately two-thirds of the range with the majority of frequencies allowed in the red direction for flow toward the brain, which will display higher arterial mean frequency shifts without aliasing artifacts. The color PRF and zero baseline may also need to be readjusted throughout the examination to allow for changes in velocity that may occur if carotid tortuosity or stenosis is present. Adjustments in the PRF are generally needed in the examination of the carotid bulb where the color differentiation scale should be set to visualize the slower flow in the boundary separation zone. The PRF range is generally adjusted higher to detect increased velocity in the region adjacent to the flow divider. Similarly, the color PRF should be increased to display higher velocities detected in the presence of carotid stenosis and to avoid aliasing. In the poststenotic zone, the color PRF should be decreased to observe the lower velocities and flow direction changes in the region of turbulent flow just distal to the stenosis. Color PRF should also be decreased when occlusion is suspected to detect the preocclusive, low velocity, high resistant signal associated with tight stenosis or carotid occlusion, and to confirm absence of flow at the sight of the occlusion. The color PRF should also be decreased in the presence of a carotid bruit to detect the lower frequencies associated with a bruit.

Color sensitivity (ensemble length) should be around 12 in systems where there is an adjustable control. The ensemble length can be increased in regions where more sensitive color representation is needed. Keep in mind that the frame rate will decrease when the ensemble length is increased. The color wall filter should also be set as low as possible, and you may need to decrease the wall filter manually when decreasing the color PRF. The color wall filter may automatically increase as the PRF is increased.

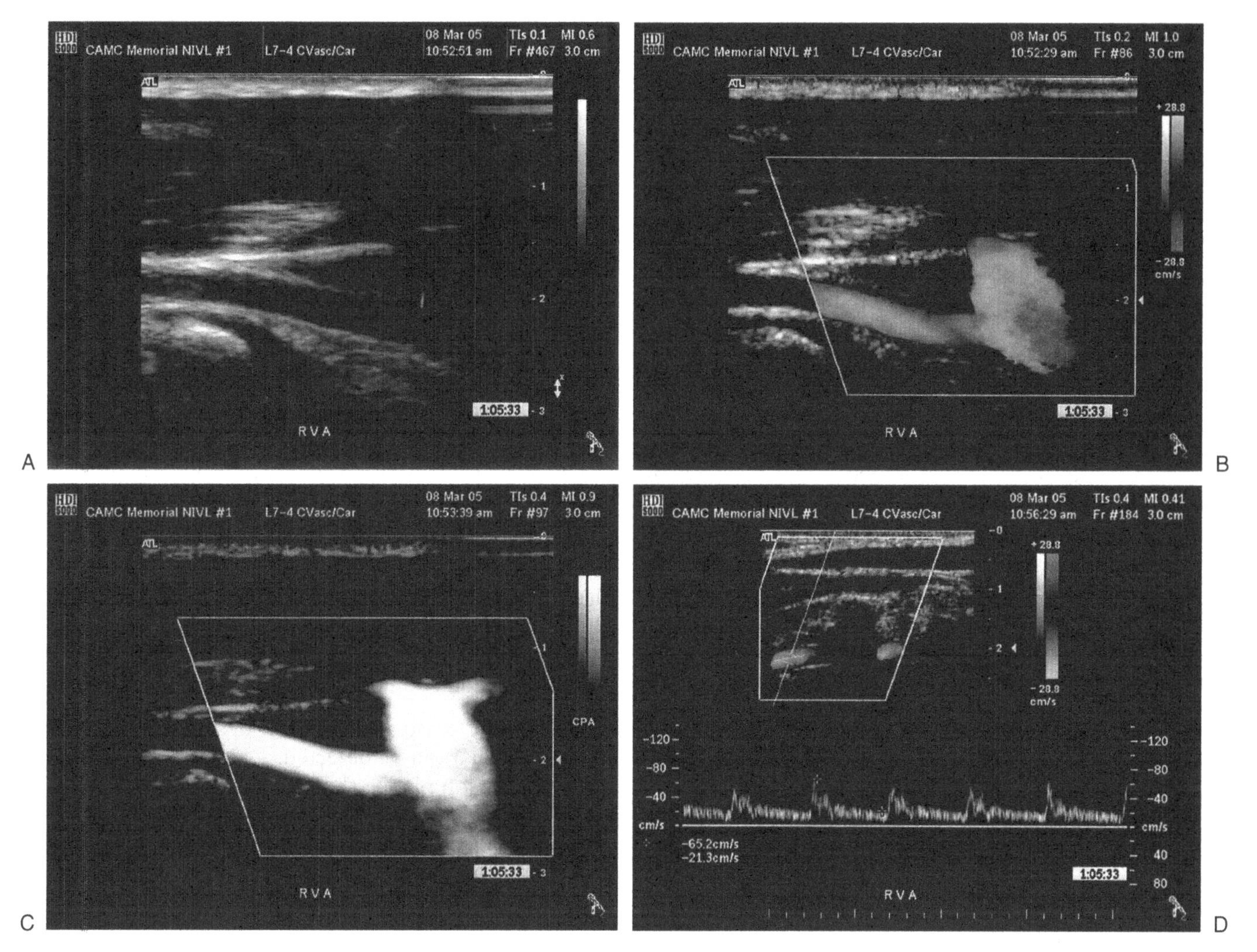

FIGURE 3–11. (A) Origin of right vertebral artery in grayscale. (B) Origin of right vertebral artery using color duplex ultrasound. (C) Origin of right vertebral artery using power Doppler. (D) Mid right vertebral artery (series of H appearance).

The angle of the color box should also be changed to obtain the most accurate Doppler angle between the scan lines and the direction of the blood flow. This will yield a better color display, secondary to better Doppler angle. The color box should be kept to a size that is adequate for visualizing the area of interest, and should be kept small enough to keep the frame rate at a reasonable number. The color gain should be adjusted throughout the examination to detect the changing signal strength. If this is not properly adjusted, too much color may be displaced or some color information may be lost, which may result in seeing color in areas where there is no flow. In patients with very low flow or questionable carotid occlusion, an overgained level may be advantageous to show any flow that may be present.

The desaturation of the color from darker to lighter hues on the color bar indicates increasing velocities. The colors are darkest close to the zero baseline, and as the velocities increase, the colors become lighter. Color should be selected so that the highest frequency shifts in each direction are of high contrast to each other so that you can easily detect aliasing, e.g., the color selection can be set so that low to high velocities are seen as dark blue to light green to aqua in one direction and red to orange to yellow in the opposite direction. Aliasing in these circumstances would appear as aqua, adjacent to yellow.

Since the frame rate is affected by the PRF, ensemble length, depth, and width of the color box, it should be kept as high as possible to capture the rapid change in flow dynamics that occurs with carotid stenosis, particularly in the carotid bulb region. The frame rate decreases with decreasing PRF and increasing the color ensemble length will also decrease the frame rate. Increased color box width and deep insonation will also decrease the frame rate.

Limitations of Duplex Technology

Duplex technology of the carotid arteries may be adversely affected by the following: acoustic shadowings from calcification, soft tissue edema or hematoma, the depth or course of the vessel, the size of the neck, and the presence of sutures or skin staples.

Duplex ultrasonography may also overestimate or underestimate the degree of stenoses or plaquing. Underestimation of disease can be noted if it fails to appreciate very low level echoes of soft plaque, or the examiner does not carefully interrogate the vessel and misses accelerated flow; or in patients with long, smooth plaque formation, which does not have the accelerated, turbulent flow pattern usually associated with the hemodynamically significant stenoses, or if an inappropriate Doppler angle is used (e.g., above 60°). Stenoses can also be overestimated when an artifact is mistaken for a carotid plaque, if accelerated flow is mistakenly attributed to stenosis, if there is vessel tortuosity or kinking, and in the presence of significant stenoses or occlusion on the contralateral side.

Due to the varying filling phases of the cardiac cycle, cardiac arrhythmia makes it more difficult to evaluate the flow spectra. Also, the flow velocity will be lower in a wider vessel and higher in a narrower vessel at the same flow intensity. Therefore, the flow in a wide carotid sinus can easily be disturbed, and may incorrectly suggest pathological findings.

Interpretation and Determination of Disease Severity

A complete extracranial carotid duplex examination should include the following data.

1. The peak systolic and end diastolic velocities of common carotid, internal carotid, and external carotid arteries, right and left subclavian arteries, and vertebral arteries.
2. The internal carotid artery to common carotid artery peak systolic velocities ratio.
3. Flow direction of the vertebral artery (antegrade or retrograde).
4. Analysis of the Doppler spectral waveform of the examined vessels.
5. The presence or absence of plaque and description of its morphology.

B-Mode Imaging Interpretation

An echoic area should be evident between the walls of the vessel, indicating the absence of pathology, i.e., plaquing, whose density usually differs from that of the blood. An echoic line indicating the endothelium may be evident at the vessel lumen. The following abnormalities can be noted on B-mode imaging:

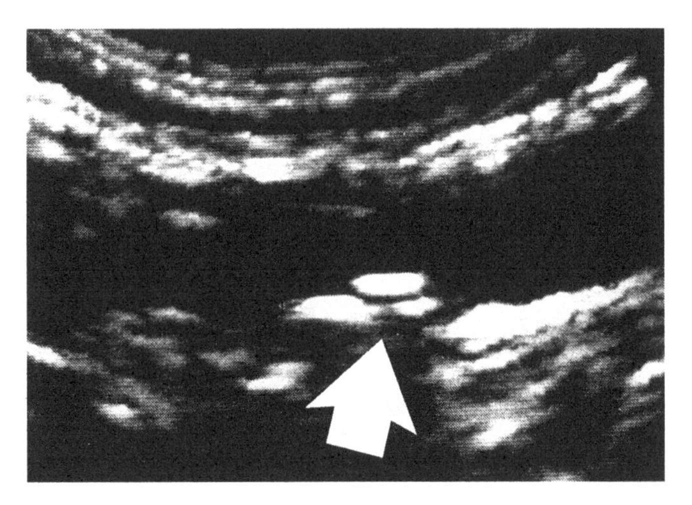

FIGURE 3–12. Duplex ultrasound image of the carotid artery showing homogeneous plaque (arrow).

1. Fatty streaks, low level echoes of similar appearance (homogeneous) can be detected.
2. Fibrous soft plaque (homogeneous): low to medium level echoes of similar appearance (Figure 3–12).
3. Complex plaque (heterogeneous): low, medium, and high level echoes indicating soft and dense areas (Figure 3–13). This plaque is a mixture of isoechoic, hyperechoic, or hypoechoic plaque.
4. Calcification: very bright, highly reflected echoes are noted. The acoustic shadowing from calcifications prevents a thorough evaluation of the vessel and may result in the calculation of an erroneous percentage of stenosis (Figure 3–1).
5. Vessel thrombosis: fresh carotid thrombosis may not be detected without using Doppler flow sampling since fresh thrombus has the same echogenicity of flowing blood.

Carotid plaque morphology is generally characterized into smooth (Figure 3–14) or irregular plaques (Figure 3–15) according to surface, and homogeneous (Figure 3–12) versus heterogeneous (Figure 3–13) according to plaque structure. An ulcerative plaque is usually an irregular plaque with a cleft within the plaque that can be seen on B-mode imaging (Figure 3–16).

Estimation of Stenosis Based on B-Mode Imaging

Ideally, carotid plaque should be visible from at least two of the longitudinal, or sagittal projections, and in the transverse view to give a rough estimate of stenosis.

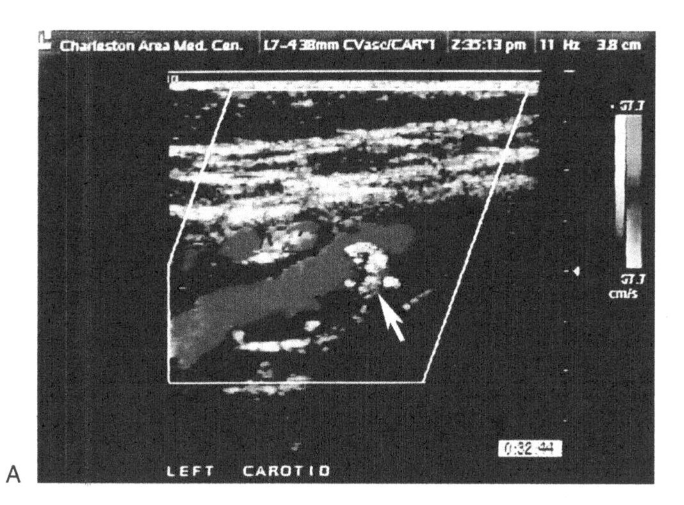

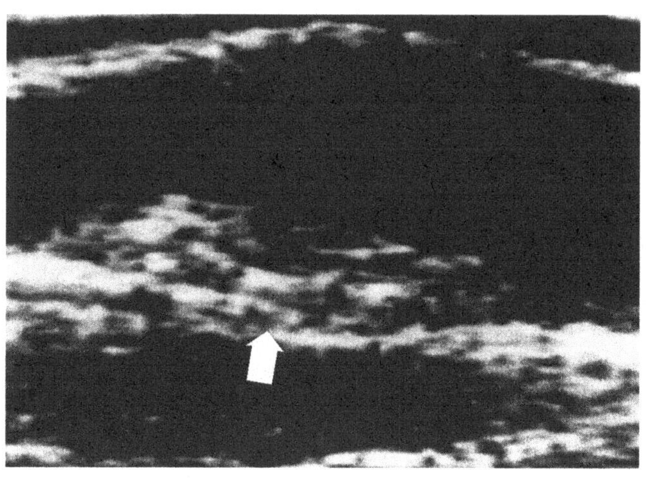

FIGURE 3–13. (A) Color duplex ultrasound image of the carotid bifurcation showing a complex heterogeneous plaque at the origin of the internal carotid artery (arrow). (B) A duplex ultrasound image of the carotid artery showing a heterogeneous plaque (arrow).

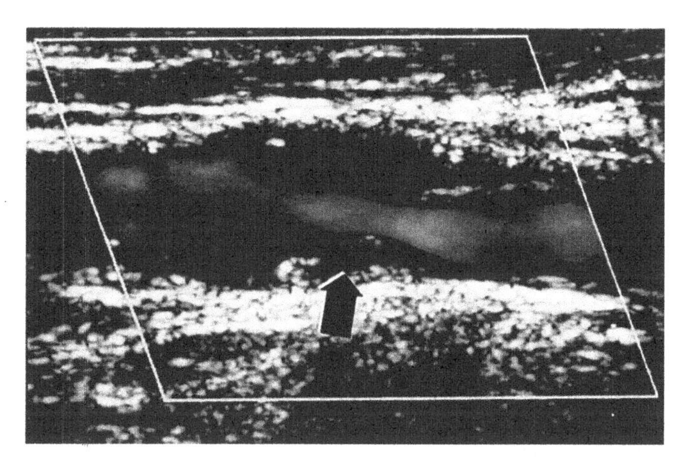

FIGURE 3–14. A color duplex ultrasound image of the carotid artery showing a smooth heterogeneous plaque (arrow). The dark center of the plaque may represent intraplaque hemorrhage.

Percent diameter stenosis equals the ratio of the residual diameter to vessel lumen diameter minus 1 multiplied by 100. Percentage of area of stenosis is calculated similarly, except you substitute the area for the diameter. The vessel lumen diameter (in longitudinal view) or area (in transverse view) is measured from intima to intima. Then the residual lumen diameter, or area, is measured (Figure 3–17). The percent reduction is calculated using the above formula. The approximate relationship between diameter and area of stenosis is shown in Table 3–1. These values are applicable to circular geometry.

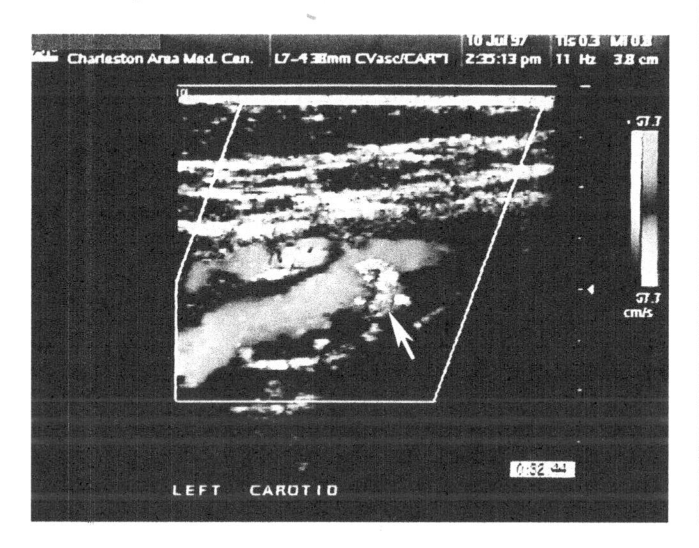

FIGURE 3–15. A carotid color duplex ultrasound image showing an irregular plaque of the proximal internal carotid artery (arrow).

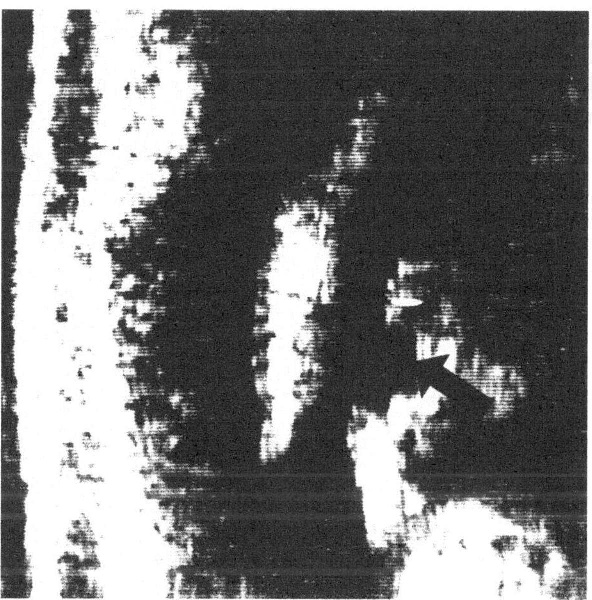

FIGURE 3–16. A duplex ultrasound image of the carotid bifurcation showing an ulcerative lesion of the proximal internal carotid artery (arrow).

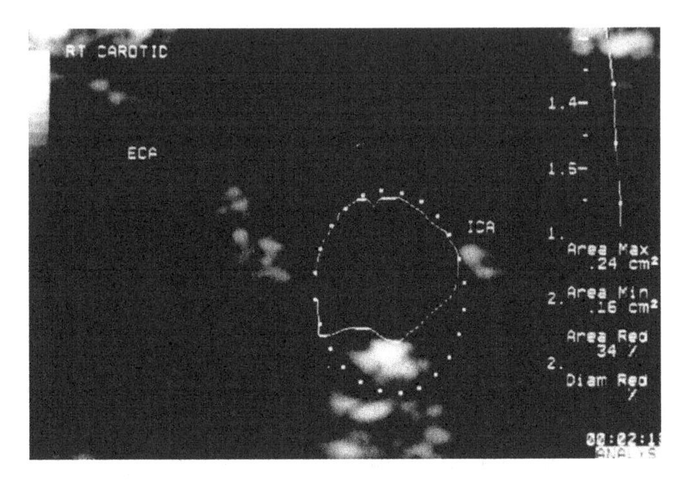

FIGURE 3–17. Calculation of area reduction percent stenosis. This image reflects the greatest stenosis in transverse diameter. An elliptical measurement of the arterial lumen is taken. Then an elliptical trace of the residual lumen is made. The percent area reduction is calculated by the duplex machine. To calculate the diameter reduction percent stenosis, a similar calculation is performed with the vessel in longitudinal view.

A chronic arterial occlusion may be diagnosed using B-mode imaging, although Doppler interrogation is essential to this diagnosis. Depending on the type of occlusive process, the artery may be filled with highly echogenic material or be anechoic.

Determination of Disease Severity Using Doppler Spectral Analysis

Identification of disease in the carotid system uses both qualitative and quantitative data. Careful attention to unusual echoes on the image serves as a qualitative guide to the presence of disease at sites where careful scrutiny with a Doppler component should be performed. The changes in spectra obtained from the common, internal, and external carotid arteries provide quantitative information for the determination of the severity of disease in these locations. This is probably best considered by describing the normal and abnormal spectra generated in various anatomical locations by disease of varying severity, according to the University of Washington criteria.[11]

These original criteria by the University of Washington are described in the following sections since they are still commonly used in the United States, and they have been the foundation for interpretation of carotid artery stenosis. However, later is this chapter you will find that other authorities modified these criteria to be compatible with the indication for carotid endarterectomy as proposed by the North American Symptomatic Carotid Endarterectomy Trial (NASCET) and Asymptomatic Carotid Artherosclerosis Study (ACAS) trials.

TABLE 3–1. % Diameter stenosis vs. % area stenosis.[a,b]

% Stenosis by	
Diameter stenosis	Area reduction
0	0
10	19
11	36
30	51
40	64
50	75
60	84
70	91
80	96
90	99
100	100

[a]% Diameter stenosis (%Ds) = 100 × [1 − (inner diameter/outer diameter)]. % Area stenosis (%As) = 100 × [1 − (inner area/outer area)]. $\%As = 100 - 100 \times [1 - \%Ds/100)]^2$.
[b]Assuming concentric circle.

Normal Internal Carotid Spectra or Minimal Disease (0–15% Stenosis)

The characteristic features of normal internal carotid artery spectra are shown in Figure 3–3. The peak frequency at systole is less than 4kHz (a peak systolic velocity of <125cm/s) with minimal degrees of spectral broadening during the initial deceleration phase of systole, followed by mild spectral broadening during diastole. The velocities are always in the forward direction and, therefore, the frequencies depicted on the scale are always above the zero line. The velocity envelope during systole is relatively narrow and displays a large clear window area under the systolic curve. Correlation with arteriographic findings has supported the view that this type of waveform may also be generated with minimal disease up to 15–20% diameter reduction and, therefore, identification of this type of waveform confirms the presence of either a normal vessel or one in which only minimal disease is present. Figure 3–18 is a color duplex imaging of a normal common carotid artery, an internal carotid artery, and an external carotid artery.

Mild Stenosis (16–<50%)

As noted in the discussion regarding findings with animal studies, it is over the range of mild stenosis that spectral broadening changes in both magnitude and timing, and it is the presence of spectral broadening in systole, particularly during the deceleration phase, which is characteristic of the spectra generated by the presence of mild disease. As shown in Figures 3–19 and 3–20, the peak

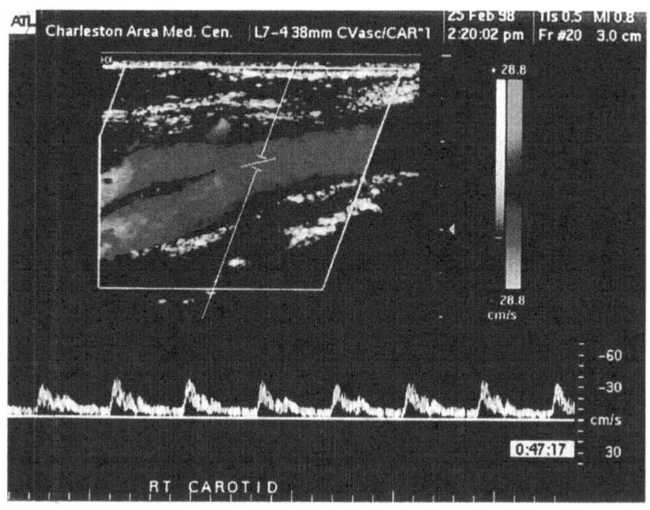

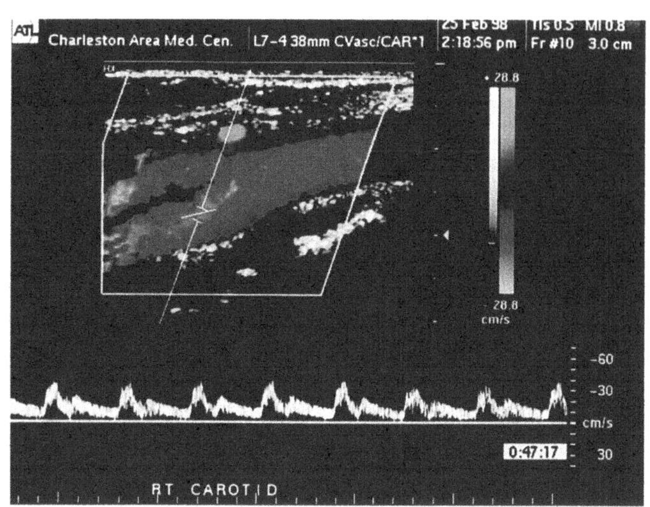

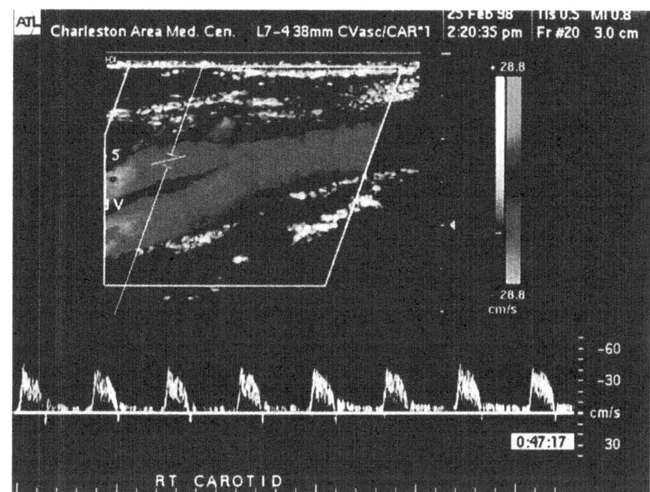

FIGURE 3–18. (A) A color duplex ultrasound image showing a normal common carotid artery with a normal Doppler spectra (bottom of figure). (B) A color duplex ultrasound image of the carotid bifurcation showing a normal internal carotid artery with a normal Doppler spectra (bottom of figure). (C) A color duplex ultrasound image of the carotid bifurcation showing a normal external carotid artery with a normal Doppler spectra (bottom of figure).

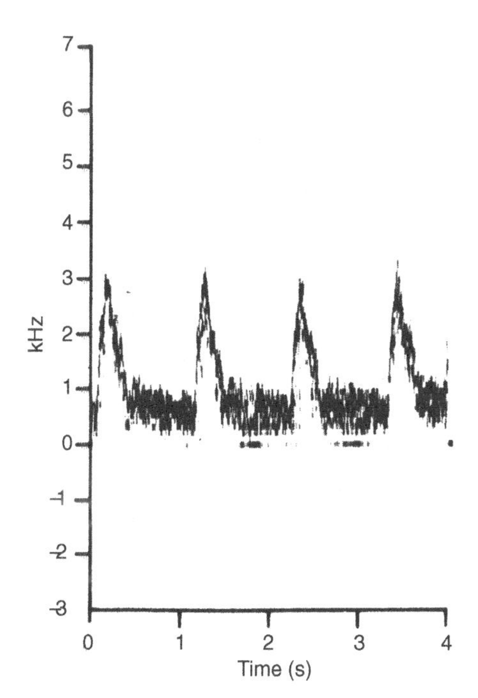

FIGURE 3–19. Internal carotid artery Doppler spectra associated with mild stenosis (15% to <50%).

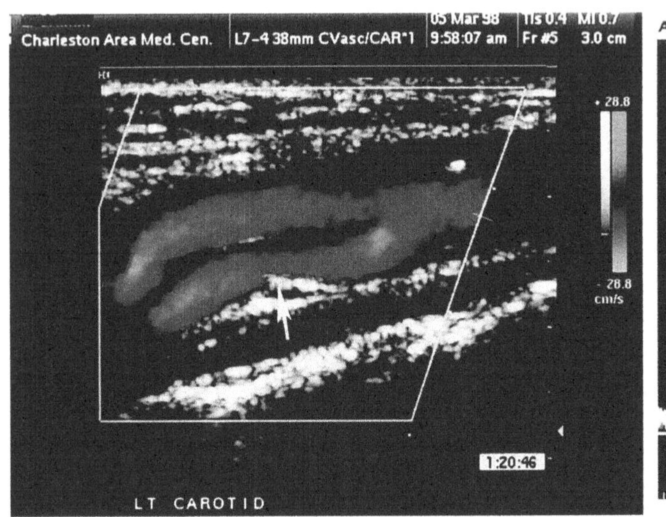

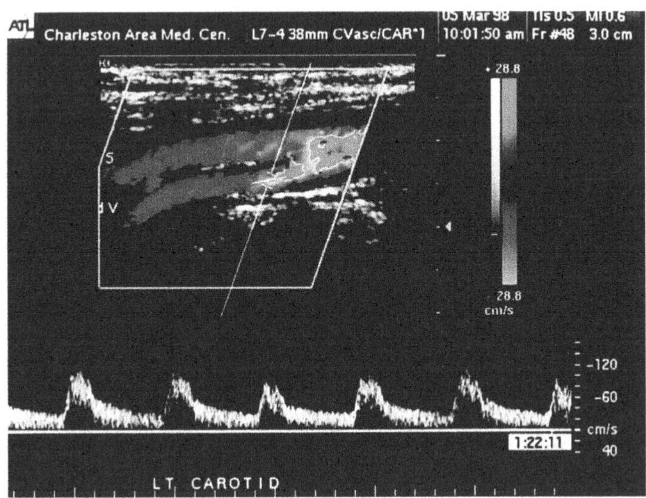

FIGURE 3–20. (A) A color duplex ultrasound image showing mild plaquing (15% to <50% stenosis) of the internal carotid artery (arrow). (B) The same patient in (A) showing internal carotid artery Doppler spectra associated with mild stenosis.

frequency remains below 4 kHz (a peak systolic velocity of <125 cm/s) and spectral broadening is also present during diastole, although it may be of greater magnitude than seen in the normal. Again, velocity is always in the forward direction, and therefore the frequencies, even during diastole, are above the zero frequency line.

Moderate to Severe Disease (50–<80% Stenosis)

As the lesion becomes progressively more occlusive (50–<80% diameter reduction), the velocity of the red blood cells traversing the stenosis increases, producing an increase in peak frequency or velocity at systole (Figures 3–21 and 3–22). Frequencies above 4 kHz in systole (a peak systolic velocity of >125 cm/s and an end diastolic velocity of <125 cm/s) are characteristic of this stenosis.

Tight Stenosis (80–99%)

With the development of high-grade lesions in excess of 80% diameter reduction, the end diastolic frequency increases (>4 kHz, or a peak systolic velocity of ≥125 cm/s and an end diastolic velocity of ≥125 cm/s) so that the ratio between peak frequency at systole and peak frequency at diastole falls, providing an accurate method of identifying these high-grade lesions. Diffuse spectral broadening is also present during the whole of the cycle, and with these lesions, the diastolic velocity at the lower frequencies approaches zero (Figures 3–23 and 3–24).

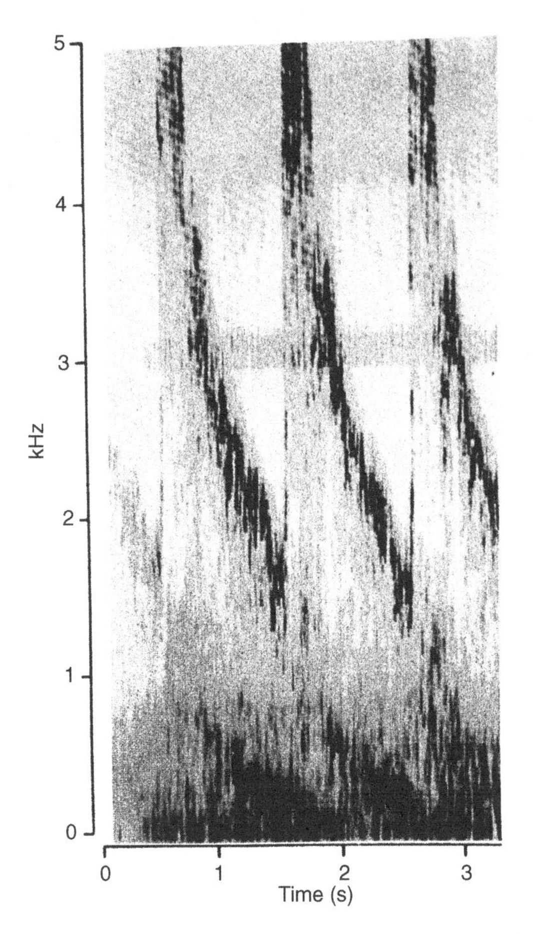

FIGURE 3–21. Internal carotid artery Doppler spectra of severe stenosis (50% to <80%).

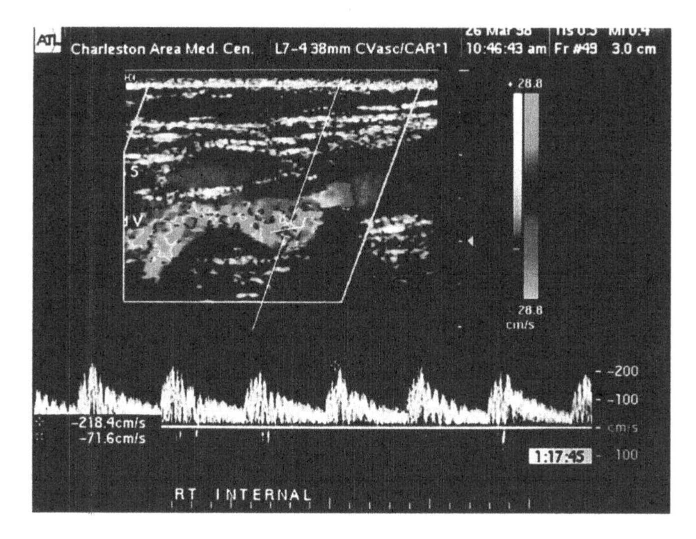

FIGURE 3–22. A color duplex ultrasound image of an internal carotid artery showing Doppler spectra of severe stenosis (50% to <80%). The peak systolic velocity on this patient was 218.4 cm/s with an end diastolic velocity of 71.6 cm/s.

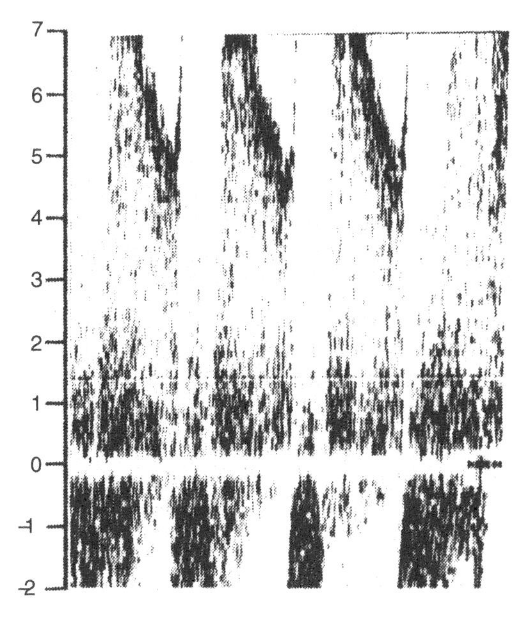

FIGURE 3–23. Internal carotid artery Doppler spectra of tight stenosis (80–99%).

Internal Carotid Occlusion

Occlusion of the internal carotid artery (Figure 3–25) is recognized by imaging a vessel in the characteristic anatomical location of the internal carotid artery with no detectable Doppler signal. It is important to ensure that the internal carotid artery is being examined, and as part of this evaluation, visualization of the external carotid artery is mandatory. The differentiation between the internal and external carotid arteries is made by visualization of the superior thyroid artery branch. Changes in the real-time spectra produced by compression of the superficial temporal artery that increases the outflow resistance usually result in a decrease in peak systolic frequency. Other features characteristic of occlusion are the presence of frequencies to the zero baseline, or even

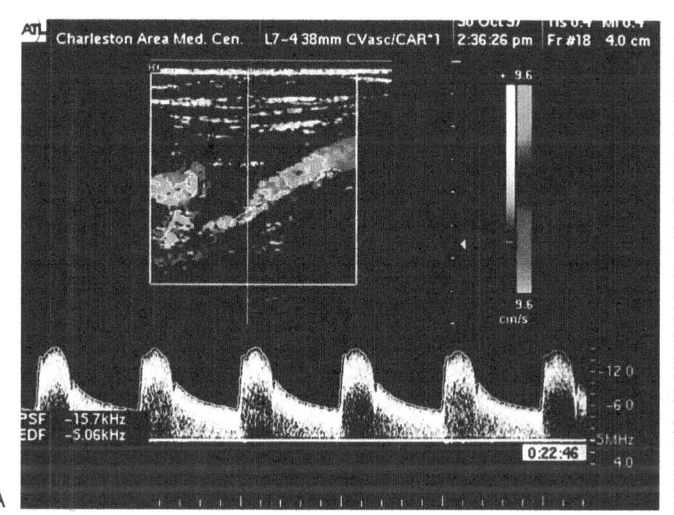

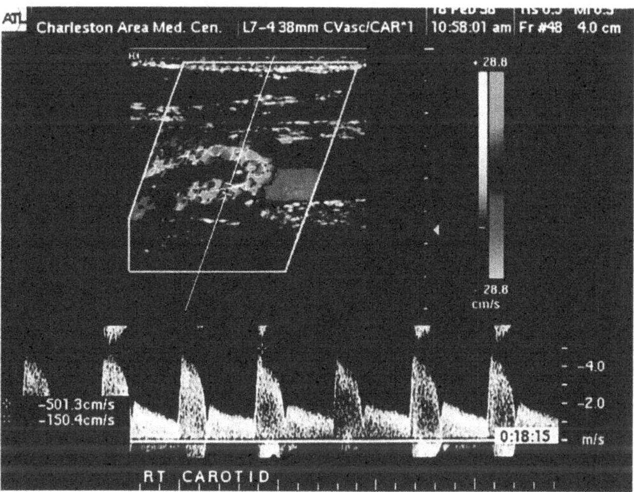

FIGURE 3–24. (A) A color duplex ultrasound image of the internal carotid artery showing Doppler spectra of tight stenosis (80–99%). The peak systolic frequency was 15.7 kHz with an end diastolic frequency of 5.06 kHz. (B) A color duplex ultrasound image of an internal carotid artery showing Doppler spectra of tight stenosis (80–99%). The peak systolic velocity was 501.3 cm/s with an end diastolic velocity of 150.4 cm/s.

negative frequencies, indicative of flow reversal obtained from the common carotid artery low in the neck.[12] When the internal carotid artery is occluded, the ipsilateral common carotid artery assumes a velocity pattern similar to that of the external carotid artery and the external carotid artery may assume flow characteristics of the internal carotid artery, i.e., high diastolic component.

Common carotid artery occlusion can also be diagnosed by color duplex ultrasound. Figure 3–26 shows retrograde flow of the external carotid artery and antegrade flow of the internal carotid artery.

Occlusions are periodically missed due to changes in physiologic parameters attendant upon the presence of internal carotid artery occlusions. Figure 3–27 shows the arteriogram and spectra obtained from a patient in whom internal carotid occlusion was missed because the external carotid artery was a major source of collateral blood flow to the middle cerebral artery, and, as such, developed the spectral changes characteristic of a high-grade internal carotid stenosis. Errors such as this can be avoided by careful evaluation of the image for the presence of branches originating from the vessel being examined and the change in the velocity profile induced by superficial temporal artery compression.

The Role of Power Doppler and Carotid Artery Occlusion

Power Doppler ultrasound displays an estimate of the entire power contained in that part of the received radio

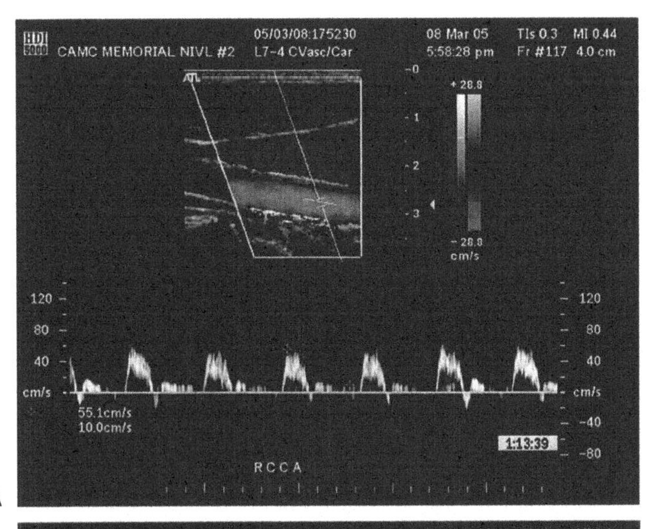

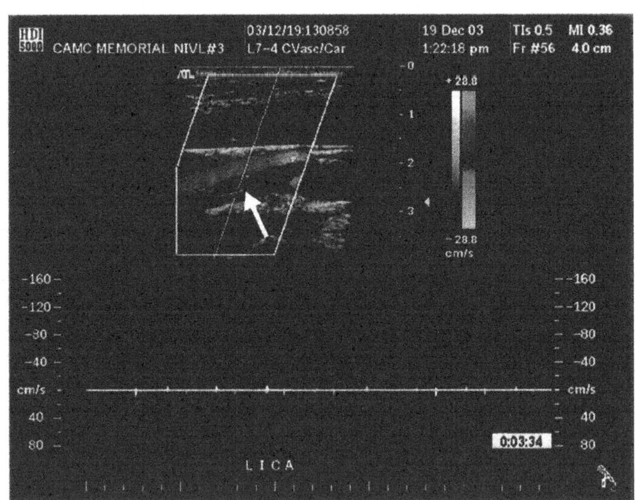

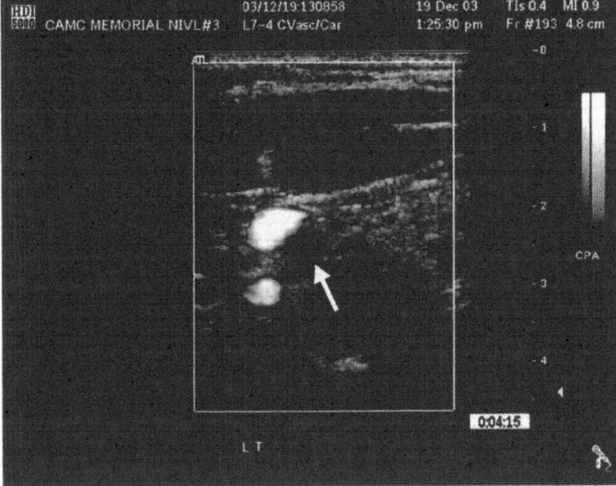

FIGURE 3–25. (A) A common carotid artery Doppler spectra produced by occlusion of the ipsilateral internal carotid artery. Peak frequency is not abnormally high, but the characteristic feature is the presence of reverse flow in diastole. (B) Internal carotid artery occlusion in longitudinal view (no color flow). (C) Internal carotid artery occlusion in transverse view [no color flow in power Doppler (arrow); color flow is seen in the external carotid artery].

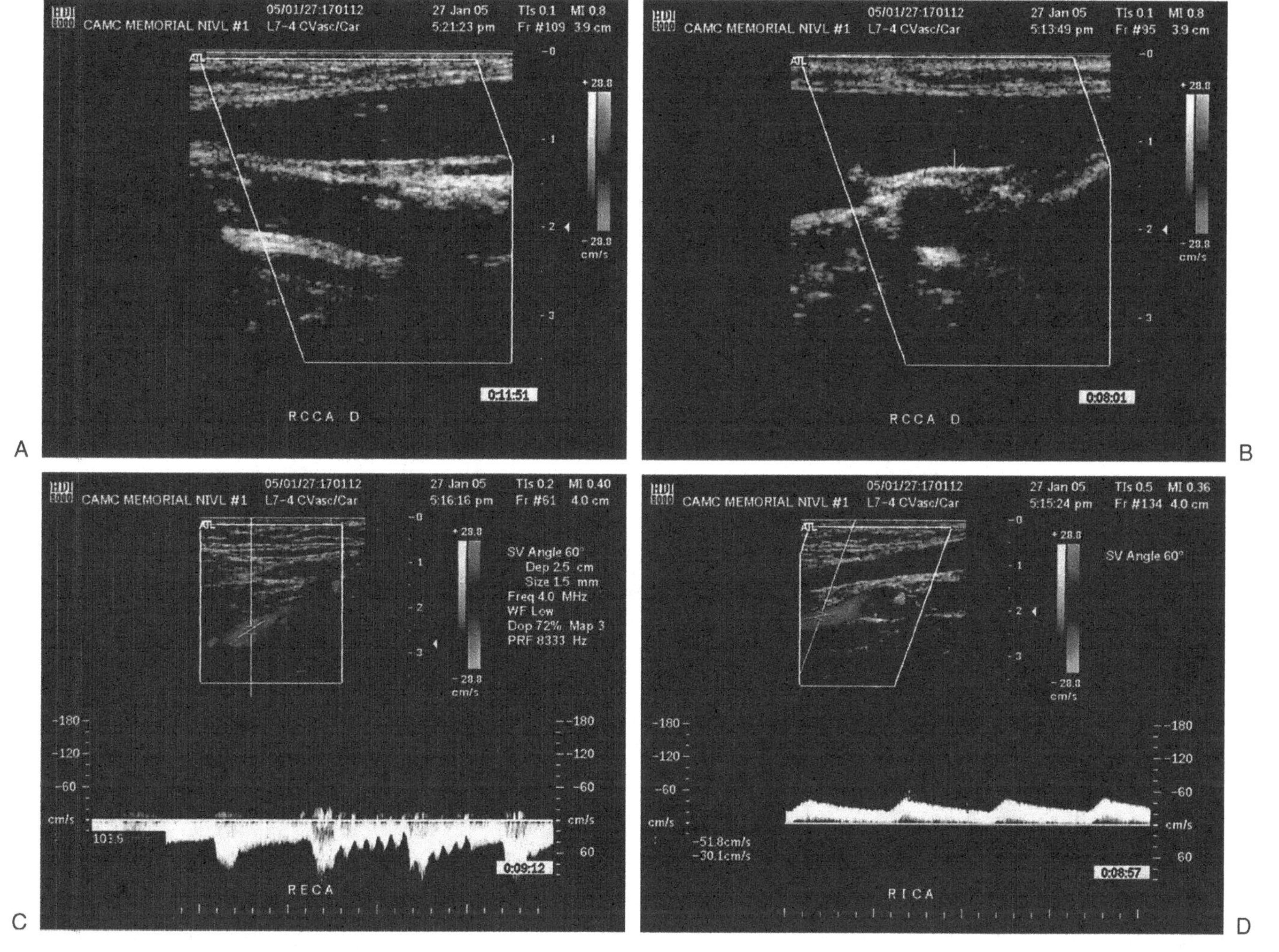

FIGURE 3–26. (A) Right common carotid artery occlusion in longitudinal view. (B) Right common carotid artery occlusion in transverse view. (C) Retrograde flow in external carotid artery. (D) Antegrade flow in internal carotid artery.

frequency ultrasound signal for which a phase shift corresponding to motion of the target is detected; in contrast, conventional color Doppler imaging displays Doppler frequency shift information. In a recent study by us,[13] five out of six patients (83%) who were felt to have total carotid occlusion by conventional color duplex were confirmed to have subtotal occlusion by adding power Doppler imaging (Figure 3–28).

External Carotid Artery Disease (High-Grade Stenosis)

Lesions producing a greater than 50% diameter reduction of the external carotid artery are identified by the presence of peak frequencies in excess of 4.5 kHz associated with diffuse spectral broadening (Figure 3–29). The overall shape of the waveform with frequencies in the negative range remains normal.

Proposed New Duplex Classification for Threshold Stenoses Used in Various Symptomatic and Asymptomatic Carotid Endarterectomy Trials[14]

Based on the duplex criteria, many laboratories, including our own, classified internal carotid artery stenosis into categories patterned after those used at the University of Washington:[11] normal, 1–15% stenosis, 16–49% stenosis, 50–79% stenosis, 80–99% stenosis, and total

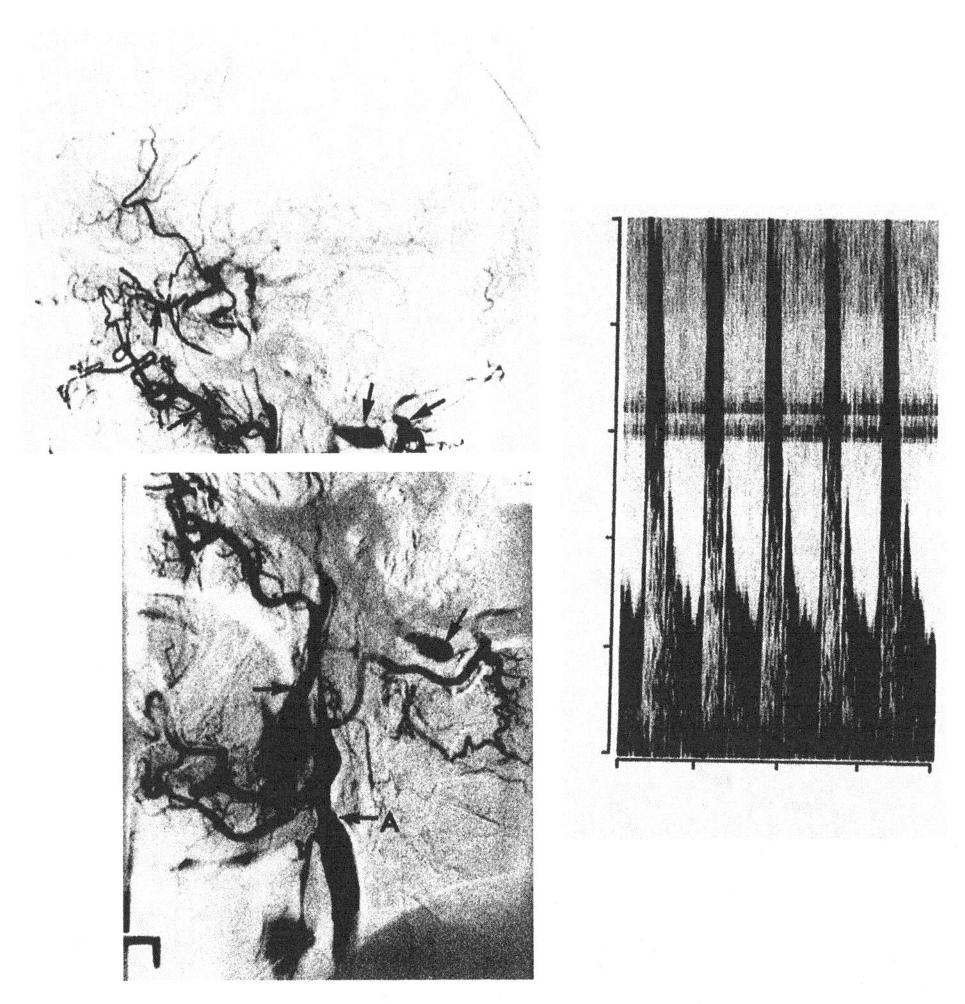

FIGURE 3–27. Arteriogram (left) and Doppler spectra (right) obtained from a missed internal carotid occlusion showing the external carotid artery functioning as a major collateral to the middle cerebral vessels. The spectra show peak frequencies in excess of 4.5 kHz in association with spectral broadening and no flow reversal. This appearance is produced by the low resistance outflow bed of the external carotid into the middle cerebral artery.

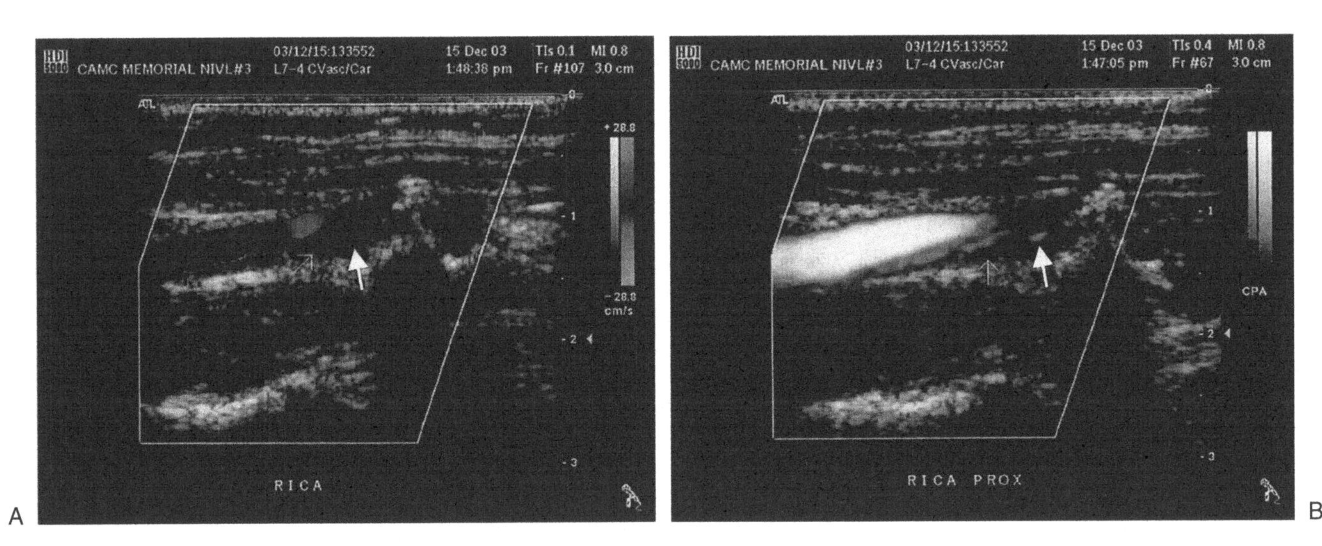

FIGURE 3–28. (A) Color duplex imaging of a right internal carotid artery suggesting total occlusion. (B) Power Doppler image of same artery showing string sign (arrow), i.e., subtotal occlusion.

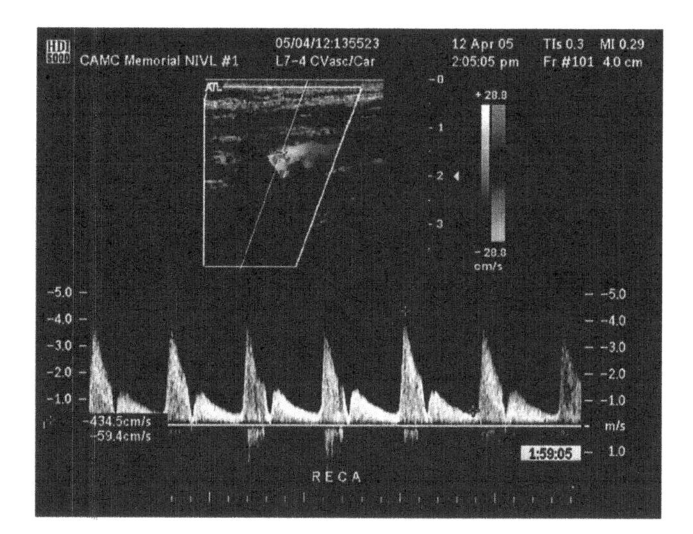

FIGURE 3–29. Doppler spectra produced by high-grade stenosis of external carotid arteries. This patient has a peak systolic velocity of 434.5 cm/s. Flow in diastole reaches the zero baseline.

occlusion. While these classifications have been useful clinically in the past, they do not correlate with threshold stenoses utilized in the recent trials investigating symptomatic (NASCET)[15] and asymptomatic (ACAS[16] and Veteran's Administration Asymptomatic Carotid Stenosis Trial Investigators[17]) carotid artery disease. With the publication of the NASCET findings showing conclusive benefit of carotid endarterectomy for symptomatic patients with 70–99% stenosis, several recent studies have attempted to develop duplex criteria to identify patients with ≥70% carotid stenosis.[18–21] With the subsequent report from the ACAS group[22] showing significant benefit of carotid endarterectomy in asymptomatic patients with ≥60% stenosis, others[23–26] reported optimal duplex criteria for detecting ≥60% stenosis.

It should be noted that the 5-year absolute risk reduction rate for ipsilateral stroke in the ACAS study was only 5.8%. Therefore, the duplex criteria for screening ≥60% internal carotid artery stenosis should have a high positive predictive value since these patients are likely to undergo invasive carotid angiography and/or carotid endarterectomy. This, along with increasing reports advocating carotid endarterectomy based on carotid duplex results alone, without preoperative arteriography,[27,28] prompted us to identify and evaluate new duplex velocity criteria for threshold stenoses used in various symptomatic and asymptomatic carotid endarterectomy trials (NASCET, ACAS, and VA studies). In addition, we identified the best duplex criteria that yielded a high positive predictive value (≥95%) for the threshold level of asymptomatic internal carotid artery stenosis of ≥60%, therefore minimizing unnecessary arteriography with its associated risk of stroke. We also identified the best duplex criteria that provided a high negative predictive value for the threshold level of symptomatic internal carotid artery stenosis of ≥70% to minimize missing patients who would benefit the most from a carotid endarterectomy.

Patient Population and Methods

Two hundred and thirty-one patients (462 arteries) who underwent both carotid color duplex scanning and arteriography from January 1992 to December 1994 were studied. Carotid color duplex scanning was performed using high-resolution real-time imaging (7.5 mHz) and a pulsed Doppler (5.0 mHz) duplex scanner (Ultramark-9, HDI system, Advanced Technology Laboratories, Bothel, WA) in standard fashion.[29]

Results

Four hundred and four carotid arteries had systolic and diastolic velocity measurements available for comparison with arteriography results.

Data derived from receiver operator curves were used to calculate the sensitivity, specificity, positive predictive value, negative predictive value, and overall accuracy of selected internal carotid artery peak systolic velocities, internal carotid artery end-diastolic velocities, and ratio of the peak systolic velocity of the internal carotid artery to the peak systolic velocity of the common

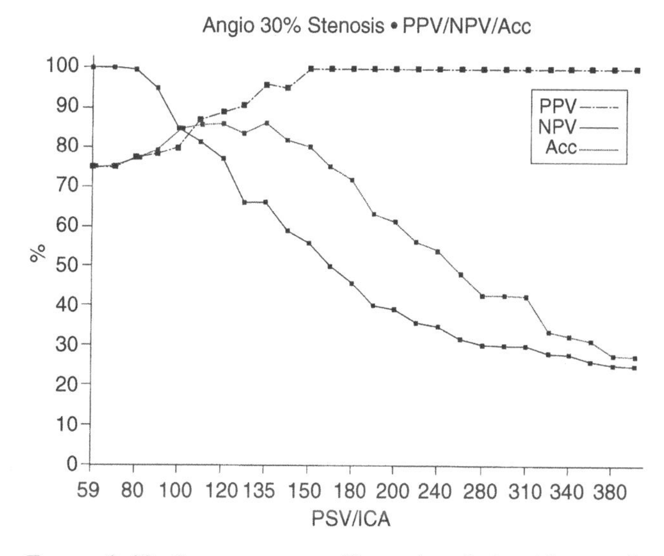

FIGURE 3–30. Response curve illustrating the positive predictive value, negative predictive value, and overall accuracy of various peak systolic velocities of the internal carotid artery in diagnosing ≥30% angiographic internal carotid artery stenosis.

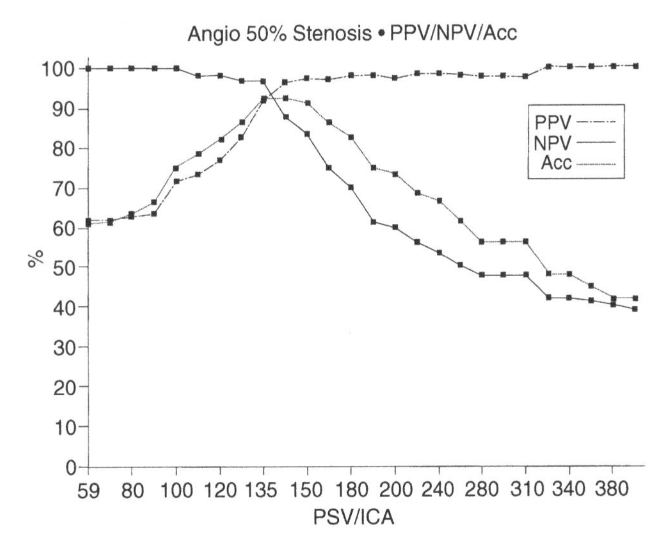

FIGURE 3–31. Response curve illustrating the positive predictive value, negative predictive value, and overall accuracy of various peak systolic velocities of the internal carotid artery in diagnosing ≥50% angiographic internal carotid artery stenosis.

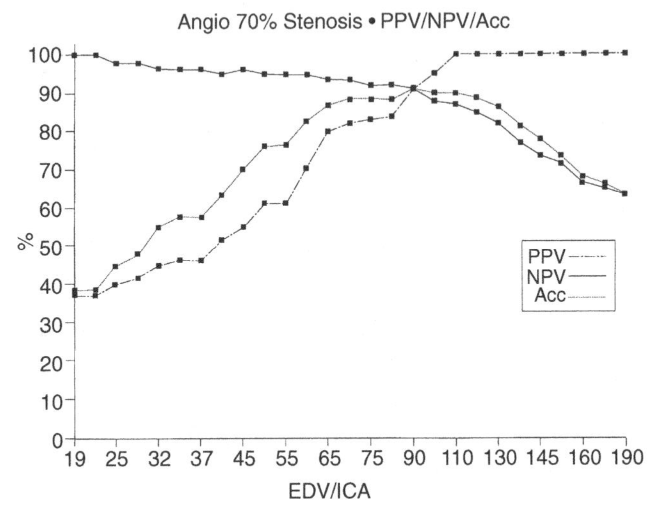

FIGURE 3–33. Response curve illustrating the positive predictive value, negative predictive value, and overall accuracy of various end diastolic velocities of the internal carotid artery in diagnosing ≥70% angiographic internal carotid artery stenosis.

carotid artery in detecting ≥30%, ≥50%, ≥60%, and ≥70–99% angiographic internal carotid artery stenosis. Figures 3–30 through 3–34 show the response curves for the positive predictive value, negative predictive value, and the overall accuracy for diagnosing various angiographic internal carotid artery stenoses for various internal carotid artery peak systolic velocities or end diastolic velocities.

Table 3–2A and B correlates the results obtained with the new proposed criteria to the percentage of angiographic stenoses in 404 carotid arteries.

The optimal duplex values that provide the best positive predictive value (≥95%) and have a good overall accuracy in detecting ≥60–99% and ≥70–99% internal carotid artery stenoses are listed in Table 3–3A and the optimal duplex values that provide the best negative pre-

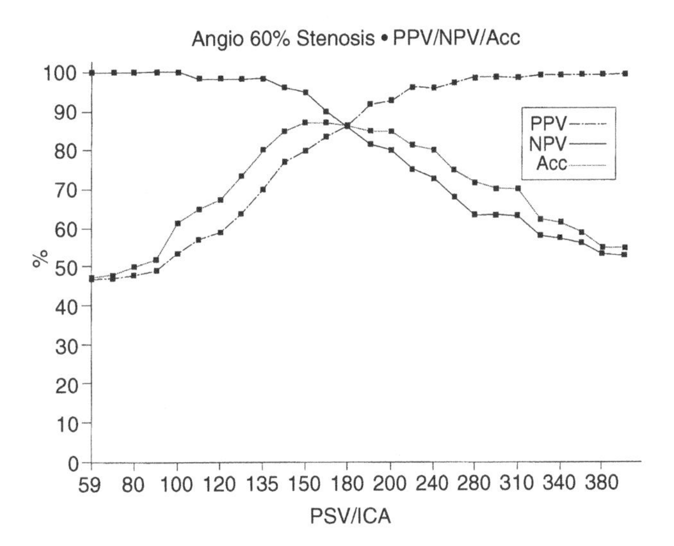

FIGURE 3–32. Response curve illustrating the positive predictive value, negative predictive value, and overall accuracy of various peak systolic velocities of the internal carotid artery in diagnosing ≥60% angiographic internal carotid artery stenosis.

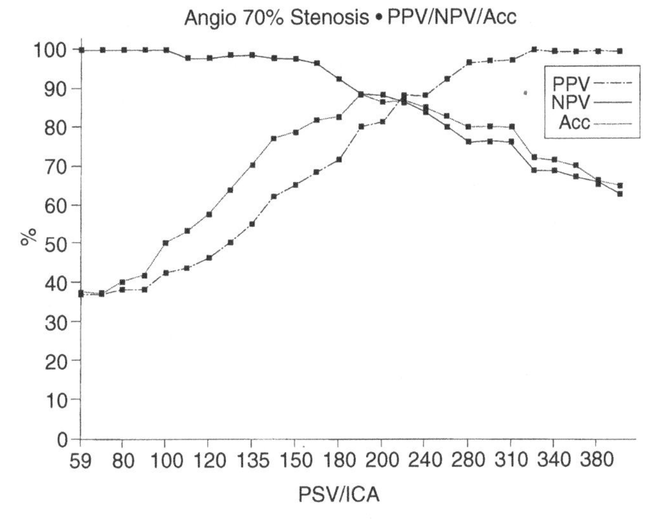

FIGURE 3–34. Response curve illustrating the positive predictive value, negative predictive value, and overall accuracy of various peak systolic velocities of the internal carotid artery in diagnosing ≥70% angiographic internal carotid artery stenosis.

TABLE 3–2A. Carotid duplex velocity criteria versus angiography: sensitivity, specificity, PPV, NPV, and overall accuracy according to the newly proposed categories of ICA stenosis.[a]

Duplex criteria (cm/s)	% Stenosis per angiogram 0–29%	30–49%	50–59%	60–69%	>70–99%	Total
ICA PSV <120	68	19	0	0	1	88
ICA PSV ≥ 120	32	30	13	4	1	80
ICA PSV ≥ 140	1	5	39	16	12	73
ICA PSV ≥ 150 and EDV ≥ 65	0	0	4	12	8	24
ICA PSV ≥ 150 and EDV ≥ 90	0	2	1	9	127	139
Total	101	56	57	41	149	404

[a]Kappa = 0.58 ± 0.03, perfect agreement = 68.32%. ICA, internal carotid artery; PSV, peak systolic velocity; EDV, end diastolic velocity.

TABLE 3–2B. Accuracy of color duplex ultrasound based on the new criteria.[a]

Duplex criteria overall	% Stenosis Sensitivity	Specificity	PPV	NPV	Accuracy
ICA PSV > 120 cm/s (<30% vs. ≥30% stenosis)	93%	67%	90%	77%	87%
ICA PSV ≥ 140 cm/s (<50% vs. ≥50% stenosis)	92%	95%	97%	89%	93%
ICA PSV > 150 and EDV ≥ 65 cm/s (<60% vs. ≥ 60% stenosis)	82%	97%	96%	86%	90%
ICA PSV > 150 and EDV ≥ 90 cm/s (<70% vs. ≥70% stenosis)	85%	95%	91%	92%	92%

[a]ICA, internal carotid artery; PSV, peak systolic velocity; EDV, end diastolic velocity.

TABLE 3–3A. Selected optimal criteria with best PPV (> or equal to 95%) and overall accuracy in detecting > or equal to 60–99% and 70–99% ICA stenosis.[a]

Best PPV for ≥60% ICA stenosis	PPV	Overall accuracy	Sensitivity	Specificity	NPV
ICA PSV ≥220 cm/s	96%	82%	64%	98%	76%
ICA EDV ≥80 cm/s	96%	87%	79%	97%	84%
ICA/CCA PSV ratio ≥4.25	96%	71%	41%	99%	65%
ICA PSV and EDV 150 and 65[b]	96%	90%	82%	97%	86%
Best PPV for ≥70% ICA stenosis					
ICA PSV ≥300 cm/s	97%	80%	48%	99%	76%
ICA EDV ≥110 cm/s[b]	100%	91%	75%	100%	87%
ICA/CCA PSV ≥ none	—	—	—	—	—
ICA PSV and EDV 150, 110[b]	100%	91%	75%	100%	87%

[a]PPV, positive predictive value; NPV, negative predictive value; ICA, internal carotid artery; PSV, peak systolic velocity; CCA, common carotid artery; EDV, end diastolic velocity.
[b]These values have the best PPV and overall accuracy.

TABLE 3–3B. Selected optimal criteria with best NPV (> or equal to 95%) and overall accuracy in detecting > or equal to 60–99% and 70–99% ICA stenosis.[a]

Best NPV for ≥60% stenosis	NPV	Overall accuracy	Sensitivity	Specificity	PPV
ICA PSV ≥135 cm/s[b]	99%	80%	99%	64%	71%
ICA EDV—none	—	—	—	—	—
ICA/CCA PSV ratio ≥1.62	95%	71%	97%	47%	62%
ICA PSV and EDV—none	—	—	—	—	—
Best NPV for ≥70% ICA stenosis					
ICA PSV ≥150 cm/s[b]	99%	80%	99%	69%	65%
ICA EDV ≥60 cm/s	96%	83%	94%	77%	71%
ICA/CCA PSV ≥ none	—	—	—	—	—
ICA PSV and EDV—none	—	—	—	—	—

[a]NPV, negative predictive value; PPV, positive predictive value; ICA, internal carotid artery; PSV, peak systolic velocity; CCA, common carotid artery; EDV, end diastolic velocity.
[b]These values have the best NPV and overall accuracy.

dictive value (≥95%) and a good overall accuracy in detecting ≥60–99% and≥70–99% internal carotid artery stenoses are shown in Table 3–3B.

In choosing our criteria for peak systolic velocity and end diastolic velocity, we chose the values that gave the highest overall accuracy. Which criteria to use is, therefore, dependent on the "outcome" desired by the clinician. Although some surgeons have advocated carotid endarterectomy based on duplex criteria alone,[27,28] the decision to proceed with an arteriogram is based on the duplex findings in the majority of patients. The mortality and morbidity of arteriography vary from institution to institution, but can be significant.[22,30] We propose that vascular laboratories at institutions with significant mortality and morbidity in relation to carotid arteriography use duplex criteria with a ≥95% positive predictive value and the best overall accuracy in order to minimize the number of patients undergoing unnecessary arteriography (Table 3–3A). These criteria can also be utilized when carotid endarterectomy is performed without preoperative arteriography. In those institutions where arteriography does not significantly add to the mortality and morbidity of the overall treatment of carotid disease, we suggest using the criteria described in Table 3–3B. These criteria have the highest negative predictive value to ensure that only a minimum number of patients with ≥60% or ≥70% stenoses is missed.

The new classification that we are proposing would consist of lesions <30%, ≥30–49%, ≥50–59%, ≥60–69%, and ≥70%. This new duplex classification would fit into the existing trials (NASCET, ACAS, and VA), and may be of benefit as new conclusions are released. By reporting results using these criteria, the clinician will be better able to make decisions regarding the need for carotid endarterectomy or arteriogram based on the risks and benefits for individual patients. With the added risks of arteriography, decisions to operate would be better based on duplex findings alone. Having positive predictive values ranging from 90 to 97% and accuracies of 87–93% can eliminate many unnecessary arteriograms.

It is important to note that the data obtained by individual vascular laboratoriess will vary across the country. Differences in equipment, abilities and consistencies of vascular technicians, and reader interpretations will cause variabilities from laboratory to laboratory.[31] Therefore, each laboratory must adapt a method that employs the equipment it uses and has validated its method when using proposed new duplex criteria.

Other studies have sought to reconcile these trials [NASCET, European Carotid Surgery Trialists (ECST), and ACAS] with duplex criteria.[18–21] A summary of these studies can be found in Table 3–4. As noted in this table, different overall accuracies were reported according to each technique and according to specific duplex criteria. This can be partially explained by the differences in scanning techniques, technologists' experience, angle of insonation, or different ultrasound systems. It has been shown that linear array transducers may overestimate peak systolic velocity in a flow phantom.[32]

Consensus Panel on Diagnostic Criteria for Grading Carotid Artery Stenosis Using Color Duplex Ultrasound

A multidisciplinary panel of experts was invited by the Society of Radiologists and Ultrasound in 2002 to attend a consensus conference on diagnostic criteria to grade carotid artery stenosis using duplex ultrasound. The consensus panel agreed on a specific set of criteria that would be helpful in grading focal proximal internal carotid artery stenosis, which is noted in Table 3–5. These criteria were to be used for new laboratories requesting applicable criteria for prospective validation. It was also recommended for established laboratories, which had previously developed their own criteria that were outdated.

Validation of ultrasound criteria can be difficult since different scanners are used in various laboratories. Therefore, it is important for each laboratory to validate its own criteria, and use these accordingly.

Accuracy of Duplex Scanning in the Detection of Carotid Disease

Various clinical studies have reported an overall accuracy of 80–97% in diagnosing carotid artery stenosis.[14,18–21,33–40] Table 3–4A and B summarizes some of these studies.

Effect of Contralateral Stenosis or Occlusion on Ipsilateral Carotid Stenosis Duplex Criteria

A number of studies in the recent literature have reported decreased accuracy of duplex scanning in predicting the degree of ipsilateral internal carotid stenosis in the presence of contralateral high-grade stenosis or carotid occlusion.[29,41–46] When conventional standard criteria[11] were applied in this circumstance, the result was an overestimation of the degree of iplsilateral stenosis (up to 48%),[45] often resulting in incorrect assignment to a higher category of disease and thus creating a false-positive interpretation.[29,41–46] It has been proposed that this phenomenon occurs because of a compensatory increase in flow velocity in the ipsilateral carotid system to maintain a stable cerebral circulation via the Circle of Willis.[42]

TABLE 3–4A. Comparison of several studies correlating angiographic 50–69%, 60–99%, and 70–99% ICA stenosis with duplex scanning.[a]

Criteria (reference)	Number of ICAs	Ultrasound System	Accuracy (%)	Sensitivity (%)	Specificity (%)	PPV (%)	NPV (%)
30–49% stenosis							
PSV ≥120cm/s[14]	462	ATL, UM9 (HDI)	87	93	67	90	77
50–69% stenosis							
PSV >140cm/s[14]	462	ATL, UM9 (HDI)	93	92	95	97	89
PSV ≥130cm/s and EDV ≤100cm/s[18]	120	Acuson 128	97	92	97	93	99
60–99% stenosis							
PSV ≥150cm/s and EDV ≥65cm/s[14]	462	ATL, UM9 (HDI)	90	82	97	96	86
PSV ≥130cm/s and EDV ≥40cm/s[19]	120	Acuson 128	80	97	72	62	98
PSV ≥260cm/s and EDV ≥70cm/s[23]	352	Acuson 128, ATL, UM9	90	84	94	92	88
PSV ≥290cm/s and EDV ≥80cm/s[23]			88	78	96	95	84
70–99% stenosis							
PSV ≥150cm/s and EDV ≥90cm/s[14]	462	ATL, UM9 (HDI)	92	85	93	91	92
PSV ≥130cm/s and EDV ≥100cm/s[18]	770	QAD 1, QAD 2000	95	81	98	89	96
PSV ≥270cm/s and EDV ≥110cm/s[19]	120	Acuson 128	93	96	91	—	—
PSV ≥325cm/s[20]	184	Acuson 128	88	83	91	80	92
ICA/CCA PSV ratio ≥4.0[20]			88	91	87	76	96
PSV ≥130cm/s and EDV ≥100cm/s[21,b]	914	QAD 2000 Phillips P700	95	87	97	89	96
PSV ≥130cm/s and EDV ≥100cm/s[21,c]			93	78	97	88	94

[a]PPV, positive predictive value; NPV, negative predictive value; PSV, peak systolic velocity; ICA, internal carotid artery; CCA, common carotid artery; EDV, end diastolic velocity.
[b]Prospective validation of criteria developed in Faught *et al.*,[18] including ICA occlusions.
[c]Analysis of criteria developed in Faught *et al.*,[18] excluding ICA occlusion.

TABLE 3–4B. Accuracy of carotid duplex ultrasound compared to arteriography in recent series.

Author	Year	Carotids/ patients	Stenosis (%)	Sensitivity/ specificity (%)	PPV/NPV (%)	Overall accuracy (%)
Patel[33]	1995	176/88	70–99	94/83		86
Hood[21]	1996	457/457	70–100	87/97	89/96	95
Huston[34]	1998	100/50	70–99	97/75	67/98	83
AbuRahma[14]	1998	462/231	70–99	85/95	91/92	92
Belsky[35]	2000	92/46	0–100	79/96	94/87	89
Anderson[36]	2000	80/40	50–69	35/87	50/78	73
			70–99	82/71	38/95	73
Back[37]	2000	74/40	50–100	100/72	88/100	91
			75–100	90/74	72/91	81
Johnston[38]	2001	452	50–99	87	46/73	68
Nederkoorn[39]	2002	313/313	70–90	88	76/75	88
MacKenzie[40]	2002	375/192	70–99	81/89	66/95	87

TABLE 3–5. Ultrasound consensus criteria for carotid stenosis.[a]

Stenosis range	ICA PSV	ICA EDV	ICA/CCA PSV ratio	Plaque
Normal	<125cm/s	<40cm/s	<2.0	None
<50%	<125cm/s	<40cm/s	<2.0	<50% diameter reduction
50–69%	125–230cm/s	40–100cm/s	2.0–4.0	≥50% diameter reduction
70—near occlusion	>230cm/s	>100cm/s	>4.0	≥50% diameter reduction
Near occlusion	May be low or undetectable	Variable	Variable	Significant, detectable lumen
Occlusion	Undetectable	Not applicable	Not applicable	Significant, no detectable lumen

[a]ICA, internal carotid artery; PSV, peak systolic velocity; EDV, end diastolic velocity; CCA, common carotid artery.

Fujitani *et al.*[45] were the first to recommend modification of the standard duplex criteria in patients with contralateral internal carotid occlusion. However, in this study, only the effect of the contralateral total carotid occlusion was studied. Patients with less than total occlusion of the contralateral artery were excluded from the study population.

The recognition of this phenomenon as consistent and clinically significant led us to undertake a retrospective study to compare the accuracy of various existing duplex criteria [standard,[11] Fujitani,[45] internal carotid/common carotid artery ratio (ICA/CCA)[47]] used in grading ipsilateral carotid stenosis in patients with contralateral high-grade stenosis or occlusion. In addition, we propose a new modified duplex criteria that we believe to be superior to the existing criteria in terms of overall accuracy.

These new criteria were developed because of our dissatisfaction with the results of the standard method in grading ipsilateral stenosis in the presence of severe contralateral disease. We had observed that most patients with ≥50% stenosis on arteriography had a peak systolic frequency of the internal carotid artery of ≥4.5kHz in the presence of severe contralateral disease.

Patient Population and Methods

From January 1992 to December 1993, 178 patients (356 arteries) were identified as having significant (>50%) internal carotid artery stenosis by carotid duplex ultrasonography, and they subsequently underwent carotid arteriography within 6 weeks.

Criteria for duplex ultrasonography classification of the degree of stenosis are shown in Table 3–6. Four different sets of criteria for each patient were analyzed: (1) the standard criteria (University of Washington),[11] (2) Fujitani criteria,[45] (3) ICA/CCA ratio criteria,[47] and (4) the new revised criteria that we are proposing. These criteria were used to assign each artery to one of five

TABLE 3–6. Doppler frequency spectral or velocity criteria for carotid artery stenosis.[a]

Classification	Arteriographic lesion	Spectral criteria
Standard method		
Grade I	1–15% diameter reduction	PSF <4kHz (<125cm/s), minimal SB
Grade II	16–49% diameter reduction	PSF <4kHz (<125cm/s), increased SB
Grade III	50–79% diameter reduction	PSF ≥4kHz (≥125cm/s) EDF <4.5kHz (<140cm/s)
Grade IV	80–99% diameter reduction	PSF >4kHz (>125cm/s) EDF >4.5kHz (>140cm/s)
Grade V	Occlusion	No internal carotid flow signal Low or reversed diastolic component in common carotid artery
New method (AbuRahma) similar to standard method except for the following		
Grade II	16–49% diameter reduction	PSF <4.5kHz (<140cm/s) EDF <4.5kHz (<140cm/s)
Grade III	50–79% diameter reduction	PSF ≥4.5kHz (≥140cm/s) EDF <4.5kHz (<140cm/s)
Grade IV	80–99% diameter reduction	PSF >4.5 kHz (>140cm/s) EDF >4.5kHz (>140cm/s)
Fujitani method—same as standard method except for the following		
Grade II	16–49% diameter reduction	PSF >4kHz (>125cm/s) EDF <5kHz (<155cm/s)
Grade III	50–79% diameter reduction	PSF >4.5kHz (>140cm/s) EDF <5kHz (<155cm/s)
Grade IV	80–99% diameter reduction	PSF >4.5kHz (>140cm/s) EDF >5kHz (>155cm/s)
ICA/CCA ratio method		
Grade I and II	1–49% diameter reduction	SVR <1.5
Grade III	50–79% diameter reduction	SVR ≥1.5, PEDV <100cm/s
Grade IV	80–99% diameter reduction	SVR ≥1.8, PEDV >100cm/s
Grade V	Occlusion	No internal carotid artery flow signal

[a]PSF, peak systolic frequency; EDF, end diastolic frequency; SB, spectral broadening; SVR, systolic velocity ratio (ICA/CCA peak systolic velocity ratio); PEDV, peak end diastolic velocity.

TABLE 3–7. Comparison of duplex grades to arteriogram grades.

	Arteriogram grades					
Duplex grades	Grade I (%)	Grade II (%)	Grade III (%)	Grade IV (%)	Grade V (%)	Total
Standard method						
Grade I	38 (100)	0	0	0	0	38
Grade II	0	17 (100)	0	0	0	17
Grade III	2 (1)	52 (30)	111 (64)	8 (5)	0	173
Grade IV	0	0	0	87 (100)	0	87
Grade V	0	0	0	2 (5)	39 (95)	41
($k = 0.760$, 95% confidence interval = 0.708–0.812)						
New method						
Grade I	38 (100)	0	0	0	0	38
Grade II	2 (3)	63 (93)	3 (4)	0	0	68
Grade III	0	6 (5)	108 (88)	8 (7)	0	122
Grade IV	0	0	0	87 (100)	0	87
Grade V	0	0	0	2 (5)	39 (95)	41
($k = 0.923$, 95% confidence interval = 0.891–0.955, $p < 0.001$)						
Fujitani method						
Grade I	38 (64)	20 (34)	1 (2)	0	0	59
Grade II	2 (4)	43 (78)	9 (16)	1 (2)	0	55
Grade III	0	6 (4)	101 (58)	66 (38)	0	173
Grade IV	0	0	0	28 (100)	0	28
Grade V	0	0	0	2 (5)	39 (95)	41
($k = 0.608$, 95% confidence interval = 0.547–0.668)						
ICA/CCA ratio method[a]						
Grades I and II	27 (48)	21 (38)	4 (7)	1 (2)	3 (5)	56
Grade III	13 (8)	48 (30)	93 (58)	7 (4)	0	161
Grade IV	0	0	14 (14)	87 (86)	0	101
Grade V	0	0	0	2 (5)	36 (95)	38
Total	40	69	111	97	39	356
($k = 0.642$, 95% confidence interval = 0.542–0.742)						

[a]ICA, internal carotid artery; CCA, common carotid artery.

categories: grade I, 1–15% stenosis; grade II, 16–49% stenosis; grade III, 50–79% stenosis; grade IV, 80–99% stenosis; and grade V, total occlusion.

Results

The standard method overestimated 56 (16%) of 356 stenoses in contrast to 3% for the new method ($p < 0.001$), and this effect was most evident in the 50% to <80% stenosis category (30%). The Fujitani method underestimated 97 (27%) of 356 stenoses, and the ICA/CCA ratio overestimated stenoses in 77 (22%) of 356. The overall exact correlation was 94, 82, 70, and 75% for the new, standard, Fujitani, and ICA/CCA ratio, respectively. The x^2 statistic and corresponding confidence intervals for the new method ($x^2 = 0.923$, ±0.016) are significantly higher ($p < 0.001$) than those for the standard method ($x^2 = 0.760$, ±0.027), the Fujitani method ($x^2 = 0.608$, ±0.031), and the ICA/CCA ratio method ($x^2 = 0.642$, ±0.051). The overall accuracy in diagnosing ≥50% ipsilateral stenosis in the whole series was 85% for the standard method, 97% for the new method, 95% for the Fujitani method, and 81% for the ICA/CCA ratio. The new method was superior to the standard and ICA/CCA ratio methods ($p < 0.001$) and the Fujitani method ($p = 0.024$).

Table 3–7 compares the results of duplex grades with those of arteriography on the basis of four different criteria. Tables 3–8 to 3–10 summarize the results of the study.

The new proposed criteria fared very well in the analysis, with only 3% overall overestimation of the disease and 3% overall underestimation of the disease. The overall exact correlation between duplex and arteriographic grading was 94% and was superior to the other criteria in each case ($p < 0.001$).

The new criteria yielded sensitivity, specificity, positive and negative predictive values, and overall accuracy values superior to those of the other three criteria in predicting ≥50% ipsilateral stenosis, when all patients with 0–100% contralateral stenosis were included ($p < 0.001$) in each case. When divided into 50% to <80% contralateral stenosis and 80–99% contralateral stenosis or total occlusion, the new criteria proved once again to be

TABLE 3–8. Comparison of duplex methods versus arteriography for sensitivity/specificity in diagnosis of > or equal to 50% ipsilateral stenosis in patients with arteries of 50% to <80% stenosis on contralateral side.[a]

Carotid arteriogram	<50% stenosis (%)	>50% stenosis (%)	Total	Sensitivity (%)	Specificity (%)	PPV (%)	NPV (%)	Overall accuracy (%)
Standard method[b]								
<50% stenosis	24 (100)	0	24	100	56	78	100	83
≥50% stenosis	19 (22)	68 (78)	87					
New method								
<50% stenosis	42 (95)	2 (5)	44	97	98	99	95	97
≥50% stenosis	1 (1)	66 (99)	67					
Fujitani method[c]								
<50% stenosis	42 (91)	4 (9)	46	94	98	98	91	96
≥50% stenosis	1 (1)	64 (99)	65					
ICA/CCA ratio method[d]								
<50% stenosis	19 (86)	3 (14)	22	96	44	73	86	76
≥50% stenosis	24 (27)	65 (73)	89					
Total	43	68	111					

[a]PPV, positive predictive value; NPV, negative predictive value; ICA, internal carotid artery; CCA, common carotid artery.
[b]New method versus standard method, $p < 0.001$ (Z statistics for proportion).
[c]New method versus Fujitani method, $p > 0.05$ (Z statistics for proportion).
[d]New method versus ICA/CCA ratio method, $p < 0.001$ (Z statistics for proportion).

superior to the standard and ICA/CCA ratio criteria ($p < 0.001$). The differences between the new criteria and Fujitani criteria in these patients did not reach statistical significance. This finding is not surprising, because the Fujitani criteria were developed from a study in which the contralateral artery was totally occluded and were designed to be used in such cases, rather than to be applied to all vessels studied, as they were in this series.

Some clinicians believe that the most important clinical issue is accuracy in detecting stenoses of greater than or less than 80%, contralateral to a tight stenosis or occlusion. The standard method results were very comparable to the new method and somewhat comparable to the ICA/CCA ratio method in all parameters examined, including overall accuracy. This finding is not surprising, because both the standard and new methods require an end diastolic frequency of the internal carotid artery of

TABLE 3–9. Comparison of duplex methods versus arteriography for sensitivity/specificity in diagnosis of >50% ipsilateral stenosis in patients with arteries with 80–99% stenosis of the contralateral side.[a]

Carotid arteriogram	<50% stenosis (%)	>50% stenosis (%)	Total	Sensitivity (%)	Specificity (%)	PPV (%)	NPV (%)	Overall accuracy (%)
Standard method								
<50% stenosis	26 (100)	0	26	100	53	68	100	76
≥50% stenosis	23 (32)	48 (68)	71					
New method								
<50% stenosis	45 (100)	0	45	100	92	92	100	96
≥50% stenosis	4 (8)	48 (92)	52					
Fujitani method								
<50% stenosis	45 (96)	2 (4)	47	96	92	92	96	94
≥50% stenosis	4 (8)	46 (92)	50					
ICA/CCA ratio method								
<50% stenosis	23 (92)	2 (8)	25	96	47	64	92	71
≥50% stenosis	26 (36)	46 (64)	72					

[a]PPV, positive predictive value; NPV, negative predictive value; ICA, internal carotid artery; CCA, common carotid artery.
[b]New method versus standard method, $p < 0.001$ (Z statistics for proportion).
[c]New method versus Fujitani method, not significant (Z statistics for proportion).
[d]New method versus ICA/CCA ratio method, $p < 0.001$ (Z statistics for proportion).

TABLE 3–10. Comparison of duplex methods versus arteriography for sensitivity/specificity in diagnosis of equal to or >50% stenosis in patients with total occlusion on contralateral side.[a]

Carotid arteriogram	<50% stenosis (%)	>50% stenosis (%)	Total	Sensitivity (%)	Specificity (%)	PPV (%)	NPV (%)	Overall accuracy (%)
Standard method[b]								
<50% stenosis	5 (100)	0	5	100	33	71	100	74
≥50% stenosis	10 (29)	24 (71)	34					
New method								
<50% stenosis	15 (94)	1 (6)	16	96	100	100	94	97
≥50% stenosis	0	23 (100)	23					
Fujitani method[c]								
<50% stenosis	15 (83)	3 (17)	18	88	100	100	83	92
≥50% stenosis	0	21 (100)	21					
ICA/CCA ratio method[d]								
<50% stenosis	6 (100)	0	6	100	40	73	100	77
≥50% stenosis	9 (27)	24 (73)	33					

[a]PPV, positive predictive value; NPV, negative predictive value; ICA, internal carotid artery; CCA, common carotid artery.
[b]New method versus standard method, $p < 0.01$ (Z statistics for proportion).
[c]New method versus Fujitani method, $p = 0.15$ (Z statistics for proportion).
[d]New method versus ICA/CCA ratio method, $p < 0.01$ (Z statistics for proportion).

>4.5 kHz for the diagnosis of ≥80% stenosis. However, the Fujitani method had a poorer sensitivity and an overall accuracy of only 85% in contrast to an overall accuracy of 98% for the new and standard methods in this group of patients (80–99% contralateral stenosis). This finding can be explained by the requirement of an end diastolic frequency of the internal carotid artery of >5 kHz for the diagnosis of ≥80% stenosis for the Fujitani method. Similar observations were noted in patients with a total contralateral occlusion. Our results were comparable to data previously reported by others.[41–46]

Table 3–11 summarizes the duplex accuracy of various criteria in the presence of contralateral stenosis or occlusion.

TABLE 3–11. Accuracy of duplex criteria with contralateral severe stenosis or occlusion.[a]

Criteria and reference	Accuracy (%)	Sensitivity (%)	Specificity (%)	PPV (%)	NPV (%)
>50% stenosis					
Fujitani[45]	74	97	57	62	96
AbuRahma[29]					
Fujitani	92	88	100	100	83
Standard	74	100	33	71	100
AbuRahma	97	96	100	100	94
Ratios	77	100	40	73	100
50–79% stenosis					
Fujitani: PSV >140 cm/s, EDV <155 cm/s[45]	71	84	70	28	97
AbuRahma[29]					
Fujitani: PSV >140 cm/s, EDV <155 cm/s	97	99	98	98	95
Standard: PSV >125 cm/s, EDV <140 cm/s	83	100	56	78	100
AbuRahma: PSV ≥140 cm/s, EDV <140 cm/s	97	97	98	99	95
Ratios: ICA/CCA ratio ≥1.5, EDV <100 cm/s	76	96	44	73	86
80–99% stenosis					
Fujitani: PSV >140 cm/s, EDV >155 cm/s[45]	96	91	97	89	98
AbuRahma[29]					
Fujitani: PSV >140 cm/s, EDV >155 cm/s	94	96	92	92	96
Standard: PSV >125 cm/s, EDV >140 cm/s	76	100	53	68	100
AbuRahma: PSV >140 cm/s, EDV >140 cm/s	96	100	92	92	100
Ratios: ICA/CCA ratio ≥1.8, EDV >100 cm/s	71	96	47	64	92

[a]PPV, positive predictive value; NPV, negative predictive value; PSV, peak systolic velocity; EDV, end diastolic velocity; ICA, internal carotid artery; CCA, common carotid artery.

Clinical Use of Carotid Duplex Scanning

Carotid duplex ultrasound reports routinely include flow velocities and the degree of stenoses. However, several carotid reports, particularly those from nonaccredited vascular laboratories, have several inconsistencies that can be extremely critical in clinical decision making. A carotid duplex ultrasound examination should be termed "inconclusive" if the findings are uncertain, and it cannot be ensured that the carotid artery does not have significant carotid artery disease.[48,49] Calcification and shadowing, high bifurcation, short neck, or any other circumstances that prevent adequate interrogation of the carotid artery can result in an inconclusive examination. In this scenario, other diagnostic modalities must be recommended to delineate the proper pathology. Inconsistent carotid examination is used when the imaging and velocity determination of the color duplex ultrasound are not consistent with each other, and additional tests are also required in these circumstances. Significant carotid artery stenosis may be present without associated increased flow velocities. This can be partially explained by complex or calcified lesions or dampened flow by an extremely high-grade lesion.

The accuracy of duplex scanning in the examination of the carotid artery bifurcation has resulted in its use in symptomatic patients for the detection of disease, the evaluation of patients with neck bruits, postoperative studies of endarterectomized vessels, and the sequential examination of asymptomatic patients to document progression of disease.[50] Other clinical implications include carotid endarterectomy without angiography, intraoperative assessment of carotid endarterectomy, long-term follow-up after carotid endarterectomy, plaque morphology and outcome, and carotid duplex scanning following trauma. The clinical implications of duplex ultrasound technology will be discussed in detail in Chapter 13.

References

1. Kossoff G. Gray Scale Echography in Obstetrics and Gynecology. Report No. 60. Sydney, Australia, Commonwealth Acoustic Laboratories, 1973.
2. Olinger CP. Ultrasonic carotid echoarteriography. Am J Roentgenol 1969;106:282–295.
3. Hartley DJ, Strandness DE Jr. The effects of atherosclerosis on the transmission of ultrasound. J Surg Res 1969;9:575–582.
4. Barber FE, Baker DW, Nation AWC, *et al.* Ultrasonic duplex echo-Doppler scanner. IEEE Trans Biomed Eng 1974;81:109–113.
5. Blackshear WM, Phillips DJ, Chikos RM, *et al.* Carotid artery velocity patterns in normal and stenotic vessels. Stroke 1980;11:67–71.
6. Reilly LM. Importance of carotid plaque morphology. In: Bernstein EF (ed). *Vascular Diagnosis*, 4th ed., pp. 333–340. St. Louis, MO: Mosby-Year Book, 1993.
7. AbuRahma AF, Kyer PR, Robinson P, *et al.* The correlation of ultrasonic carotid plaque morphology and carotid plaque hemorrhage: Clinical implications. Surgery 1998;124:721–726.
8. AbuRahma AF, Thiele S, Wulu J. Prospective controlled study of the natural history of asymptomatic 60% to 69% carotid stenosis according to ultrasonic plaque morphology. J Vasc Surg 2002;36:437–442.
9. Gronholdt M, Nordestgaard B, Schroeder T, *et al.* Ultrasonic echolucent carotid plaques predict future strokes. Circulation 2001;104:68–73.
10. Thiele BL, Hutchison KJ, Green RM, *et al.* Pulsed Doppler waveform patterns produced by smooth stenosis in the dog thoracic aorta. In: Taylor DEM (ed). *Blood Flow Theory and Practice*, pp. 85–104. New York: Academic Press, 1983.
11. Zierler RE, Strandness DE Jr. Noninvasive dynamic and real-time assessment of extracranial cerebrovasculature. In: Wood JH (ed). *Cerebral Blood Flow: Physiologic and Clinical Aspects,* pp. 311–323. New York: McGraw-Hill, 1987.
12. Bodily KC, Phillips DJ, Thiele BL, *et al.* Noninvasive detection of internal carotid artery occlusion. Angiology 1981;32:517–521.
13. AbuRahma AF, Jarrett K, Hayes JD. Clinical implications of power Doppler three-dimensional ultrasonography. Vascular 2004;12:293–300.
14. AbuRahma AF, Robinson, PA, Stickler, DL, *et al.* Proposed new duplex classification for threshold stenoses used in various symptomatic and asymptomatic carotid endarterectomy trials. Ann Vasc Surg 1998;12:349–358.
15. North American Symptomatic Carotid Endarterectomy Trial Collaborators. Beneficial effect of carotid endarterectomy in symptomatic patients with high-grade carotid stenosis. N Engl J Med 1991;325:445–453.
16. Asymptomatic Carotid Atherosclerosis Study Group. Study design for randomized prospective trial of carotid endarterectomy for asymptomatic atherosclerosis. Stroke 1989;20:844–849.
17. Veteran's Administration Cooperative Study. Role of carotid endarterectomy in asymptomatic carotid stenosis. Stroke 1986;17:534–539.
18. Faught WE, Mattos MA, van Bemmelen PS, *et al.* Color-flow duplex scanning of carotid arteries: New velocity criteria based on receiver operator characteristic analysis for threshold stenoses used in the symptomatic and asymptomatic carotid trials. J Vasc Surg 1994;19:818–828.
19. Neale ML, Chambers JL, Kelly AT, *et al.* Reappraisal of duplex criteria to assess significant carotid stenosis with special reference to reports from the North American Symptomatic Carotid Endarterectomy Trial and the European Carotid Surgery Trial. J Vasc Surg 1994;20:642–649.
20. Moneta GL, Edwards JM, Chitwood RW, *et al.* Correlation of North American Symptomatic Carotid Endarterectomy Trial (NASCET) angiographic definition of 70% to 99% internal carotid artery stenosis with duplex scanning. J Vasc Surg 1993;17:152–159.

21. Hood DB, Mattos MA, Mansour A, *et al.* Prospective evaluation of new duplex criteria to identify 70% internal carotid artery stenosis. J Vasc Surg 1996;23:254–262.
22. Executive Committee for the Asymptomatic Carotid Atherosclerosis Study. Endarterectomy for asymptomatic carotid artery stenosis. JAMA 1995;273:1421–1428.
23. Moneta GL, Edwards JM, Papanicolaou G, *et al.* Screening for asymptomatic internal carotid artery stenosis: Duplex criteria for discriminating 60% to 99% stenosis. J Vasc Surg 1995;21:989–994.
24. Carpenter JP, Lexa FJ, Davis JT. Determination of sixty percent or greater carotid artery stenosis by duplex Doppler ultrasonography. J Vasc Surg 1995;22:697–705.
25. Burnham CB, Liguish J Jr, Burnham SJ. Velocity criteria redefined for the 60% carotid stenosis. J Vasc Technol 1996;20(1):5–11.
26. AbuRahma AF, Pollack JA, Robinson, PA, *et al.* New duplex criteria for threshold stenoses used in the asymptomatic carotid atherosclerosis study (ACAS). Vasc Surg 1999;33:23–32.
27. Marshall WG Jr, Kouchoukos NT, Murphy SF, *et al.* Carotid endarterectomy based on duplex scanning without preoperative arteriography. Circulation 1988;78(Suppl I):I-1–I-5.
28. Geuder JW, Lamparello PJ, Riles TS, *et al.* Is duplex scanning sufficient evaluation before carotid endarterectomy? J Vasc Surg 1989;9:193–201.
29. AbuRahma AF, Richmond BK, Robinson PA, *et al.* Effect of contralateral severe stenosis or carotid occlusion on duplex criteria of ipsilateral stenoses: Comparative study of various duplex parameters. J Vasc Surg 1995;22:751–762.
30. AbuRahma AF, Robinson PA, Boland JP, *et al.* Complications of arteriography in a recent series of 707 cases: Factors affecting outcome. Ann Vasc Surg 1993;7:122–129.
31. Haynes B, Thorpe K, Raylor W, *et al.* Poor performance of ultrasound in detecting high-grade carotid stenosis (Abstract). Can J Surg 1992;35:446.
32. Daigle RJ, Stavros AT, Lee RM. Overestimation of velocity and frequency values by multi-element linear array Dopplers. J Vasc Tech 1990;14:206–213.
33. Patel MR, Kuntz KM, Klufas RA, *et al.* Preoperative assessment of the carotid bifurcation: Can magnetic resonance angiography and duplex ultrasonography replace contrast arteriography? Stroke 1995;26:1753–1758.
34. Huston J, Nichols DA, Luetmer PH, *et al.* MR angiographic and sonographic indications for endarterectomy. AJNR 1998;19:309–315.
35. Belsky M, Gaitini D, Goldsher D, *et al.* Color-coded duplex ultrasound compared to CT angiography for detection and quantification of carotid artery stenosis. Eur J Ultrasound 2000;12:49–60.
36. Anderson GB, Ashforth R, Steinke DE, *et al.* CT angiography for the detection and characterization of carotid artery bifurcation disease. Stroke 2000;31:2168–2174.
37. Back MR, Wilson JS, Rushing G, *et al.* Magnetic resonance angiography is an accurate imaging adjunct to duplex ultrasound scan in patient selection for carotid endarterectomy. J Vasc Surg 2000;32:429–440.
38. Johnston DC, Goldstein LB. Clinical carotid endarterectomy decision-making. Neurology 2001;56:1009–1015.
39. Nederkoorn PJ, Mali WP, Eikelboom BC, *et al.* Preoperative diagnosis of carotid artery stenosis: Accuracy of noninvasive testing. Stroke 2002;33:2003–2008.
40. MacKenzie KS, French-Sherry E, Burns K, *et al.* B-mode ultrasound measurement of carotid bifurcation stenoses: Is it reliable? Vasc Endovasc Surg 2002;36:123–135.
41. Spadone DP, Barkmeier LD, Hodgson KJ, *et al.* Contralateral internal carotid artery stenosis or occlusion: Pitfall of correct ipsilateral classification. A study performed with color flow imaging. J Vasc Surg 1990;11:642–649.
42. Forconi S, Johnston KW. Effect of contralateral internal carotid stenosis on the accuracy of continuous wave Doppler spectral analysis results. J Cardiovasc Surg 1987; 28:715–718.
43. Hayes AC, Johnston KW, Baker WH, *et al.* The effect of contralateral disease on carotid Doppler frequency. Surgery 1988;103:19–23.
44. Beckett WW Jr, Davis PC, Hoffman JC Jr. Duplex Doppler sonography of the carotid artery: False positive results in an artery contralateral to an artery with marked stenosis. AJR 1990;155:1091–1095.
45. Fujitani RM, Mills JL, Wang LM, *et al.* The effect of unilateral internal carotid arterial occlusion upon contralateral duplex study: Criteria for accurate interpretation. J Vasc Surg 1992;16:459–468.
46. Fisher M, Alexander K. Influence of contralateral obstructions on Doppler-frequency spectral analysis of ipsilateral stenoses of the carotid arteries. Stroke 1985;16:846–848.
47. Bluth EI, Stavros AT, Marich KW, *et al.* Carotid duplex sonography: A multicenter recommendation for standardized imaging and Doppler criteria. RadioGraphics 1988;8: 487–506.
48. Lovelace TD, Moneta GL, Abou-Zamzam AM Jr, Edwards JM, Yeager RA, Landry GJ, Taylor LM Jr, Porter JM. Optimizing duplex follow-up in patients with an asymptomatic internal carotid artery stenosis of less than 60%. J Vasc Surg 2001;33:56–61.
49. Lavensen GS. The carotid artery ultrasound reports: Considerations in evaluation and management. J Vasc Ultrasound 2004;28:15–19.
50. Roederer GO, Langlois MD, Jager MD, *et al.* The natural history of carotid arterial disease in asymptomatic patients with cervical bruits. Stroke 1984;15:605–613.

4 The Role of Color Duplex Scanning in Diagnosing Diseases of the Aortic Arch Branches and Carotid Arteries

Clifford T. Araki, Bruce L. Mintz, and Robert W. Hobson II

Introduction

Extracranial cerebrovascular disease is most commonly diagnosed at the carotid bifurcation/proximal internal carotid artery. While ultrasound is excellent at detecting the bifurcation lesion, it has been limited in its application to disease in other cerebrovascular segments.

Atherosclerotic disease in the truncal branches of the aortic arch typically occurs at the origin of the branch vessels. The clinical consequences of these lesions include hypoperfusion and thromboembolic events that can impact the anterior or posterior cerebrovascular circulation and circulation to the upper extremities. Their potential for atheroembolic strokes in the anterior circulation and subclavian steal from the posterior circulation is sufficient for surgeons to consider intervention when significant lesions are detected.[1]

The incidence of atherosclerotic disease in the branches of the arch is much lower than it is for the carotid bifurcation but is not well documented. Studies performed in the 1960s and 1970s estimated disease in the arch branches to account for no more than 17% of symptomatic extracranial cerebrovascular disease.[2–4] In 1968, Hass *et al.* reported a severe lesion in one or more of the aortic arch branches in one-third of patients examined by cerebrovascular arteriography. In 101 autopsy patients, a similar percentage was ascribed to ulcerative disease in the arch branches, second only to the carotid sinus.[6]

The incidence of arch lesions has not been systematically evaluated by arteriography and ultrasound has not been considered sufficient to evaluate the arch and its branches. The lack of an adequate assessment has made the natural history of these lesions unclear and indications for repair have not been well established. With endovascular surgery poised to treat these once difficult lesions, the availability of a reliable noninvasive assessment of the arch lesion now becomes clinically significant.

There are no data available to indicate how many arch lesions are missed in a typical carotid ultrasound examination and yet the perceived limitations of ultrasound testing may be due to technique more than hardware. New ultrasonic approaches to these poorly assessed structures should be made to extend the characterization of the extracranial cerebrovascular examination for the potential benefit of this subset of patients.

Anatomy of the Aortic Arch and Brachiocephalic Veins

Aortic Arch

To ultrasonically evaluate the arch and its branches, the orientation of the arch has to be recognized as it projects from the left ventricle to the descending aorta. The aorta ascends to the right of midline as it leaves the left ventricle. The pericardium attaches to the ascending aorta and pulmonary artery as they leave the heart, just beyond their origination. The arch itself becomes an extrapericardial structure. The aorta ascends from the heart to the right of the pulmonary artery. It arches around and above the right branch of the pulmonary artery, anterior to the trachea; it then forms an oblique trajectory from the right anterior mediastinum to the left posterior mediastinum. It forms the descending thoracic aorta to the left of the trachea and esophagus. As the descending aorta, it continues its course along the posterior wall of the chest, toward the left side of the vertebral column.

The aortic arch is approximately 4.5 cm in length. At 2.5–3 cm, it has a slightly larger diameter than the abdominal aorta that we are accustomed to seeing. Three truncal branches arise from the arch: innominate (brachiocephalic trunk), the left common carotid artery, and the left subclavian artery (Figure 4–1). All arise perpendicular to the flow axis of the arch and ascend through the mediastinum to carry blood to the upper extremities and head.

A.F. Aburahma, J.J. Bergan (eds.), *Noninvasive Cerebrovascular Diagnosis*, DOI 10.1007/978-1-84882-957-2_4,

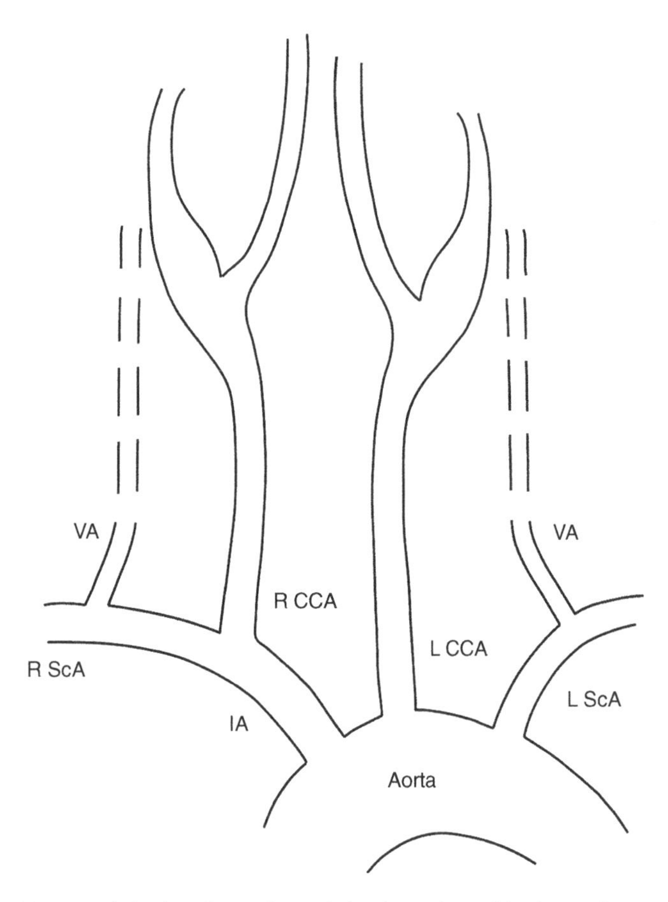

FIGURE 4–1. Aortic arch and its branches. IA, innominate artery; R ScA, right subclavian artery; VA, vertebral artery; R CCA, right common carotid artery; L CCA, left common carotid artery; L ScA, left subclavian artery.

The innominate artery is the first and largest arch branch. It arises near midline, anterior to the trachea, and courses gently to the right. Just below the base of the right neck, it bifurcates to form the right subclavian and right common carotid arteries.

The left common carotid artery is typically the second branch from the aortic arch. Arising immediately after the innominate artery, it also originates in front of the trachea and curves gently toward the left side of the neck. Both the innominate and left common carotid arteries start near midline, then curve gently laterally. The common carotid arteries course to the right and left of midline, where both right and left common carotid arteries approach the carotid bifurcation in a posterior position on either side of the trachea.

The left subclavian artery is the third arch branch, ascending toward the neck but bending laterally to course through the thoracic outlet. In some, the right subclavian artery may originate from the innominate slightly higher in the chest to take a more downward projection to enter the thoracic outlet.

The arch rises in the superior mediastinum fairly high in the chest but lies protected by the sternum. The truncal branches also arise behind the sternum and sternoclavicular joints at about the level of the third and fourth thoracic vertebra. This protected position makes a direct transthoracic ultrasonic approach to the arch impossible.

The basic branch anatomy is shared by two-thirds (65%) of the population.[7] The remaining one-third has a variant anatomy. The most frequent variant lies in a common origin shared by the innominate and left common carotid arteries, the so-called brachiocephalic branch or bovine configuration. This occurs in 27% of the population. Much less frequently, the vertebral artery originates from the aorta between the left common carotid and the left subclavian arteries (2–6% of cases). Rarely (less than 1%), the right subclavian artery originates from the arch distal to the left subclavian or the right vertebral originates from the right common carotid artery or the arch.

Brachiocephalic Veins

The central veins demonstrate greater symmetry than the supraaortic arteries (Figure 4–2). The internal jugular

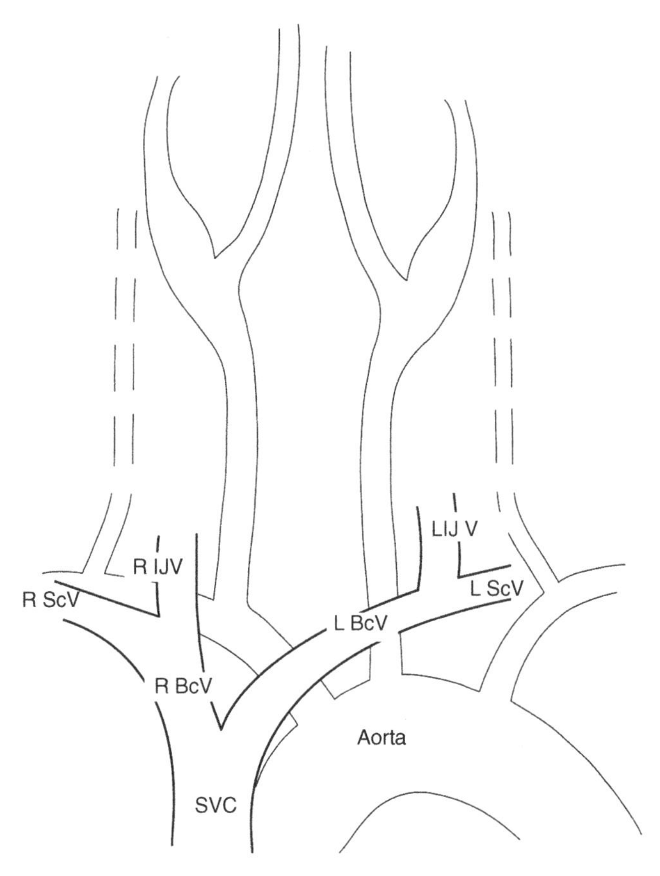

FIGURE 4–2. Brachiocephalic veins and superior vena cava. RScV, right subclavian vein; R IJV, right internal jugular vein; R BcV, right brachiocephalic vein; LBcV, left brachiocephalic vein; L ScV, left subclavian vein; L IJV, left internal jugular vein; SVC, superior vena cava.

veins of the neck and subclavian veins from the upper extremities are confluent, forming the right and left brachiocephalic veins. The external jugular veins also drain into the subclavian veins bilaterally, near the originations of the brachiocephalic veins. The right and left brachiocephalic veins converge to form the superior vena cava (SVC) at about the level of the aortic arch. The SVC lies to the right of the arch, causing a bit of asymmetry. The right brachiocephalic vein descends directly into the SVC as a short venous segment but the left brachiocephalic vein is longer and sharply angulated because of the position of the SVC. The left brachiocephalic vein courses obliquely from the left internal jugular (IJ) vein to the right chest, lying anterior to the branch arteries of the arch. Both brachiocephalic veins converge to form the SVC. Approximately 7 cm in length, the SVC is in contact with the pleura of the right lung, the trachea, and aorta. There are no valves in the brachiocephalic trunks or SVC.

Imaging the Aortic Arch and Brachiocephalic Veins

The arch and branches are a neglected area that is seldom imaged with ultrasound because of dense ultrasound reflections produced by bone and lung air. It is, however, described as part of a standard echocardiographic assessment made through a suprasternal approach.[8]

The suprasternal notch is the midline depression that lies at the base of the neck, between the sternum and larynx. Echocardiography uses the notch to visualize the ascending aorta, arch, and descending thoracic aorta as a means for evaluating the aorta for valvular insufficiency, dissection, aneurysm, or coarctation.[9] Though it is described as a standard echo approach, the image is often less than satisfactory, and is seldom used in adult echocardiography.

The echocardiographer uses a 2- to 5-MHz transducer to visualize the ascending aorta, arch, and descending aorta. The transducer produces a small footprint for the more superficial arch branches and is less suited for branch vessel assessment. For the neck, vascular sonographers use high-frequency (5–10 MHz) linear probes to image the extracranial cerebrovascular branches at the carotid bifurcation. The examination approaches the cervical carotid arteries from the lateral neck, alongside the sternocleidomastoid muscle. The scan typically ends centrally at the right common carotid origin and left common carotid artery at the neck base.

As a compromise, the midline, suprasternal approach should be our approach to the supraaortic vessels, using a low-frequency curvilinear probe rather than the small footprint echo or the high-frequency linear probe. The obvious drawbacks to imaging the arch and its branches from this angle include (1) interference from the sternum and claviculae that severely limits access. The ultrasound beam is projected downward through a narrow acoustic window that limits the anterior–posterior projection by the sternum and neck; (2) the truncal arteries project directly toward the probe and veins project directly away from the probe. The resulting B-mode echoes are weakly reflective and poorly illuminate the walls of the central branches; (3) color Doppler compensates for the weak B-mode image, but the number of large vessel flows and color artifacts picked up from the bright echo-reflective surfaces of the mediastinum and pleura produces a confusing image with large swaths of color.

To overcome these problems, recognizing the anatomy of the arch and brachiocephalic veins is important to scanning the central vessels. It is also important to maintain an orientation that is based upon the known ultrasonic anatomy. The examination can be performed by first placing the curvilinear transducer above the sternum and positioning the probe to produce a panoramic view of both common carotid arteries and IJ veins at the base of the neck (Figure 4–3). With this view as the reference point, the scan can be extended centrally by grayscale and color. The right common carotid artery will be seen to rapidly converge with the subclavian artery to become the innominate artery. On the left, the common carotid artery will be seen to simultaneously continue uninterrupted toward the arch. As the probe is projected centrally, both innominate and left common carotid artery will approach one another. The larger innominate artery will approach midline from the patient's right and the left common carotid artery will course obliquely from the left. From further left, the left subclavian artery will course toward the arch from the clavicle.

The arteries and veins of interest lie in front of the trachea. Because the arch projects obliquely from right to left, anterior to posterior, the probe, positioned for a transverse view of the innominate and left common carotid artery, will also capture the aorta in near transverse. The aorta will be seen in grayscale as a 2–3 cm pulsatile mass. By color, flow in the aorta will be notably disturbed. Flow in the innominate and left common carotid will be much more uniform and easily traced as tracks of color flow directed toward the probe. Both arteries can be interrogated by spectral Doppler as they approach the aorta.

Once the relative positions of the arteries are identified, the innominate artery (Figure 4–4) and left common carotid artery (Figure 4–5) may be imaged individually in longitudinal view by rotating the ultrasound probe on the neck base to the left of midline.

The left subclavian artery may be the most difficult to follow. To visualize the subclavian, the transducer probe will be positioned above the clavicle, projecting the heel of the probe toward the left posterior aspect of the notch (Figure 4–6). Ultrasound reflections will capture bright

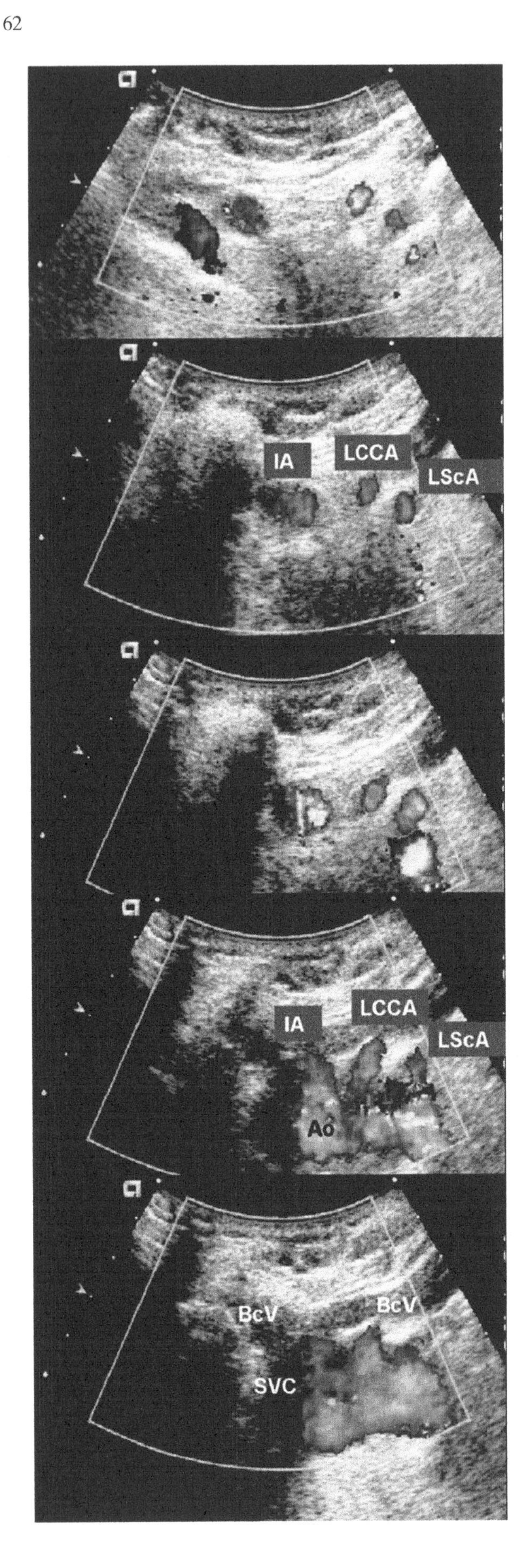

FIGURE 4–3. Imaging the aortic arch and its branches. Branches of the arch from the neck base (top) to aorta (bottom) are scanned with a 4-MHz curvilinear probe placed horizontally above the suprasternal notch. The innominate artery (IA), left common carotid artery (LCCA), and left subclavian artery (LScA) are shown in oblique slices. Scanning centrally, the supraaortic branches enter the aorta (Ao). With greater probe angulation (bottom), the convergence of the right and left brachiocephalic veins (BcV) can be imaged to form the superior vena cava (SVC). The right sternoclavicular joint produces an acoustic shadow alongside the SVC.

reflections from the pleura and left lung. Artifactual duplication of the left subclavian artery by B-mode and color could then result from mirror imaging reverberation (Figure 4–6).

The subclavian artery should be identified as the color flow pattern that lies superficial to any color artifact. To avoid further confusion, the left subclavian artery could be followed from the axillary artery, below the clavicle, through the thoracic outlet to the subclavian artery.

Difficulties in imaging may be associated with configuration of the arch. The arch has been described in coiled and uncoiled configurations with the supraaortic trunks

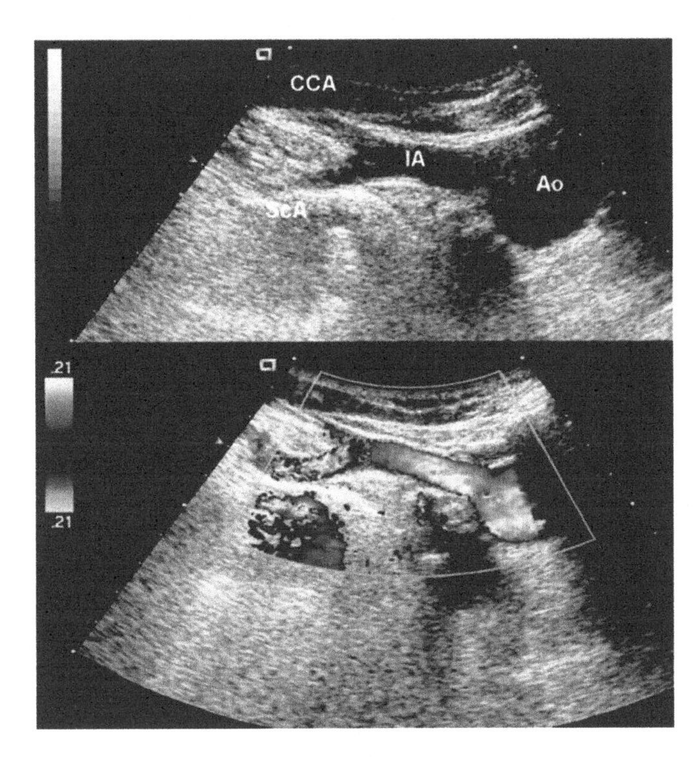

FIGURE 4–4. Longitudinal view of the innominate artery from the aorta (Ao) to the innominate artery (IA), right common carotid artery (CCA), and right subclavian artery (ScA), using a 4-MHz curvilinear probe. The probe is placed toward the left of midline. A shadow is cast from the left clavicle at the sternoclavicular joint. A mirror imaging reverberation artifact can be noted below the bright reflector and right subclavian artery.

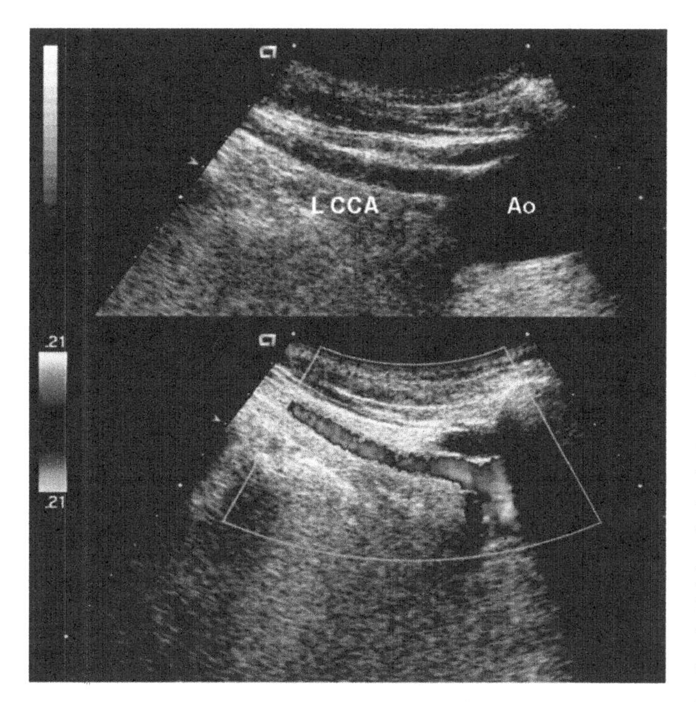

FIGURE 4–5. Longitudinal view of the left common carotid artery (L CCA) and aorta (Ao) scanned with a 4-MHz curvilinear probe, demonstrating the origin of the left common carotid artery, internal jugular vein, and shadowing from the sternoclavicular joint.

Brachiocephalic Veins

Imaging the brachiocephalic veins follows the same reference points as the arterial scan, with a view of the IJ veins bilaterally at the base of the neck. From that point both veins can be followed to their confluence with the subclavian veins and traced to the SVC (Figures 4–3 and 4–7). The left brachiocephalic vein lies anterior to the left common carotid and innominate arteries as it approaches the SVC. Visualization requires a greater anterior angulation, and may be more difficult than visualizing the truncal arterial branches.

The SVC lies to the right of the aorta. This causes some dissymmetry between the right and left brachiocephalic veins that join to form the SVC. The right brachiocephalic vein is short and descends vertically to the SVC. The left brachiocephalic vein will be seen to curve from the patient's left to right as it descends centrally. It is approximately 6 cm in length and will be seen coursing anterior to the branch arteries of the arch. Because the right brachiocephalic vein and SVC are in contact with the pleura of the right lung, there may be substantial color artifact that must be sorted out to identify the confluence.

originating from different points of the arch.[10] The better configuration positions the innominate on the right edge of the apex and the left subclavian artery on the left edge. The take-off points, located on the superior wall of the arch, are optimally positioned for ultrasound imaging and endovascular cannulation. The more difficult imaging configuration occurs when the innominate artery arises from the aorta, before the apex, and its origin lies below the level of the apex. In this "uncoiled" position the left common carotid and subclavian arteries may be similarly displaced to the right. The deeper take-off of the innominate artery may prevent adequate ultrasonic visualization as well as increase the difficulty of endovascular cannulation.

Difficulties caused by anomalous anatomy and inaccessible origination of any arch branch due to coiling or confusing color artifacts may be overcome by continually backtracking the scan to familiar territory at the neck base. Retracing the path of each branch should then allow normal anatomy to be separated from variants and artifacts. The lack of branches central to the innominate, left common, and left subclavian arteries should allow indirect spectral Doppler evidence of a hemodynamically significant stenosis or occlusion when the orificial lesion is not accessible.

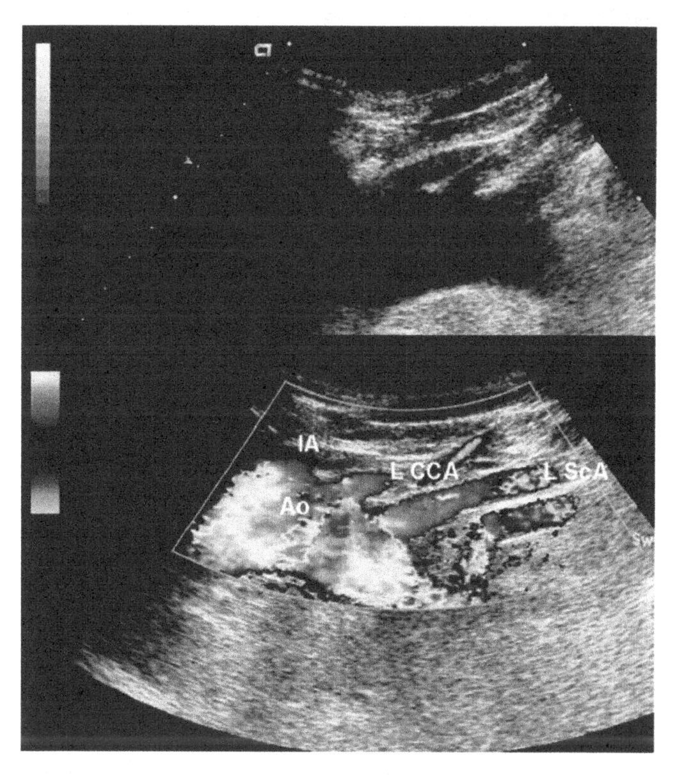

FIGURE 4–6. Longitudinal view of the left subclavian artery (LScA) and originations of the left common carotid artery (LCCA) and innominate artery (IA) from the aorta (Ao). A mirror imaging reverberation artifact can be noted below the bright reflector and left subclavian artery.

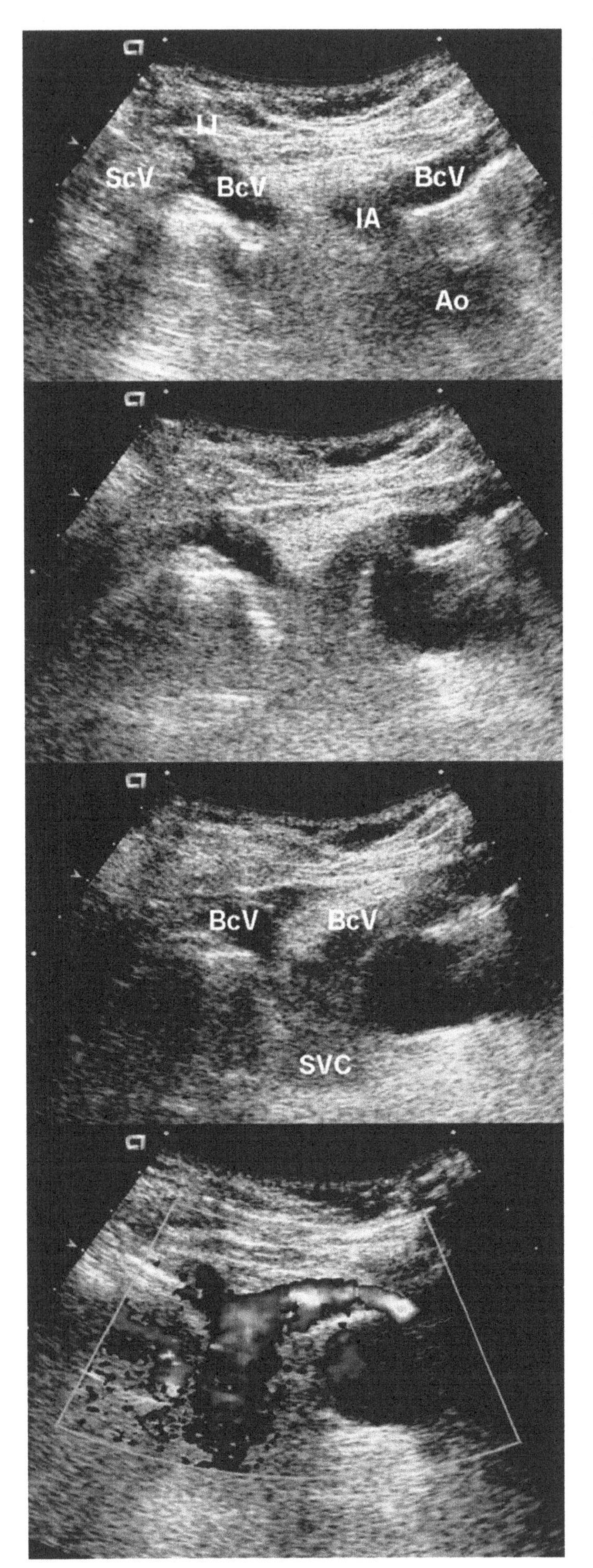

FIGURE 4–7. Imaging the brachiocephalic veins and superior vena cava. From the neck base (top), the right subclavian vein (ScV) and right internal jugular vein (IJ) can be seen to enter the right brachiocephalic vein (BcV). The left brachiocephalic vein crosses from left to right anterior to the innominate artery (IA), above the aorta (Ao). When scanning centrally (bottom), the confluence of both brachiocephalic veins (BcV) can be seen to form the superior vena cava (SVC).

Using Color Flow to Assess the Central Vessels

B-mode imaging does not provide an optimal view of the great vessels and color imaging is important for confirming the relevant structures and guiding the spectral Doppler interrogation. Advantages and limitations of color flow imaging are worth discussing.

Color Doppler technology is the main form of color flow imaging used in commercial instrumentation. Activation of the color Doppler mode displays flow-related color within the borders of a box that is superimposed on the B-mode image. Color Doppler slows the frame rate. While B-mode information can be acquired from single pulses, color Doppler information for a scan line requires multiple insonation pulses. The number of pulses required to collect the Doppler information is called a pulse train or packet.[11] More pulses in a packet provide a better estimate of flow velocities but requires more time. Hence, turning color on decreases the frame rate.

The frame rate also decreases because the color is written within a large number of color gates that are present in the color box. While spectral Doppler uses one gate in one scan line to sample the Doppler shifted frequencies, color Doppler packs the color box with multiple gates in multiple scan lines to display colorized flow anywhere within the box. The vertical dimension of the box determines the number of sample gates along each scan line and the lateral dimension determines the number of scan lines.[12] The frame rate decreases because the same calculation is made for all gates in the box, whether color is applied to the pixel or not. The operator is able to select the color box size and, to a certain extent, the number of gates in a scan line and the number of scan lines. This affects the size of the color pixel and allows the operator to trade-off color resolution for frame rate.[13]

Color Doppler

Color adds an obvious advantage to standard B-mode/spectral Doppler duplex if it rapidly identifies blood flow and guides the placement of the spectral Doppler. Limitations in color may hinder diagnosis and extend the examination time if it is used as a crutch rather than an aid. Color may do the following:

- Overwhelm subtle grayscale shadings of the B-mode image that may be more important than the color information.
- Slow the frame rate to below real-time imaging. Scan times will improve if most of the scan is performed in B-mode and color is activated only when necessary.
- Mislead the inexperienced sonographer. Color sensitivity adjustments are subjective, experience based, and instrument specific. Color registration may be difficult to achieve.
- Have difficulty demonstrating the presence of flow. Echoes received from moving red blood cells are much weaker than the reflections returned for the B-mode image. A relatively good B-mode image of an artery may not be matched by a good velocity signal by color or spectral Doppler simply because of a lack of adequate signal strength. Overreliance on the presence or absence of color may be misleading.
- Overflow the edge of the vessel. The size of a color pixel is variable and can be much larger than the grayscale pixel. Color overflowing the vessel edge may misrepresent the tightness of a stenosis.
- Demonstrate flow where there is none. Mirror image reverberation artifact can occur when a bright reflector lies below the insonated vessel. The result is a false duplication of flow by spectral and color Doppler below the bright interface. A reverberation color artifact may also occur within bright stationary reflectors with the vibration of stiff calcified surfaces.

To the inexperienced sonographer, who does not recognize the potential pitfalls and the necessary adjustments for optimization, color can be a major frustration. This is particularly true when the dependence on color has limited the person's recognition of grayscale morphology and spectral Doppler waveform characteristics. However, once the limits are recognized, there is a distinct advantage to using color to guide the examination. Among the benefits are the following:

- Setting the pulse repetition frequency (PRF) about the expected average velocity will provide good luminal color fill.
- Higher velocity flows produce color aliasing that displays a mixture of hues in adjacent pixels. Within the area of aliasing, color mixing occurs over the top of the color bar scale. There is a scattering of color progressions from light red to light blue that occurs through the unsaturated hues, passing through white. Aliasing can be distinguished from physiologic flow reversals, which cause the color to change in adjacent pixels from uniformly saturated reds to saturated blues, passing through black rather than white.
- Turbulence can produce a color bruit. Flow turbulence produces a high-frequency vibration in the vessel wall. This vibration is transmitted to the skin surface as an audible bruit or palpable thrill and is also picked up by color Doppler as intense speckling of color that spills over the wall of the vessel around the point of greatest turbulence.
- If a stenosis is suspected, possibly with color aliasing or bruit, the point of highest velocity can be located by increasing the PRF. With a tight stenosis or arteriovenous fistula, it is not unusual to find a color hotspot in a tight stenosis or arteriovenous fistula that is continuously lit, indicating continuous forward flow across the stenosis. This is presumably the result of a pressure drop that is maintained throughout the cardiac cycle, indicating that the pressure distal to the stenosis remains lower than the diastolic pressure.
- Color is helpful for distinguishing ulcerations from hypoechoic plaque. For this purpose, it would be worth increasing spatial resolution over frame rate to increase the number of sample gates and decrease the size of the color pixel. It is also advisable to decrease the PRF, increase the filter, and increase persistence. The latter adjustments will detect the slower flows filling the ulcerations and smooth the color fill throughout the cardiac cycle.

Through these characteristics, color flow imaging provides an excellent adjunctive modality for assessing the central vessels of the chest. The relatively simple branch anatomy of the large vessels and the lack of potential small branch collaterals and the assessment made distal to an arterial stenosis or occlusion make the evaluation more straightforward.

Conclusions

The prevalence and clinical significance of arch branch disease will be recognized only through routine evaluation. Unfortunately, suprasternal ultrasonic imaging of the aortic arch and brachiocephalic veins will probably not be a routine part of the standard carotid evaluation. It can, however, prove especially useful in identifying an arch lesion that is suggested by flow disturbances in the common carotid artery, flow reversals in the vertebral artery, or asymmetrical brachial pressures. Identifying these lesions at the time of a cerebrovascular ultrasound examination can be especially important now that catheter-based intervention may be an easy next step.

Suprasternal imaging of the brachiocephalic veins may also be a valuable tool for an upper extremity venous examination, which tends to be limiting above the clavicle. Ultrasonic imaging may even be useful in determining the placement of central venous catheters.

Used correctly, color Doppler is capable of greatly improving the scan time for a cerebrovascular examination and can be critical for the examination of the aortic arch branches and the quality of a difficult examination. It is still an adjunctive component of the examination and for the typical patient, color flow imaging may not add to the final outcome.

References

1. Berguer R. Reconstruction of the supraaortic trunks and vertebrobasilar system. In: Moore WS (ed). *Vascular Surgery: A Comprehensive Review*, 6th ed., pp. 627–642. Philadelphia: WB Saunders Co, 2002.
2. Tyras DH, Barner HB. Coronary-subclavian steal. Arch Surg 1977;112:1125–1127.
3. Fields WS, Lemak NA. Joint study of extracranial arterial occlusion. Subclavian Steal—a review of 168 cases. JAMA 1972;222:1139–1143.
4. Hadjipetrou P, Cox S, Piemonte T, Eisenhauer A. Percutaneous revascularization of atherosclerotic obstruction of aortic arch vessels. J Am College Cardiol 1999;33:1238–1245.
5. Hass WK, Fields WS, North RR, *et al.* Joint study of extracranial arterial occlusion-II: arteriography, techniques, sites, and complications. JAMA 1968;203:159–164.
6. Khatibzadeh M, Sheikhzadeh A, Gromoll B, Stierle U. Topographic pattern of advanced atherosclerotic lesions in carotid arteries. Cardiology 1998;89:235–240.
7. Uflacker R. Thoracic aorta and arteries of the trunk. In: Uflacker R (ed). *Atlas of Vascular Anatomy: An Angiographic Approach*, pp. 143–188. Baltimore: Williams & Wilkins, 1997.
8. Allen MN. The transthoracic exam. In: Allen MN (ed). *Echocardiography,* 2nd ed., pp. 181–206. London: Lippincott, Williams & Wilkins, 1999.
9. Peters PJ. Echocardiographic evaluation of the aorta in echocardiography. In: Allen MN (ed). *Echocardiography,* 2nd ed., pp. 599–614. London: Lippincott, Williams & Wilkins, 1999.
10. Eisenhauer AC. Subclavian and innominate revascularization: Surgical therapy versus catheter-based intervention. Curr Interv Cardiol Rep 2000;2:101–110.
11. Zagzebski JA. Color Doppler and color flow imaging. In: *Essentials of Ultrasound Physics,* pp. 109–122. St Louis, MO: Mosby, 1996.
12. Hedrick WR, Hykes DL, Starchman DE. *Color-Flow Imaging in Ultrasound Physics and Instrumentation,* 3rd ed., pp. 162–177. St. Louis, MO: Mosby, 1995.
13. Miele FR. Doppler. In: Miele FR (ed). *Ultrasound Physics and Instrumentation,* Vol. 2, pp. 7-1–7-28. Miele Enterprises, LLC, 2003.

5 Vertebral Artery Ultrasonography

Marc Ribo and Andrei V. Alexandrov

Introduction

Although the vertebrobasilar system accounts for up to 20% of the total cerebral blood flow and a proportionate share of strokes,[1] many cases of vertebrobasilar disease remain undiagnosed or diagnosed incorrectly. Some common symptoms, such as dizziness or transient loss of consciousness, do not always prompt detailed examination of the posterior circulation vessels. A simple, fast, noninvasive ultrasound examination of the extra- and intracranial portions of the vertebrobasilar system can yield valuable information for diagnosis and treatment.[2–10]

Noninvasive ultrasound can differentiate normal from diseased arteries, identify all categories of stenosis, localize the disease process including occlusions, detect progression of the disease, detect and quantify cerebral embolism, and assess collateral circulation to maintain cerebral blood flow.

Mastering cerebrovascular ultrasound requires knowledge of anatomy, physiology of cardiovascular and nervous systems, fluid dynamics, pathological changes in a variety of cerebrovascular disorders,[11–21] as well as basic ultrasound physics and instrumentation.[22–28]

The aim of this chapter is to describe the methods of cerebrovascular ultrasound testing of the vertebrobasilar system, practical criteria for interpretation, and relevance of these findings to patient management. Rapid bedside evaluation by an expert sonographer with a portable ultrasound unit is an excellent screening test that can provide an immediate impact on patient management at a lower cost and no time delays compared to other imaging methods.

Anatomy of the Vertebrobasilar Arterial System

When performing a vascular ultrasound examination, it is necessary to think about generated images with respect to transducer position, i.e., a sonographer should "think in 3-D" or three dimensions about the vessel being investigated. A sonographer should further imagine how this arterial segment would look on an angiogram. We strongly encourage those learning and interpreting ultrasound to be familiar with cerebral angiograms[11] since invasive angiography is the gold standard for assessment of accuracy of ultrasound testing.

The vertebral arteries arise from the subclavian arteries and pass cephalad in the neck to enter the bony canal at the C6 vertebrae. They course through the transverse processes of the vertebrae (Figure 5–1), and enter the base of the skull through the foramen magnum. At this point, the right and left vertebral arteries join together to form the basilar artery. The trunk of the basilar artery courses for about 3 cm or more before terminating in the posterior cerebral arteries (Figure 5–1), which make up the posterior portion of the circle of Willis.

Extracranial Duplex Ultrasound Examination Technique and Scanning Protocol

The extracranial vertebrobasilar duplex examination includes longitudinal B-mode scans of the vertebral artery mid-cervical portion followed by the origin and the most distal portion accessible on the neck. To optimize the grayscale image, set the dynamic range to 40–50 dB and the time-gain compensation (TGC) as appropriate to the depth of the vertebral arteries.

Duplex ultrasound allows segmental assessment of the vertebral artery flow between transverse processes in 96–100% of cases (Figure 5–2), and visualization of the vertebral artery origins in 65–90% of the patients. These segments should be thoroughly evaluated in patients with strokes or transient ischemic attacks in the posterior circulation. Vertebral duplex provides not only

A.F. Aburahma, J.J. Bergan (eds.), *Noninvasive Cerebrovascular Diagnosis*, DOI 10.1007/978-1-84882-957-2_5,

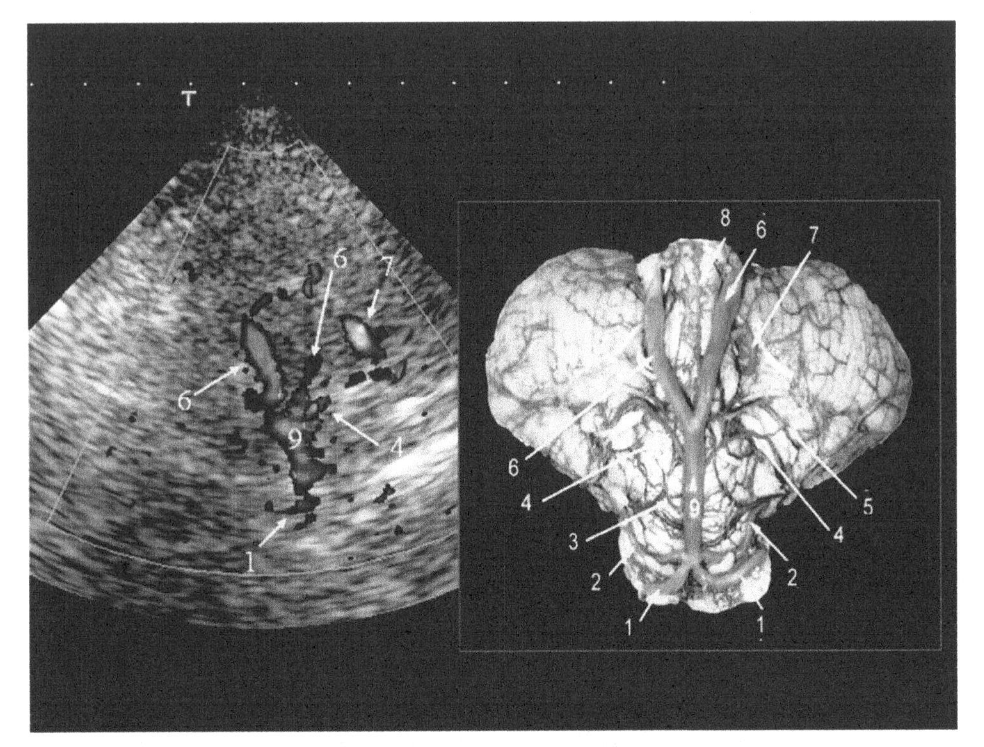

FIGURE 5–1. Anatomy of the vertebrobasilar system. Comparison between the display observed by transcranial color-coded duplex and an anatomopathologic specimen.1: Left posterior cerebral artery; 4: anterior inferior cerebellar artery; 6: vertebral arteries; 7: posterior inferior cerebellar artery.

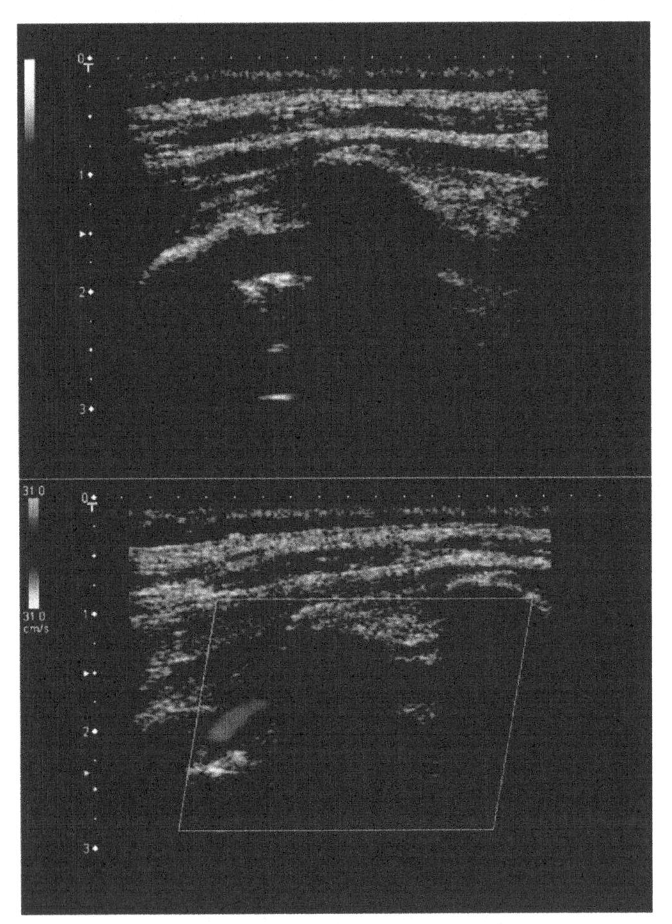

FIGURE 5–2. (A) Longitudianal view of the vertebral artery between the vertebral "shadows" on B-mode. (B) Superimposed color flow image.

information about the portion insonated directly, but indirect information about the proximal and distal vessel segments. The spectrum of vertebral pathology detectable by duplex scanning includes

1. vertebral artery stenosis (origin, V2, V3, and V4 segments) (Figure 5–3),
2. vertebral artery occlusion or absence of flow due to congenital aplasia,
3. hypoplastic vertebral artery, and
4. subclavian steal (Figure 5–4).

Unfortunately there are no established criteria for grading various degrees of extracranial vertebral artery stenosis, however, normal peak systolic velocity is approximately 40–50 cm/s. The velocity may be low in a subdominant or hypoplastic vertebral artery. If duplex shows a significant, i.e., ≥50% vertebral stenosis, the velocity doubles compared to prestenotic or poststenotic segments or the contralateral side. A greater than 70% stenosis will triple the velocity. Generally, most significant focal stenoses in the vertebral artery produce a peak systolic velocity elevation above 100 cm/s. Large vessel atheromatous disease that could be responsible for posterior circulation symptoms usually presents with vertebral artery stenosis or occlusion with preexisting plaque formation (Figure 5–3).

Infrequently, duplex examination may show findings consistent with vertebral artery dissection,[28] and further testing needs to be done to determine if it is an isolated vertebral dissection or an extension of aortic arch dissection. Further consideration should be given as to whether this dissection is spontaneous or trauma related.

Finally, the finding of subclavian steal (Figure 5–4), often a harmless hemodynamic phenomenon, indicates the presence of atherosclerotic stenosis or occlusion in the subclavian artery.[29] Occasionally, subclavian steal can produce symptoms related to transient hypoperfusion in the basilar artery.[29,30] Latent subclavian steal can be demonstrated by early systolic deceleration and the arrival of highest velocities in late systole. The "hyperemia test" can provoke flow reversal in patients with latent steal. A blood pressure cuff is inflated in the ipsilateral arm to suprasystolic values and the patient is asked to perform physical exercise of that arm to increase metabolic demand and vasodilation. Upon sudden cuff release a systolic flow reversal with low diastolic antegrade flow is seen (Figure 5–4).

The so-called alternating flow signal or a total reversal of flow at rest represents different stages of the subclavian steal phenomenon. It is called a syndrome if clinical symptoms of posterior circulation ischemia develop.

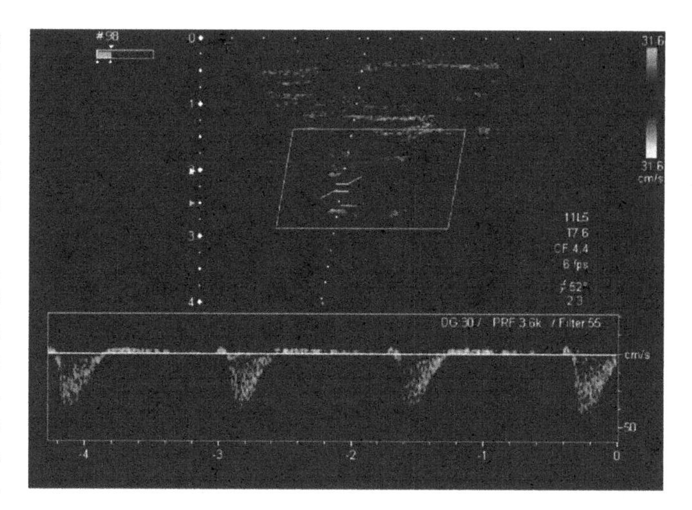

FIGURE 5–4. Subclavian steal; reversed systolic flow in the cervical portion of the vertebral artery with very low antegrade diastolic velocity.

Imaging in the Longitudinal Plane

Optimize the image so that the normal linear reflectivity of the arterial wall is apparent. To find the vertebral artery, visualize the common carotid artery (longitudinal view, transducer position anterior to the sternocleidomastoid muscle). Steer the color beam toward the proximal common carotid artery (CCA). Rock the probe slightly to the lateral aspect of the neck to image the vertebral artery as it courses through the transverse processes of the vertebrae ("shadows"). "Heel-toe" the probe above the clavicle to image the origin of the vertebral artery as it arises from the subclavian artery. Confirm that the direction of flow in the vertebral artery is the same as the CCA.

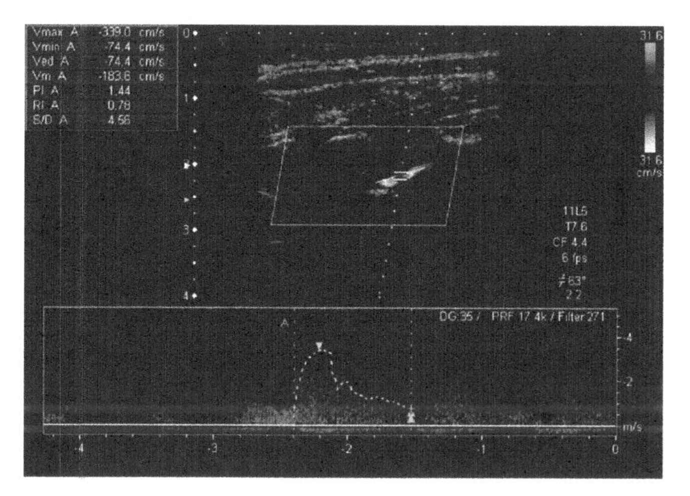

FIGURE 5–3. Vertebral stenosis in its cervical portion. Angle corrected velocity measurement shows a peak systolic velocity of 339 cm/s.

Color Flow Ultrasound Evaluation of Flow Dynamics

Choose the appropriate color pulse repetition frequency (PRF) by setting the color velocity scale for the expected velocities in the vessel. For normal adult arteries, the peak systolic velocity range is usually around or under 40–50 cm/s. Adjust the scale further to avoid systolic aliasing (low PRF) or diastolic flow gaps (high PRF or filtering) in normal vessels.

Optimize the color power and gain so that flow signals are recorded throughout the lumen of the vessel with no "bleeding" of color into the surrounding tissues.

Avoid using large or wide color boxes since this will slow down frame rates and resolution of the imaging system. Use color boxes that cover the entire vessel diameter and 1–2 cm of its length. Align the box, i.e., select an appropriate color flow angle correction, according to the vessel geometry and course.

Doppler Spectral Evaluation of Flow Dynamics

Display the longitudinal image of the vertebral artery. Use color flow image as a guide for Doppler examination (Figure 5–2). Begin the examination using a Doppler sample volume size of 1.5 mm positioned in the middle of the vessel. Consistently follow one of the choices for angle correction: parallel to the vessel walls or to the color flow jet. Adjust the Doppler spectral power and gain to optimize the quality of the signal return. Slowly sweep the sample volume throughout the different intervertebral visualized segments. Identify regions of flow disturbance or where flow is absent. Additionally, include Doppler spectral waveforms proximal, within, and distal to all areas where flow abnormalities were observed. Locate the origin or proximal segment of the vertebral artery. Record flow patterns paying careful attention to flow direction. Follow accessible cervical segments of the vertebral artery. Change angulation of the color box and Doppler sample along with the course of the artery.

Extracranial Duplex Examination Should Provide the Following Data

1. Peak systolic velocity in all vessel segments.
2. End diastolic velocity in all vessel segments.
3. Flow direction and peak systolic velocity of both vertebral arteries.
4. Views demonstrating the presence and location of pathology.

Tips to Improve Accuracy

1. Consistently follow a standardized scanning protocol.
2. Always perform a complete examination of the vertebral arteries after the carotid examination.
3. Sample velocity signals throughout all arterial segments accessible.
4. Use multiple scan planes.
5. Take time to optimize the B-mode, color, and spectral Doppler information.
6. Videotape or create a digital file of the entire study including sound recordings.
7. Always use the highest imaging frequencies to achieve higher resolution.
8. Account for any clinical conditions or medications that might affect velocity.
9. Integrate data from the right and left carotid and vertebral arteries.
10. Do not hesitate to admit uncertainty and list all causes for limited examinations.
11. Expand the Doppler examination to the intracranial vessels when possible (see Chapter 6).

Tips for Optimizing Color Flow Set-up

According to standardized protocols, the patient's head should be to the left of the image. This orientation should then clearly indicate the appropriate direction of flow in the vertebral arteries. The arterial and venous flow directions are then given color assignments with respect to flow toward or away from the transducer. Traditionally, flow toward the transducer is assigned red while flow away from the probe is assigned blue. The direction of flow relative to the probe will change if the probe is rotated 180° or if the color box is steered in the opposite direction, i.e., the vein will appear red while the artery will appear blue. When this occurs, the color should be changed back to the original assignment to avoid confusion. It must also be noted that the color will change along the course of an artery if the flow direction varies throughout the cardiac cycle (triphasic, to-from) or if the vessel changes direction relative to the orientation of the sound beam.

The zero baseline of the color bar (PRF) is set at approximately two-thirds of the range with the majority of frequencies allowed in the red direction (for flow towards the brain). This setting allows you to display higher arterial mean frequency shifts (velocities) without aliasing artifacts. Allowance should be made for some flow in the reverse (blue) direction to allow for changes in flow direction (i.e., subclavian steal). When the transducer is rotated 180°, the color will change, and the zero baseline will shift with the color changes to accommodate for flow in the forward direction. You will need to adjust both the color assignment and the zero baseline to the initial setup for consistency. The color PRF and zero baseline may need to be readjusted throughout the examination to allow for the changes in velocity that occur with tortuosity and stenosis. When bruits are encountered, the color PRF should be decreased to detect the lower frequencies associated with a bruit. Usually, the frequency of these bruits is less than 1 kHz.

When occlusion is suspected, the color PRF should be decreased to detect the preocclusive, low-velocity, high-resistance signal associated with critical stenosis or occlusion and to confirm absence of flow at the site of occlusion.

The color wall filter should be set as low as possible. Note that the color wall filter may automatically increase as you increase the PRF. You may need to decrease the wall filter manually when you decrease the color PRF.

The angle of the color box should be changed to obtain the most acute Doppler angles between the scan lines and the direction of blood flow. This will result in a better color display because of more suitable Doppler angles. The angle should always be equal or less than 60°. Because linear array transducers are steered at angles of 90° and 70° from the center of the array, this may require a "heel-toe" maneuver with the transducer on the surface of the skin to adjust the position of the vessel within the color box. An alternative would be to physically change the orientation of the transducer 180°.

The desaturation of color from darker to lighter hues on the color bar indicates increasing Doppler frequency shifts, i.e., increasing velocities. Note that close to the zero baseline, the colors are the darkest. As the velocity increases, the color becomes lighter. You should select colors so that the highest frequency shifts in each direction are of high contrast to each other so that aliasing can be readily detected. For example, you could set the color selections so that low to high velocities are seen as dark blue to light green to aqua in one direction and red to orange to yellow in the opposite flow direction. Aliasing would then appear as aqua adjacent to yellow.

The frame rate should be kept as high as possible to capture the very rapid change in flow dynamics that occurs with stenosis. Remember that frame rate is affected by

1. PRF—frame rate decreases with decreasing PRF;
2. Ensemble length—increasing the color ensemble length will decrease the frame rate;
3. Width of the color box—increased width will decrease the frame rate;
4. Depth—deep insonation decreases the frame rate.

The color box should be kept to a size that is adequate for visualizing the area of interest and yet small enough to keep the frame rate at a reasonable number, approximately 15 or more to ensure adequate filling of the vessel. The frame rate is usually displayed in Hertz on the monitor.

The color gain should be adjusted throughout the examination to detect the changing signal strength. If the color gain is not properly adjusted, some color information may be lost or too much color may be displayed. In this case, you will see color in areas where there should be no flow. The gain should initially be adjusted to an "overgained" level, with color displayed in the tissue and then turned down until the tissue noise just disappears or is minimally present. This is the level at which all color images should be assessed. In situations where there is very low flow, or questionable occlusion, an "overgained" level may be advantageous to show any flow that might be present, e.g., total occlusion versus a near occlusion or critical stenosis.

References

1. Savitz SI, Caplan LR. Vertebrobasilar disease. N Engl J Med. 2005;352:2618–26.
2. Strandness DE, McCutcheon EP, Rushmer RF. Application of a transcutaneous Doppler flowmeter in evaluation of occlusive arterial disease. Surg Gynecol Obstet 1966; 122(5):1039–45.
3. Spencer MP, Reid JM, Davis DL, Paulson PS. Cervical carotid imaging with a continuous-wave Doppler flowmeter. Stroke 1974;5(2):145–54.
4. Barber FE, Baker DW, Nation AW, Strandness DE, Reid JM. Ultrasonic duplex echo-Doppler scanner. IEEE Trans Biomed Eng 1974;21(2):109–113.
5. Budingen HJ, von Reutern GM, Freund HJ. Diagnosis of cerebro-vascular lesions by ultrasonic methods. Int J Neurol 1977;11(2–3):206–18.
6. Aaslid R, Markwalder TM, Nornes H. Noninvasive transcranial Doppler ultrasound recording of flow velocity in basal cerebral arteries. J Neurosurg 1982;57(6):769–74.
7. Spence JD, Coates RK, Pexman JA. Doppler flow maps of the carotid artery compared with the findings on angiography. Can J Surg 1983;26(6):556–8.
8. Bogdahn U, Becker G, Schlief R, Reddig J, Hassel W. Contrast-enhanced transcranial color-coded real-time sonography. Stroke 1993;24:676–684.
9. Rubin JM, Bude RO, Carson PL, Bree RL, Adler RS. Power Doppler US: A potentially useful alternative to mean frequency-based color Doppler US. Radiology 1994;190(3): 853–6.
10. Burns PN. Harmonic imaging with ultrasound contrast agents. Clin Radiol 1996;51:50–55.
11. Krayenbuehl H, Yasargil MG. *Cerebral Angiography,* 2nd ed. Stuttgart: Thieme, 1982.
12. Bernstein EF. *Vascular Diagnosis*, 4th ed. St. Louis: Mosby-Year Book, 1993.
13. Polak JF. *Peripheral Vascular Sonography: A Practical Guide*. Baltimore: Williams & Wilkins, 1992.
14. Strandness DE. *Duplex Scanning in Vascular Disorders,* 2nd ed. New York: Raven Press, 1993.
15. Zweibel WJ. *Introduction to Vascular Ultrasonography,* 4th ed. St. Louis: Harcourt Health Sciences, 2000.
16. von Reutern GM, Budingen HJ. *Ultrasound Diagnosis in Cerebrovascular Disease.* Stuttgart: Thieme, 1993.
17. Tegeler CH, Babikian VL, Gomez CR. *Neurosonology.* St. Louis: Mosby, 1996.
18. Hennerici M, Neuerburg-Heusler D. *Vascular Diagnosis with Ultrasound. Clinical Reference with Case Studies.* Stuttgart: Thieme, 1998.
19. Hennerici M, Mearis S. *Cerebrovascular Ultrasound: Theory, Practice, and Future Developments.* Cambridge: Cambridge University Press, 2001.
20. Bartels E. *Color-Coded Duplex Ultrasonography of the Cerebral Arteries: Atlas and Manual.* Stuttgart: Schattauer, 1999.
21. Babikian VL, Wechsler LR (eds). *Transcranial Doppler Ultrasonography*, 2nd ed. Woburn, MA: Butterworth Heinemann, 1999.
22. Edelman SK. *Understanding Ultrasound Physics,* 2nd ed. The Woodlands: ESP, Inc., 1997.
23. Kremkau FW. *Diagnostic Ultrasound: Principles and Instruments*, 5th ed. New York: Harcourt Health Sciences, 1998.
24. *Zagzebski JA. Essentials of Ultrasound Physics.* St. Louis: Mosby, 1997.
25. Alexandrov AV. *Cerebroavascular Ultrasound in Stroke Prevention and Treatment.* New York: Blackwell, 2004.
26. Bartels E, Fuchs HH, Flugel KA. Duplex ultrasonography of vertebral arteries: Examination, technique, normal values, and clinical applications. Angiology 1992;43(3 Pt 1): 169–80.

27. Bartels E. *Color-Coded Duplex Ultrasonography of the Cerebral Vessels*. Stuttgart: Schattauer, 1999.
28. Bartels E, Flugel KA. Evaluation of extracranial vertebral artery dissection with duplex color-flow imaging. Stroke 1996;27(2):290–5.
29. Bornstein NM, Norris JW. Subclavian steal: A harmless haemodynamic phenomenon? Lancet 1986;2(8502):303–5.
30. Toole JF. *Cerebrovascular Disorders,* 4th ed. New York: Raven Press, 1990.

6
Transcranial Doppler Sonography

Marc Ribo and Andrei V. Alexandrov

The Principles of Transcranial Doppler

Transcranial Doppler sonography (TCD) was first introduced by Rune Aaslid and colleagues in 1982 to noninvasively measure blood flow velocities in the major branches of the Circle of Willis through the intact skull.[1] A 2-MHz frequency pulse wave ultrasonic beam penetrates the skull and allows returned echo signals to be detected. The frequency shift of the returned echoes is calculated using the Doppler equation $f_D = 2\ f_o\ v\ \cos\theta/(c - \cos\theta)$, where f_D is Doppler shift, f_o is the emitting frequency, v is the scatterer speed, θ is the Doppler angle, and c is the sound propagation speed. The average speed of sound in soft tissues is 1540 m/s and the Doppler angle for TCD examination is assumed to be 0° for all arteries ($\cos 0° = 1$). Therefore the Doppler equation is rearranged to calculate the velocity of moving blood in basal cerebral arteries: $v(\text{cm/s}) = 77\ f_D(\text{kHz})/f_o(\text{MHz})$, where the 77 coefficient is valid for the frequency and velocity units shown in parentheses.

TCD allows the depth and the direction of flow relative to the transducer position and the ultrasonic beam direction to be located. The depth of insonation displayed in centimeters or millimeters is manually adjusted. This is accomplished by changing the pulse repetition frequency, which is based on the average speed of sound in soft tissues. Thus to locate the signals originating at a depth of 5 cm, the machine emits the pulse and waits for the time period necessary for ultrasound to make a round trip to and from this depth [i.e., $(0.05/1540) \times 2 = 0.00006$ s]. The direction of flow depends on the angle at which the ultrasonic beam intercepts an artery. The flow moving toward the transducer (i.e., the angle of interception is less than 90°) will increase the frequency of the returned signal compared to the emitted frequency. The flow intercepted at 90° will produce no detectable Doppler shift. And if the arterial flow is directed away from the probe (i.e., the angle >90°), the frequency of the returned signal will be less than the emitted one. Therefore the Doppler shifts are coded as positive or negative and the direction of flow is determined accordingly.

Power Motion Mode

Transcranial power motion mode Doppler (PMD) was recently invented by Mark Moehring and Merrill Spencer.[2] In its current configuration, PMD, or M-mode, uses 33 overlapping Doppler samples to simultaneously display flow signal intensity and direction over 6 cm of intracranial space. PMD provides a color-coded display of all flow signals detectable at a given position and direction of the transducer in real time (Figure 6–1). The brighter PMD colors reflect stronger intensities, and this "road map" can serve as a guide for more complete spectral analysis. PMD promises to make a standard TCD examination[1–3] easy even for an inexperienced person. Instead of lengthy acquisition of skills to find windows of insonation with a single-channel spectral TCD, a clinician can search for a window of insonation relying less on sound recognition and arm coordination and not be locked into a single spectrum depth. Furthermore, PMD flow patterns, or signatures, may have their own diagnostic significance, and these flow changes can be observed over large segments of intracranial vasculature in real time. PMD may prove helpful for thrombolysis monitoring and embolus detection by tracking the time–space path of high-intensity signals traveling simultaneously to several major intracranial vessels.

Transcranial Color Duplex

There is an increasing number of reports on the use of transcranial color coded duplex (TCCD) for intracranial vascular studies[4–6] (Figure 6–1). TCCD offers a two-dimensional B-mode image that permits the brain structures to be identified. It is particularly useful in the

A.F. Aburahma, J.J. Bergan (eds.), *Noninvasive Cerebrovascular Diagnosis*, DOI 10.1007/978-1-84882-957-2_6,

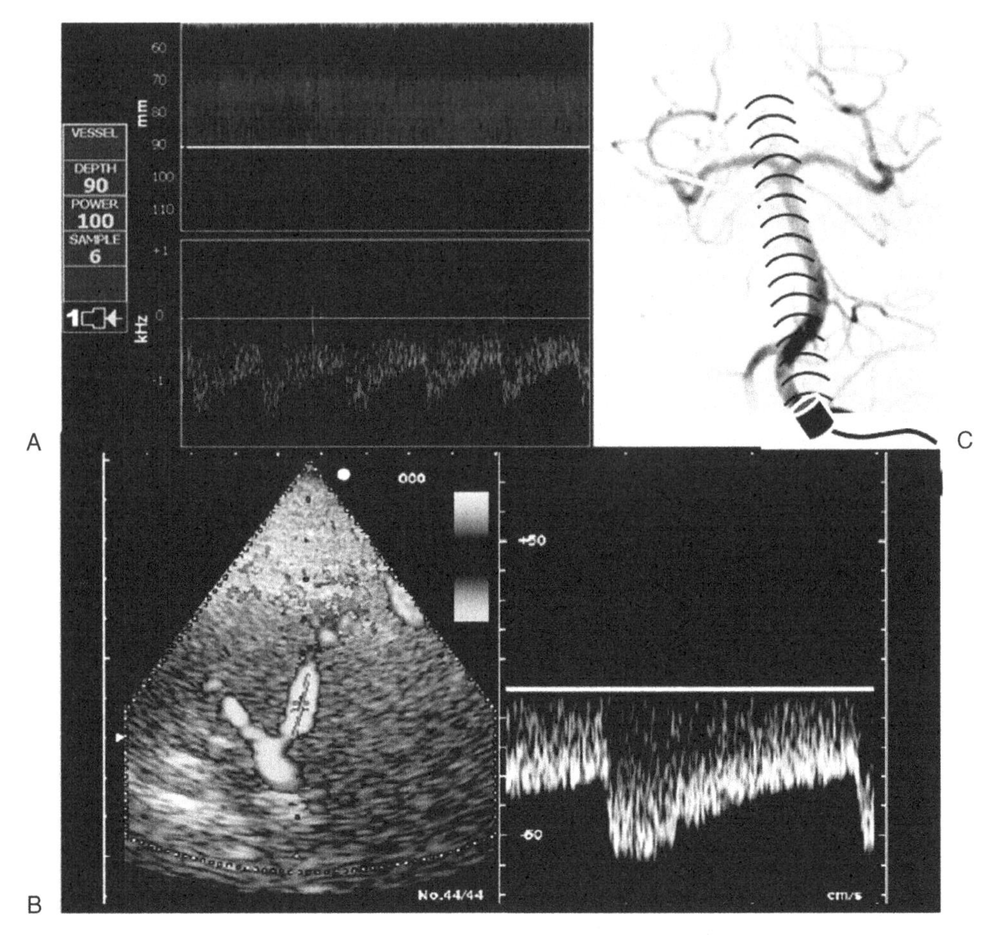

FIGURE 6–1. PMD and TCCD imaging of a normal basilar artery. On PMD display (A) the blue ribbon represents the existence of a flow away from the probe in depths between 65 and 100 mm. TCCD display (B) shows convergence of both vertebral arteries into the proximal basilar artery. (C) Insonation of vertebral and basilar arteries using a transforaminal approach.

detection of distal arterial lesions allowing angle correction in those branches parallel to the skull.[7] At bedside, B-mode imaging is able to demonstrate the midline shifting in malignant middle cerebral artery (MCA) infarctions[8] or hematoma growth with intracerebral bleeds. Duplex technology is now used in the development of brain perfusion assessment techniques with gaseous microbubble contrast agents for ultrasound imaging.[9–11]

Examination Technique

There are four "windows" for insonation (Figure 6–2): temporal, orbital, foraminal, and submandibular.[1,3] The transtemporal approach allows insonation of the middle (MCA), anterior (ACA), posterior (PCA), and communicating arteries. The transorbital approach is used to insonate the ophthalmic artery (OA) and internal carotid artery (ICA) siphon. The transforaminal approach allows the terminal vertebral and basilar arteries to be insonated through the foramen magnum. The submandibular approach is used to obtain ICA velocities as they enter the skull. To shorten the time necessary to find the window and different arterial segments, the examination should begin with the maximum power and gate settings (i.e., power 100%, gate 15 mm). Identify and store the highest velocity signals and any abnormal or unusual waveforms.

Transtemporal insonation steps:

1. Set the depth at 50 mm (distal M1-MCA) or 56 mm (mid M1-MCA).
2. Place the probe above the zygomaticus arch and aim it slightly upward and anterior to the contralateral ear/window.
3. Find any flow signal and avoid too anterior and too posterior angulation.
4. Find a flow signal directed toward the probe that resembles MCA flow.
5. Follow the signal until is disappears at shallow (40–45 mm) and deep (65–70 mm) depths.

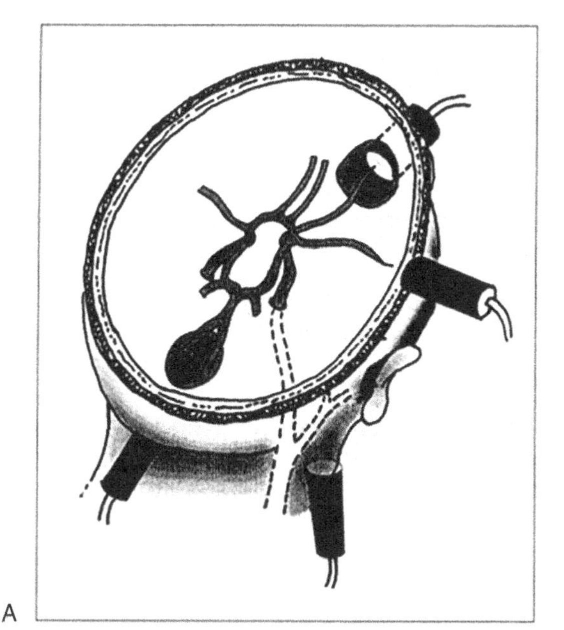

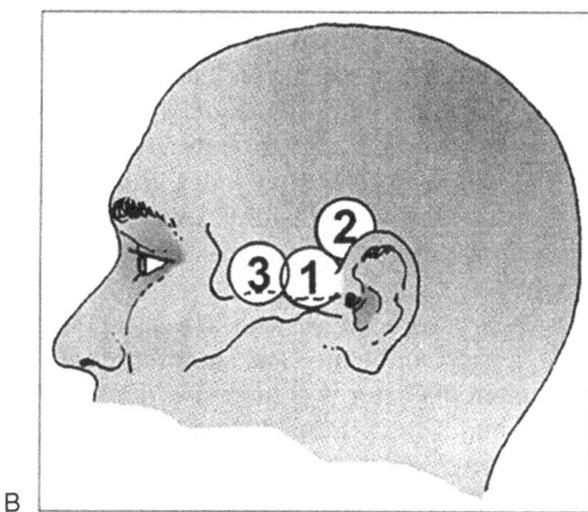

FIGURE 6–2. (A) Windows of insonation *(left to right)*: transforaminal, submandibular, temporal, and transorbital. (B) The temporal window for insonation may be found above the zygomatic arch at the middle (1), posterior (2), and anterior (3) positions.

6. Find the ICA bifurcation at 65 mm and obtain both MCA and ACA signals.
7. Find the terminal ICA signal just inferior to the bifurcation at 60–65 mm.
8. Return to the bifurcation and follow the ACA signal to 70–75 mm depths.
9. Return to the bifurcation, set the depth at 63 mm, and slowly turn the transducer posteriorly by 10–30°(usually there is a flow gap between the bifurcation and PCA signals).
10. Find PCA signals directed toward (P1) and away (P2) from the probe.

Transorbital insonation steps:

1. Decrease power to a minimum or 10%.
2. Set the depth at 52 mm and place the transducer over the eyelid and angle it slightly medially.
3. Determine flow pulsatility and direction in the distal ophthalmic artery.
4. Confirm these findings at 55–60 mm.
5. Set the depth at 60–64 mm and find the ICA siphon flow signals (usually located medially).

Transforaminal insonation steps:

1. Use full power, set the depth at 75 mm, place the transducer at midline an inch below the edge of the skull and aim it at the bridge of the nose, and identify a flow directed away from the probe.
2. Increase the depth to 80 mm [proximal basilar artery (BA)], 90 mm (mid BA), and >100 mm (distal BA).
3. Confirm these findings while decreasing the depth of insonation.
4. Set the depth at 60 mm and place the probe laterally aiming at the uni- or contralateral eye.
5. Find the vertebral artery (VA) flow directed away from the probe and follow it at 40–50 mm and 70–80 mm depths and repeat the examination on the contralateral side.

Submandibular insonation steps:

1. Set the depth at 50–60 mm, place the probe laterally under the jaw, and aim it upward and slightly medially.
2. Find a low resistance flow directed away from the probe.

The TCD interpretation consists of the assessment of (1) **velocity** changes (focal or global), (2) **asymmetry** of flow parameters (side-to-side, segmental), (3) **pulsatility** (high or low resistance), and (4) **waveform/sound** pattern recognition of flow changes. A normal transcranial Doppler examination may reveal a wide range of depths of insonation, velocity values and waveforms.

Criteria for normal TCD findings:

1. Good windows of insonation; all proximal arterial segments were found.
2. Direction of flow and depths of insonation are given in Table 6–1.
3. The difference between flow velocities in the homologous arteries is less than 30%.
4. A normal MCA mean flow velocity (MFV) does not exceed 170 cm/s in children[12] and 80 cm/s in adults.[13]
5. A normal velocity ratio: MCA > ACA ≥ siphon ≥ PCA ≥ BA > VA.
6. A positive end-diastolic flow velocity (EDV) of 20–40% of the peak systolic velocity (PSV) values and a low resistance pulsatility index (PI) of 0.6–1.1 are present in all intracranial arteries while breathing room air. A

TABLE 6–1. Normal depth, direction, and mean flow velocities in the arteries of the Circle of Willis.[a]

Artery[b]	Depth (mm)	Direction	Children	Adults
M1-MCA	45–65	Toward	<170 cm/s	32–82 cm/s
A1-CA	62–75	Away	<150 cm/s	18–82 cm/s
ICA siphon	60–64	Bidirectional	<130 cm/s	20–77 cm/s
OA	50–62	Toward	Wide range	Wide range
PCA	60–68	Bidirectional	<100 cm/s	16–58 cm/s
BA	80–100+	Away	<100 cm/s	12–66 cm/s
VA	45–80	Away	<80 cm/s	12–66 cm/s

[a]Mean flow velocity values are modified from Adams *et al.*[12] and Hennerici *et al.*[21]
[b]MCA, middle cerebral artery; ACA, anterior cerebral artery; ICA, internal carotid artery; OA, ophthalmic artery; PCA, posterior cerebral artery; BA, basilar artery; VA, vertebral artery.

high resistance flow pattern (PI ≥ 1.2) is seen in the OAs only.

7. High resistance flow patterns (PI ≥ 1.2) can be found in all arteries during hyperventilation.

Cerebrovascular Resistance and Hemodynamic Indexes

Cerebrovascular resistance (CVR) is determined by several factors that impede cerebral blood flow (CBF) and thus determine MFV: *the vessel radius, length*, and *blood viscosity*. The changes in flow resistance are mostly accomplished by arterial-arteriolar constriction/dilatation or intracranial pressure (ICP) dynamics. Under normal conditions the brain is a low-resistance arterial system and the ICA branches have considerably greater end-diastolic flow than the external carotid artery (ECA) branches. The resistance to flow is described by the PI and the resistance (RI) indexes. PI (Gosling-King) = PSV – EDV/MFV (normal values for MCA are 0.6–1.1). RI (Pourcelot) = PSV – EDV/PSV (normal values for MCA are 0.49–0.63[14]).

These indexes quantitatively reflect CVR and depend greatly on the strength of the signal recorded as well as the envelope and time averaging software. Therefore "weak signals," "poor" windows, incomplete examination, and individual variations may produce substantial drawbacks. Additional information can be gained by visual flow pattern recognition (Figure 6–3).

Pathologically increased PIs (>1.2) are seen with ICP and decreased cerebral perfusion pressure (CPP) due to decreased EDV. Pathologically low PIs (<0.5) are mainly seen in the arteries feeding arteriovenous malformations (AVM) since direct shunting of blood into the venous system results in abnormally low CVR.[15] Very low PIs may also be seen distal to a severe extra- or intracranial stenosis indicating compensatory vasodilation.[16]

Although these indexes per se may not be sufficient to diagnose extracranial disease, they should be used in a battery of TCD parameters allowing integrated assessment of intracranial circulation.[17]

Other useful indexes include the pulsatility transmission index (PTI), flow acceleration (FA), delta-MCA (δ-MCA), hemispheric index (HI), and the arterial velocities ratios.

PTI (Lindegaard) = PI (study vessel) / PI(reference vessel) × 100%; normal MCA/ICA: 93–107.[11]

FA = PSV – EDV/time differential; normal MCA: 392–592 cm/s^2.[18]

δ-MCA = Ipsi-MCA PSV – contralat-MCA PSV; normal MCA: 8.7 ± 5.9 cm/s.[19]

HI (Lindegaard) = MFV MCA/MFV ICA (normal values 1.76 ± 0.1, pathologic value ≥3).[20]

Arterial velocities ratio = VMCA/VACA (normal values 1.27 ± 0.12).[13]

PTI makes it possible to avoid the influence of changing cardiac output in patients with normal pulsatility of flow in the reference vessel. PTI is usually increased with elevated ICP and in the presence of MCA stenosis (the intracranial PI is compared to the extracranial vessel).[14,17]

The MCA flow acceleration index decreases in the presence of a severe ipsilateral extracranial carotid stenosis (229 ± 115 cm/s^2 in patients with 75–100% ICA stenosis.[14,18]

Delta-MCA also changes with increasing severity of carotid stenosis. Canthelmo *et al.* showed that if the ICA residual lumen diameter is greater than 1 mm, δ-MCA is 16.4 ± 11.7; and if the residual lumen diameter is ≤1 mm, δ-MCA is 26.6 ± 25.4; if a complete ICA occlusion is present, δ-MCA is 38.7 ± 19.4.[19] Again, note the large standard deviations that reflect between-individual differences and affect the diagnostic accuracy of these indexes if taken separately from other flow data. These indexes may be used cautiously to unmask extracranial distal ICA or siphon stenosis if other TCD and carotid duplex findings are unremarkable.

HI compares MCA MFV to the ipsilateral ICA and may help to differentiate an MCA FV increase due to spasm and/or hyperperfusion. The M1-MCA vasospasm after subarachnoid hemorrhage (SAH) is usually associated with HI values >3, while a severe (<1 mm residual lumen) M1-MCA vasospasm has been shown to correlate with HI values greater than 6.[20]

The arterial velocity ratios help to find MCA branch occlusion since higher velocities in the ACA may indicate the diversion of blood volume to the ACA due to higher resistance and/or decreased flow in the M2-MCA segment. The increased ACA velocities may reflect collateralization of flow via transcortical collaterals. However, ACA FVs can also be increased in the presence of the atretic contralateral A1-ACA segment, functioning anterior communicating artery (AComA), and the stenosis of the terminal ICA and/or unilateral A1-ACA.

Other factors that affect CBF, MFV, and the hemodynamic indexes include age, gender cardiac function, hematocrit and fibrinogen, carbon dioxide, and vasodilatory or constricting medications.[14]

TCD measurement of flow velocities, however, does not allow calculation of CBF in ml/min because of the variable and unknown arterial diameter and peripheral resistance.[9] However, the area under the waveform envelope, intensity of the signal, and relative change in the MFVs determined with the same angle of insonation are usually proportional to regional CBF changes.[10] For example, MFV changes due to vasomotor reactivity with different vasodilatory stimuli reflect CBF changes assuming that the perfused territory remains constant during investigation.[11] The use of TCD for monitoring physiological responses to vasodilatory substances is based on the concept of cerebral vasomotor reactivity (VMR) in order to identify patients at a particular risk for cerebral ischemic events.

Vasomotor Reactivity Assessment with Transcranial Doppler

The North American Symptomatic Carotid Endarterectomy Trial (NASCET), European Carotid Surgery Trialists (ECST), and Asymptomatic Carotid Atherosclerosic Study (ACAS) trials data[21–24] indicate that both hemodynamic and thromboembolic mechanisms of stroke are important in patients with carotid atherosclerosis,[25] and the emphasis is now made on identifying patients with asymptomatic severe carotid stenosis at the highest risk of stroke.[26] Therefore VMR as an index of intracranial collateralization capacity may have a prognostic value in predicting the symptomatic or asymptomatic course of carotid occlusive disease and stroke recurrence.[27]

Vasomotor reactivity assessed by TCD using vasodilating or constricting stimuli is not a measure of autoregulation. The brain autoregulation maintains CBF constant with physiological variations in blood pressure. The changes in CO_2 concentration induce a vasomotor response, which changes CBF paralleled by the velocity changes.[28] Thus, FV changes on TCD during normo-, hyper-, and hypocapnia may prove a useful index of VMR and the capacity of smaller cerebral arteries to adapt to various stimuli (Figure 6–3). Patients with ICA stenosis may be at an increased risk for stroke due to exhausted vasomotor reserve capacity on TCD.

CO_2 Reactivity

The FV modulation is most reliably and reproducibly measured by TCD at the M1-MCA segment during inhalation of different CO_2 concentrations. The end-expiratory CO_2 is measured by an infrared gas analyzer and expressed as volume percentage. The baseline TCD recording should be obtained under normocapnia, or when breathing room air, and then during steady states when air is inhaled with CO_2 concentrations ranging from 6% to 2% given for 2–3 min each. A voluntary hyperventilation is used to produce hypocapnia. TCD measurements of flow velocities should be made during each steady state and several (up to 20) cardiac cycles should be averaged to minimize variations in mean FVs. The baseline MFV is considered 100% and is compared to hyper- and hypocapnia states. VMR is expressed as percent changes of M1-MCA mean FV from hypercapnia to hypocapnia.

In normal volunteers free of cerebrovascular disease mean VMR was 86 ± 16%, n = 40, mean age 51 years.[29,30] On average, mean MCA FVs increased by 52% during hypercapnia and decreased by 35% during hypocapnia.[30]

Decreased VMR was observed in patients with ICA occlusions and symptomatic carotid artery disease in many studies, however, normal VMR could also be seen in these patients.[30] In the study reported by Ringelstein, VMR on the occluded or affected side was decreased on average by 20–25% compared to the nonoccluded side or to the normal controls.[30] The most important observation was that patients with low flow infarctions, ischemic ophthalmopathy, and hypostatic transient ischemic attacks (TIAs) had VMR of less than 38%, which is less than three standard deviations below the normal controls.[30]

VMR also decreases with the severity of carotid stenosis and increases after carotid endarterectomy on average by 20–25%, however, relatively large standard deviations allow for a considerable overlap between the subgroups of patients.[30] The most dramatic improvement of VMR was reported by Ringelstein in patients with preoperatively very low values, i.e., less than 50%. Decreased VMR may potentially identify patients with asymptomatic carotid stenosis, which carries the highest risk of stroke, and this parameter should be verified in prospective studies.[27,30,31]

Assessment of CO_2 reactivity requires special equipment that may not necessarily be available. A simpler method of VMR assessment uses voluntary breath-holding.[32] VMR is represented by the breath-holding index (BHI), which is the ratio of the percent MFV increase during hypercapnia over the time (seconds) of breath-holding. Baseline FVs are obtained during inhalation of room air followed by a 30 s breath-holding followed by a 4-s recording of the highest FVs. The efficacy of breath-holding can be assessed by a respiratory activity monitor.[32]

In normal subjects, BHI is usually greater than 1 (1.12 ± 0.3, n = 10, mean age 63 ± 11 years).[33] In

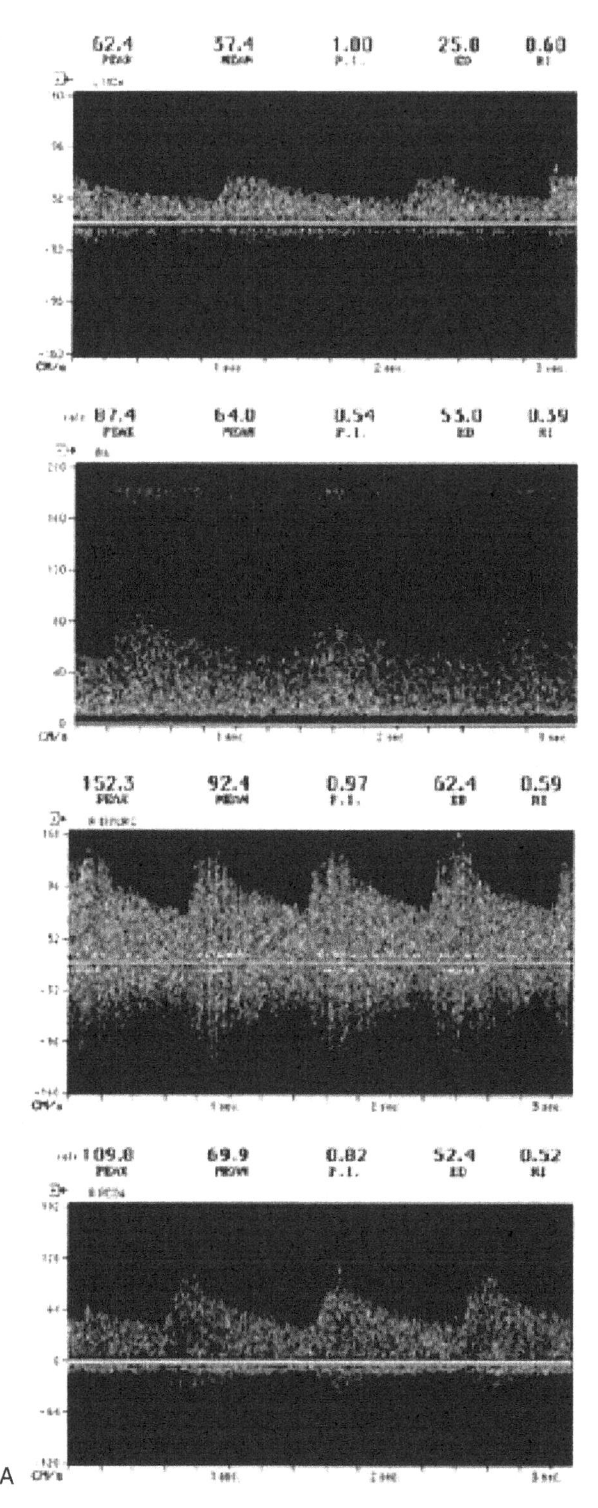

Figure 6–3. (A) Normal low-resistance flow in the Ml-MCA segment has sharp systolic flow acceleration, slow deceleration, and an end-diastolic velocity of 40% (range 20–50%) of the peak systolic values. The pulsatility index (PI) is 1.0 (range 0.6–1.1). End-diastolic flow may decrease and PI may increase with slower heart rate, hypertension, and decreased end-diastolic blood pressure (top image). Abnormally low flow resistance results in elevated velocities above age-expected limits, end-diastolic flow velocity exceeding 50% of peak systolic values, and a decreased pulsatility index of 0.54. This waveform can be seen during hypercapnia, poststenotic vasodilatation, and in partial arteriovenous malformation feeders (second image). Hyperemia typically produces abnormally high flow velocities, low-resistance PI values, and nonharmonic murmurs in the MCA and ACA as well as other intracranial arteries. The Lindegaard ratio is calculated to confirm the parallel increase in mean flow velocity in the insonated and feeding vessels (i.e., MCA/ICA < 3) (third image). Collateral flow via PComA may have elevated velocities, low resistance, a rounded shape of the peak systolic component, and a soft "wind-blowing" sound. A similar waveform may be observed in the MCA when it receives collateral flow from the posterior circulation (fourth image).

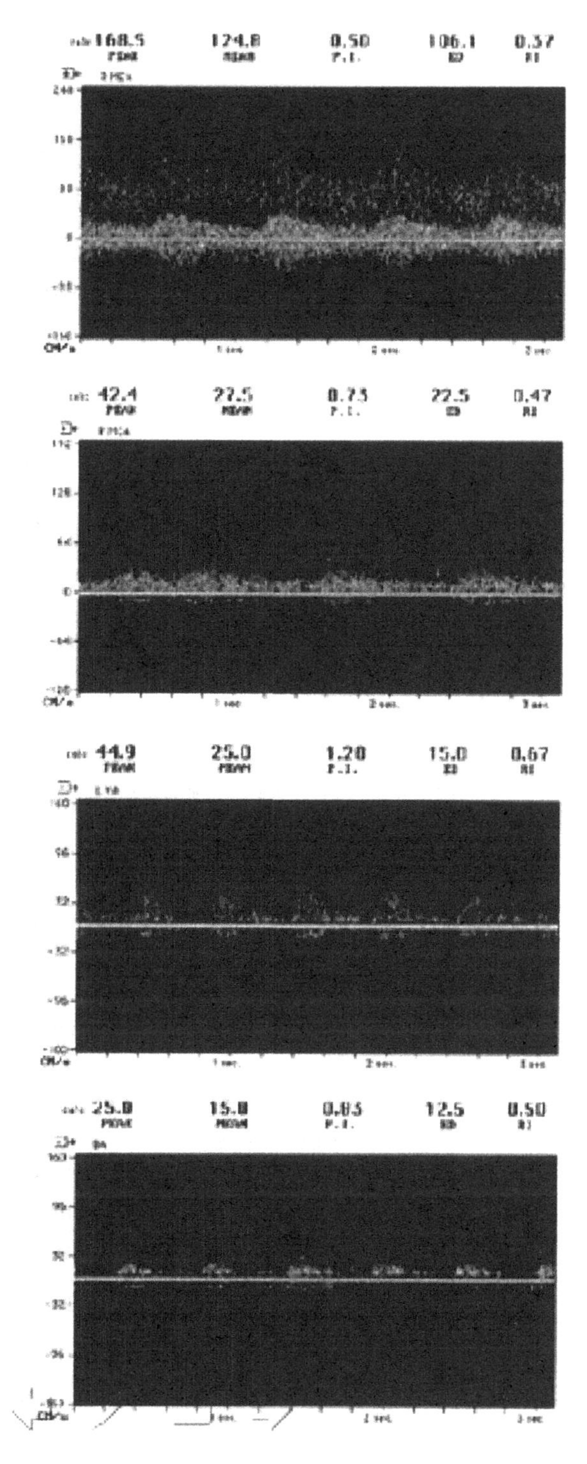

FIGURE 6–3. (B) Arterial stenosis produces a focally significant increase in flow velocities (>30% compared with other arterial segments). The "double" waveform recording shows the stenotic flow and a low-velocity, low-resistance poststenotic flow detected simultaneously using a large (>11 mm) gate of insonation (top image). Arterial near occlusion has a residual flow detected by transcranial Doppler as a "blunted" waveform. This recording shows the delayed minimal systolic flow acceleration and decreased velocities typically seen due to a flow volume decrease with near occlusion. Note the normal pulsatility of flow due to a patent vessel distal to the site of insonation (second image). Arterial occlusion distal to the site of insonation may produce increased resistance to flow in the absence of a bifurcation between these arterial segments. This high resistance (PI ~ 1.2) waveform was obtained just proximal to the basilar artery occlusion at the origin. It may be the only focal sign of a distal arterial obstruction (third image). Minimal flow signals may be a source of error responsible for false-positive and false-negative transcranial Doppler studies. False-positive results are usually obtained with poor windows of insonation, uncooperative patients, and incomplete examination. True signals have very low velocities, almost absent end-diastolic flow, and are found together with other signs of occlusion (fourth image).

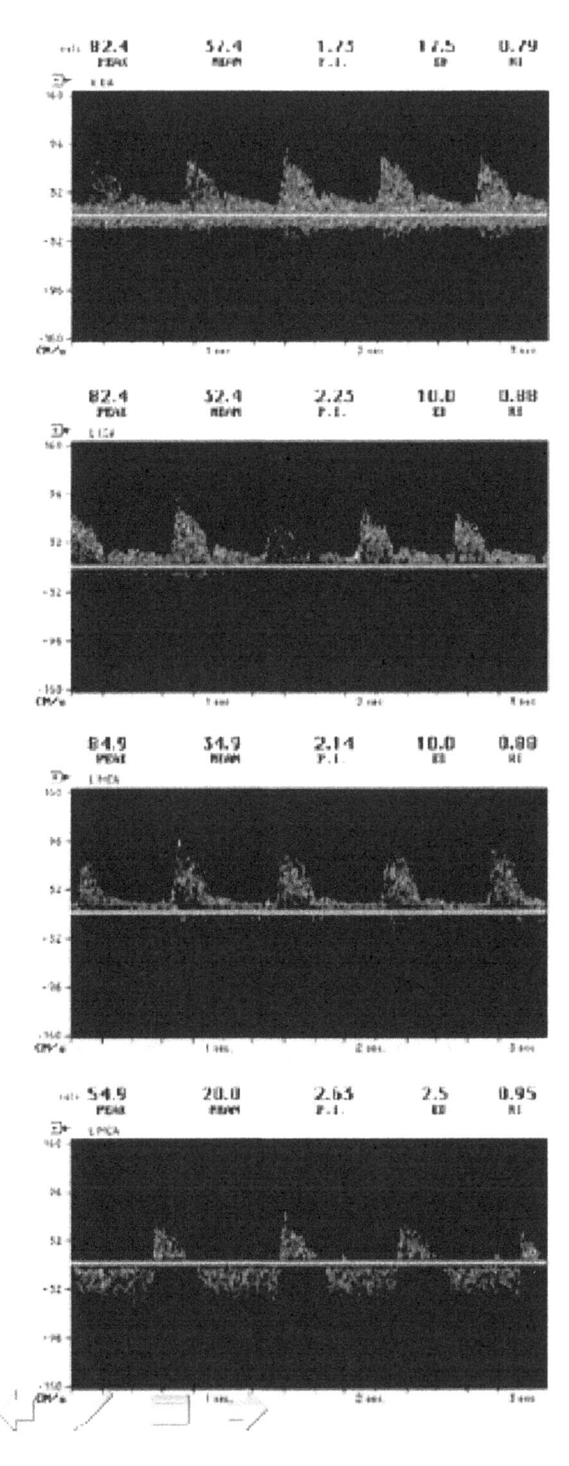

FIGURE 6–3. (C) Under normal conditions, only the ophthalmic artery (OA) has a high-resistance flow pattern with PI values 1.2 and greater. This artery carries the flow away from the brain and forms anastomoses with a high-resistance system of the external carotid artery branches. The OA velocities may vary substantially (top image). Hyperventilation induces vasoconstriction that also increases resistance to flow. The systolic component sharpens, the diacrotic notch becomes more pronounced, and the end-diastolic flow decreases. Often the triphasic waveform is observed similar to the peripheral arteries. The decrease in mean flow velocity may be proportional to the flow volume decrease caused by vasoconstriction (second image). Increased intracranial pressure decreases cerebral perfusion pressure and affects the end-diastolic flow, since blood pressure is lowest during this part of the cardiac cycle with sharp late-systolic deceleration resulting in a shorter transsystolic time (third image). When intracranial pressure exceeds cerebral perfusion pressure, reverberating flow can be detected that indicates systolic flow propagation toward the brain followed by diastolic flow reversal. If found in both MCAs and the BA for 30 min, this flow pattern indicates cerebral circulatory arrest and correlates with absent brain perfusion on a nuclear brain scan (fourth image).

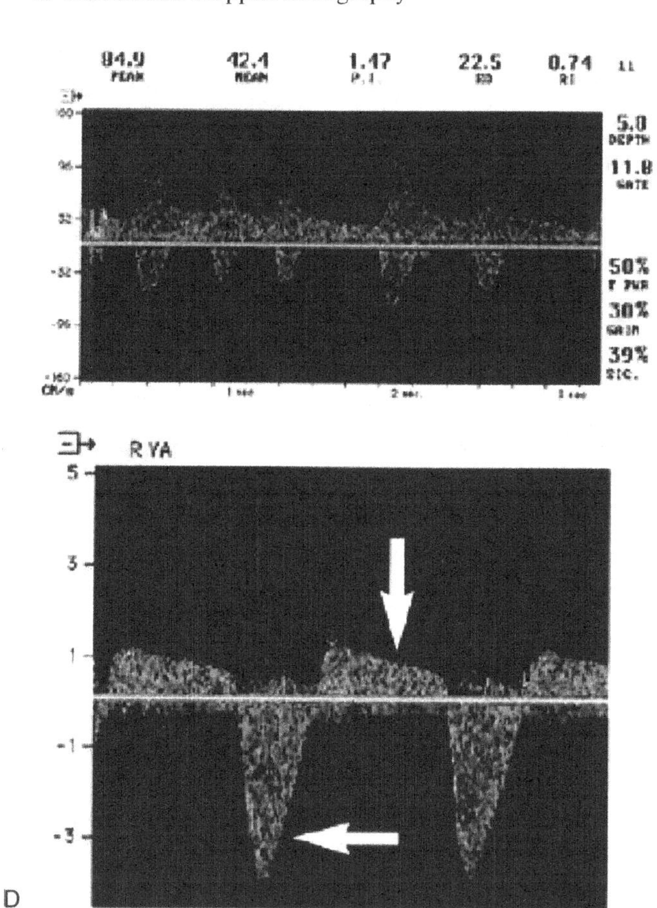

FIGURE 6–3. (D) Microembolic signals (MES) on transcranial Doppler appear as high-intensity transient signals that are primarily unidirectional (*arrow*). MES have short duration and occur randomly through the cardiac cycle. MES may be found during routine transcranial Doppler in patients with atrial fibrillation, carotid stenosis, or dissection, and may point to the pathogenetic mechanism of stroke (top image). Subclavian steal occurs when a flow-limiting lesion in the proximal subclavian artery causes flow reversal in the vertebral artery. Transcranial Doppler detects alternating flow at the junction of vertebral arteries. High-resistance flow toward the probe (*horizontal arrow*) is the reversed vertebral right artery, which now supplies a high-resistance system of the arm. Low-resistance flow (*vertical arrow*) is seen during late systole–diastole and has a normal direction since less pressure is necessary to perfuse the brain vasculature (bottom image).

asymptomatic individuals, BHI was 0.8 ± 0.4 on the stenotic side before and 1.09 ± 0.2 after carotid endarterectomy (CEA). In symptomatic individuals, BHI was 0.4 ± 0.2 on the stenotic side before and 1.06 ± 0.2 after CEA.[33] Recently, a BHI threshold of <0.69 was established in controlled prospective studies that predicts an increased risk of stroke in patients with asymptomatic severe ICA stenosis and risk of recurrent stroke in patients with symptomatic ICA stenoses or occlusion.[29]

Interpretation of CO_2 reactivity testing should be individualized with particular attention paid to the procedure employed since it requires patient cooperation and relies on the sonographer's experience. Abnormally low VMR (<50% CO_2 reactivity, or <0.5 BHI) may indicate maximal vasodilation at rest and therefore poor collateral capacity of the Circle of Willis and potentially higher risk of stroke distal to the extracranial lesion due to exhausted cerebral vasomotor reserve.[30,33] These findings, however, need to be validated in prospective outcome studies.

Vasomotor Reactivity Testing with Diamox

Diamox is a potent and reversible inhibitor of carbonic anhydrase, however, the mechanism by which it increases CBF is still disputable since cerebral metabolic rate of oxygen and arterial blood pressure remain unaffected while arterial PCO_2 increases only slightly.[27]

When administered intravenously, the effect of 1000 mg diamox (acetazolamide) bolus can be observed within 3 min with FVs reaching maximum values in 10 min, which lasts for 20 min. In normal subjects, a 35% increase in FVs is usually observed during hypercapnia.[31] Administration of diamox may be associated with minor and transient side effects: dizziness, oral dysesthesia, tinnitus, and nausea.[34] Since diamox belongs to the sulfanilamide group, any known allergy to the sulfa drugs would be a contraindication for its use.

Using xenon-133 and technetium-99 HMPAO tracers, a 30% increase in CBF was observed in normal subjects following administration of 1000 mg of diamox as well as a high dependency of CBF changes on the degree of carotid stenosis.[35,36] A good correlation was found between mean FVs on TCD and changes in CBF on SPECT or PET.[37,38] Significantly reduced VMR was seen in patients with high grade carotid stenosis suggesting that at baseline the cerebral resistance vessels are maximally dilated to maintain CBF. VMR testing with diamox shows the reduction in or even abolition of the extent to which the resistance vessels can further dilate to compensate for it.[27] However, in spite of uni- or bilateral carotid occlusion some patients have good VMR indicating a sufficient collateral capacity of the Circle of Willis and sufficient cerebral autoregulation. Therefore, VMR testing with diamox may help to differentiate patients with carotid artery disease at high and low risk of stroke and may assist in patient selection for CEA prior to cardiopulmonary bypass (CABG).

Application of Vasomotor Reactivity Testing

Major vascular risk factors for stroke have a chronic effect on the cerebral vasculature that often precedes cerebral ischemic symptoms.[31] Thus diabetes and familial hypercholesterolemia are associated with greater FV increase to vasodilatory stimuli, while chronic hypertension increases the pulsatility of flow.[39–41]

Although the degree of carotid stenosis is the strongest predictor of subsequent stroke risk,[22–24] the impaired VMR can help identify patients at a particularly high risk of stroke.[29,42]

VMR can also be impaired in patients with subarachnoid hemorrhage (SAH).[43] With increased severity of vasospasm there is a gradual reduction of VMR in response to changes in arterial CO_2.[44] Although VMR changes often parallel the course of vasospasm, nimodipine has no effect on CO_2 reactivity.[45] Whether impaired VMR has an independent prognostic value in patients with SAH and other pathologies is still unclear.[31]

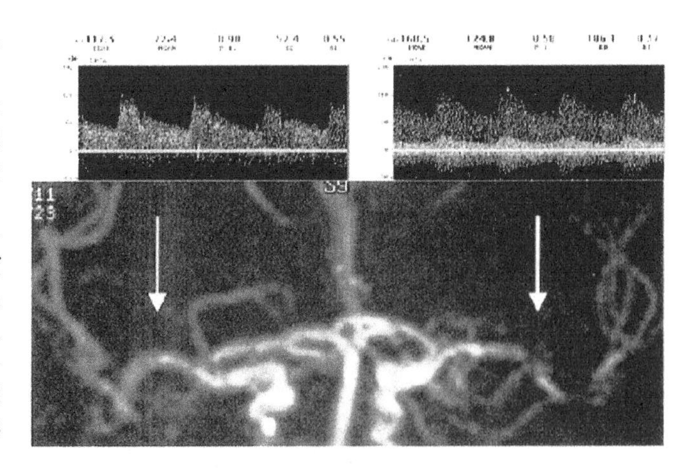

FIGURE 6–4. Left M1-MCA stenosis. A 70-year-old woman with multiple left hemispheric transient ischemic attacks. Transcranial Doppler showed a focally significant increase in the left M1-MCA flow velocities, a "double" waveform showing the stenotic flow insonated with a wide >11-mm gate. MRA shows decreased flow signals in the left mid-to-distal M1-MCA.

Diagnostic Criteria for Transcranial Doppler

The diagnostic criteria for TCD required by the Intersocietal Commission of Accreditation of Vascular Laboratories include arterial stenosis, arterial spasm and hyperemia, collateral patterns and flow direction, cerebral embolization, cerebral circulatory arrest, increased ICP, arterial occlusion, and steal syndrome. When applying for accreditation, each laboratory should accept diagnostic criteria that may include application of published criteria or the use of internally generated criteria. *Whether published or internally generated, normal values and criteria for abnormal findings have to be internally validated.*

This section provides a summary of various criteria, both previously published by other investigators[3,12–15,17,20,21] and generated internally by the STAT Neurosonology Service, University of Texas Houston Medical School.

Intracranial Arterial Stenosis

Middle Cerebral Artery

A focally significant velocity increase MFV ≥ 100 cm/s, and/or a PSV ≥ 140 cm/s, and/or an interhemispheric MFV difference of >30 cm/s in adults free of abnormal circulatory conditions are characteristic (Figure 6–4). If anemia, congestive heart failure, and other circulatory conditions associated with elevated or decreased velocities are present, then a focal MFV difference >30% between arterial segments should be applied. In general, a greater than 50% M1-MCA stenosis should double the prestenotic or homologous contralateral MCA velocity values. In children with sickle cell disease MCA MFV > 170 cm/s is considered abnormal.

Additional findings may include turbulence, or disturbed flow distal to the stenosis; increased unilateral A1-ACA MFVs (flow diversion/compensatory increase or ICA bifurcation stenosis) with a side-to-side ACA MFV ratio >1.2; a low-frequency noise produced by nonharmonic covibrations of the vessel wall; and musical murmurs due to harmonic covibrations producing pure tones (rare).

If FVs are increased throughout MCA mainstem, the differential diagnosis includes MCA stenosis, terminal ICA or siphon stenosis, hyperemia or compensatory flow increase in the presence of contralateral ICA stenosis, ACA occlusion, and incorrect vessel identification.

MCA near-occlusion or "blunted" MCA waveform presents as a focal decrease in mean flow velocities with slow systolic acceleration, slow flow deceleration, and MFV MCA < ACA or any other intracranial artery (Figure 6–5).

The decreased or minimal flow velocities with slow systolic acceleration can be due to a tight elongated MCA stenosis or thrombus causing near occlusion, or a proximal ICA obstruction. The "blunted" waveform is common in patients with acute ischemic stroke particularly presenting with hyperdense MCA on noncontrast CT scan or a flow gap on MRA (Figure 6–5).

Anterior Cerebral Artery

A focally significant ACA FV increase (ACA > MCA), and/or an ACA MFV > 80 cm/s, and/or a >30% difference between proximal and distal ACA segments, and/or a >30% difference compared to contralateral ACA with no evidence of collateralization via AcomA are characteristic. The differential diagnosis includes anterior crossfilling due to a proximal carotid artery disease. Additional

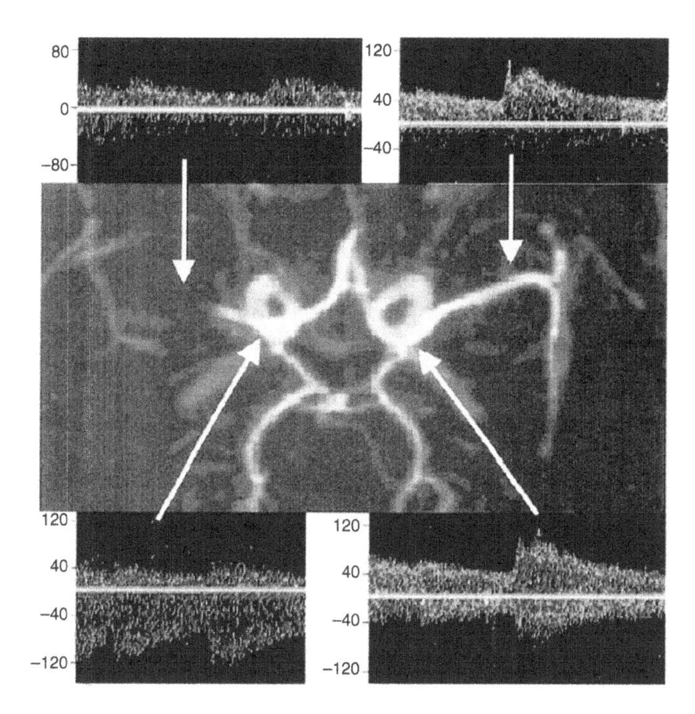

FIGURE 6–5. Right MCA near-occlusion. A 65-year-old man presented with recurrent right MCA ischemic strokes. Transcranial Doppler showed a "blunted" MCA flow signal with decreased flow velocities at the M1 origin and increased velocities in the A1-ACA indicating compensatory flow diversion. Note the decreased systolic flow acceleration in the right MCA and ACA > MCA ratio compared with the contralateral side.

findings may include turbulence and a flow diversion into MCA and/or compensatory flow increase in the contralateral ACA.

The decreased or minimal flow velocities at the A1-ACA origin may indicate a suboptimal angle of insonation from the unilateral temporal window, an atretic or tortuous A1-ACA segment, and A1-ACA near occlusion.

Common errors include incorrect vessel identification (ICA versus ACA) and velocity underestimation (suboptimal angle of insonation, poor window, weak signals).

Terminal Internal Carotid Artery/Siphon Stenosis

A focally significant FV increase in the terminal ICA bifurcation (temporal window), and/or an ICA siphon (transorbital window) resulting in an MFV ICA > MCA, and/or an MFV ICA > 70 cm/s (adults), and/or a >30% difference between arterial segments are characteristic.

The differential diagnosis includes moderate proximal ICA stenosis and/or compensatory flow increase with contralateral ICA stenosis. Additional findings may include turbulence, blunted MCA, OA MFV increase, and/or flow reversal with low pulsatility. The ICA siphon MFVs may decrease due to siphon near-occlusion (a blunted siphon signal) or distal obstruction (i.e., MCA occlusion or increased ICP).

Posterior Cerebral Artery

A focally significant FV increase presenting as an MFV PCA > ACA or ICA and/or an MFV PCA > 50 cm/s are characteristic. The differential diagnosis includes collateral flow via PcomA and siphon stenosis. Additional findings may include turbulence and a compensatory flow increase in MCA. Common sources of error include unreliable vessel identification without transcranial duplex imaging or the presence of an arterial occlusion and the top-of-the-basilar stenosis.

Basilar Artery

A focally significant FV increase presenting as an MFV BA > MCA or ACA or ICA, and/or an MFV BA > 60 cm/s, and/or a >30% difference between arterial segments are characteristic. The differential diagnosis includes the terminal VA stenosis.

Basilar artery near-occlusion is a focal FV decrease (<30% and/or BA < VA) resulting in a blunted waveform (differential with fusiform basilar with or without thrombus) or absent end-diastolic flow (differential with occlusion).

Additional findings may include turbulence, a compensatory flow increase in VAs and PICAs indicating cerebellar collateralization, and a collateral supply via PComA(s) to PCA(s) with a reversed flow in the top of the basilar artery. Common sources of error include a tortuous basilar ("not found" does not mean obstructed), elongated or distal BA stenosis, collateral flow from the posterior to anterior circulation enhancing flow changes with mild stenosis and/or tortuosity.

Terminal Vertebral Artery

A focally significant FV increase presenting as an MFV VA >> BA, and/or an MFV VA > 50 cm/s (adults), and/or a >30% difference between VAs or its segments are characteristic. The terminal VA stenosis may also present as a high resistance (PI ≥ 1.2) flow in one VA and/or a blunted or minimal flow signal. The differential diagnosis includes proximal BA or contralateral terminal VA stenoses and a compensatory flow increase in the presence of a contralateral VA occlusion. Additional findings may include turbulence, a compensatory flow increase in the contralateral vertebral artery or its branches (cerebellar collaterals), low BA flow velocities (hemodynamically significant lesion, hypoplastic contralateral VA). Common sources of error include a compensatory flow increase due to hypoplastic contralateral VA, low velocities in both VAs due to a suboptimal angle of insonation, extracranial VA stenosis or occlusion with well-developed muscular collaterals, and elongated VA stenosis/hypoplasia.

TCD can reliably detect stenoses located in M1-MCA, ICA siphon, terminal vertebral, proximal basilar arteries, and P1 PCA. The sensitivity is 85–90%, specificity 90–95%, PPV 85%, and NPV 98% with lower accuracy parameters for the posterior circulation.[3,12,15,17,20,21] TCD sensitivity is limited in patients with deep (>65 mm) stenoses due to low PRF; stenoses of M2, A2, P2 segments due to a suboptimal angle or unknown location; low flow elongated stenoses that resemble normal or low flow velocities; subtotal stenosis due to a drop in flow volume producing weak signals; tortuous vessels due to the changing angle of insonation; and collaterals and hyperemia that may mimic the stenotic flow.

Arterial Vasospasm and Hyperemia

Arterial vasospasm (VSP) is a complication of SAH, and it becomes symptomatic in more than 25% of patients by producing ischemic brain damage and delayed neurological deficit (DID). DID usually occurs when VSP results in a severe (≤1 mm) intracranial arterial narrowing producing flow depletion with extremely high velocities. It may affect the proximal stem and distal branches of intracranial arteries. VSP may coexist with hydrocephalus, edema, and infarction. The differential diagnosis with TCD should always include hyperemia, and the possibility that both spasm and hyperemia may coexist since most SAH patients routinely receive hypertension–hemodilution–hypervolemia (HHH) therapy.

Although quantitative criteria have been studied extensively,[20,46] grading VSP severity is difficult, and the interpretation of TCD findings should be individualized. Daily TCDs may detect considerable velocity/pulsatility changes that should be related to the patient's condition, medications, BP, time after onset, etc.

Proximal vasospasm in any intracranial artery results in a focal or diffuse elevation of mean flow velocities without a parallel FV increase in the feeding extracranial arteries (intracranial/extracranial vessel ratio >3).

Distal vasospasm in any intracranial artery may produce a focally pulsatile flow (PI ≥ 1.2) indicating increased resistance distal to the site of insonation. No MFV increase may be found.

Additional findings may include daily changes in velocity, ratio, and PIs anytime during the first 2 weeks but particularly pronounced during the critical 3–7 days after the onset of SAH.

MCA-specific criteria: see Table 6–2. The differential diagnosis includes hyperemia, a combination of vasospasm and hyperemia in the same vessel, residual vasospasm, and hyperemia.

TABLE 6–2. Criteria for grading M1-MCA vasospasm with or without hyperemia.[a]

Velocity	MCA/ICA ratio[b]	Interpretation
<120	≤3	Hyperemia
>80	3–4	Hyperemia + possible mild spasm
≥120	3–4	Mild spasm + hyperemia
≥120	4–5	Moderate spasm + hyperemia
>120	5–6	Moderate spasm
≥180	6	Moderate-to-severe spasm
≥200	≥6	Severe spasm
>200	4–6	Moderate spasm + hyperemia
>200	3–4	Hyperemia + mild (often residual) spasm
>200	<3	Hyperemia

[a]Optimized criteria were developed using the data from Bragoni *et al.*,[14] De Chiara *et al.*,[39] and Sugimari *et al.*[40]
[b]MCA, middle cerebral artery; ICA, internal carotid artery.

Prognostically unfavorable signs include an early appearance of MCA MFV ≥ 180 cm/s, a rapid (>20% or + >65 cm/s) daily MFV increase during critical days 3–7, an MCA/ICA ratio ≥6, and the abrupt appearance of high pulsatility (PI > 1.5) of flow in two or more arteries indicating increased ICP and/or distal vasospasm.[20,46]

Other intracranial arteries: see Table 6–3. Grading VSP severity in the arteries other than MCA is difficult. Sloan suggested reporting VSP as possible, probable, and definite.[46] The differential diagnosis includes hyperemia and its combination with vasospasm in these arteries.

An individual correlation of baseline angiography with same day TCD findings may improve the accuracy of TCD in detecting further VSP onset. A focal increase in MFVs and an increase in MFVs disproportionate to therapy will indicate the development of vasospasm. For example, an MCA MFV increase by +50 cm/s may indicate a 20% diameter reduction of the vessel[47] and since FV is inversely proportionate to the vessel radius, a 30% diameter reduction usually doubles the velocity on TCD.

TABLE 6–3. Optimized criteria for grading vasospasm (VSP) in intracranial arteries.

Artery/MFV[a]	Possible VSP[b]	Probable VSP[b]	Definite VSP[b]
ICA	>80	>110	>130
ACA	>90	>110	>120
PCA	>60	>80	>90
BA	>70	>90	>100
VA	>60	>80	>90

[a]MFV, mean flow velocity; ICA, internal carotid artery; ACA, anterior cerebral artery; PCA, posterior cerebral artery; BA, basilar artery; VA, vertebral artery.
[b]After hyperemia has been mostly ruled out by the focality of the velocity increase and by an intracranial artery/extracranial ICA ratio >3 except posterior circulation vessels. Optimized criteria were modified from Sloan MA *et al.*[46]

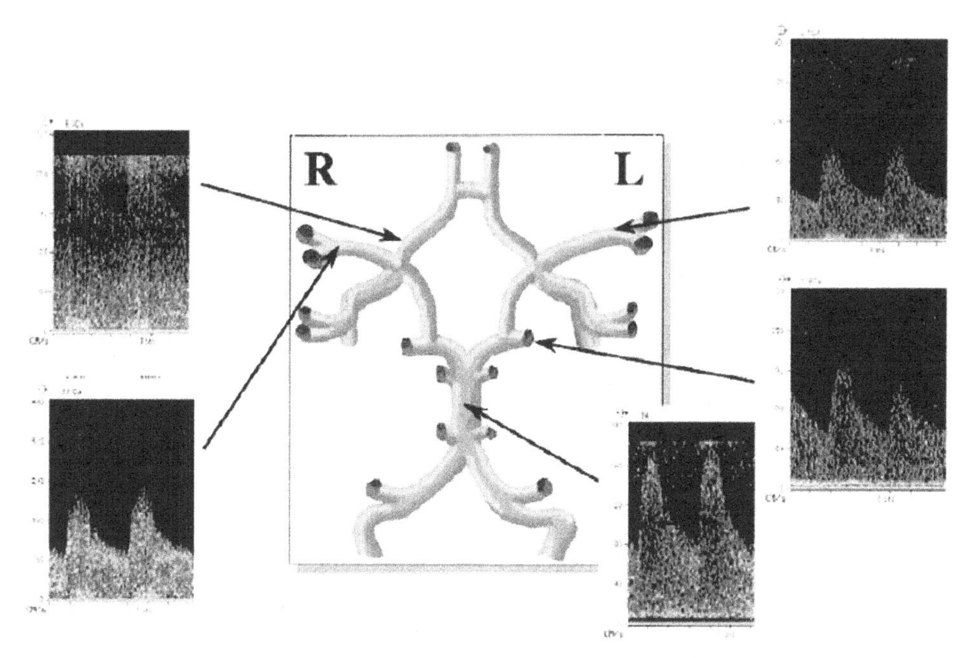

FIGURE 6–6. Severe ACA, PCA, and BA vasospasm. Arterial vasospasm. A 55-year-old woman had a subarachnoid hemorrhage and surgically clipped left PCA aneurysm. Transcranial Doppler showed an MFV/PI of 222/0.5 in the right A1-ACA with an ACA/ICA MFV ratio >6; 131/0.9 in the right M1-MCA with an MCA/ICA MFV ratio = 4; 109/0.9 in the basilar artery; 130/0.8 in the left PCA; and 103/1.0 in the left M1-MCA with an MCA/ICA MFV ratio <3. The interpretation was severe right A1-ACA vasospasm with moderate basilar and left PCA vasospasm. Digital subtraction angiography confirmed these findings.

Therefore TCD is more sensitive to changes in intracranial artery diameter than angiography. Since TCD is a screening tool, the criteria should be adjusted toward a higher sensitivity to detect any degree of vasospasm in order to institute HHH therapy. At the same time, a higher specificity threshold should be used for severe vasospasm to minimize the number of false-negative angiograms. TCD may also help to guide angiography toward the affected vessel and to select the best projection to demonstrate the lesion (Figure 6–6). Angioplasty with papaverine can be performed to restore the patency of the vessel affected by VSP (Figure 6–7).[48]

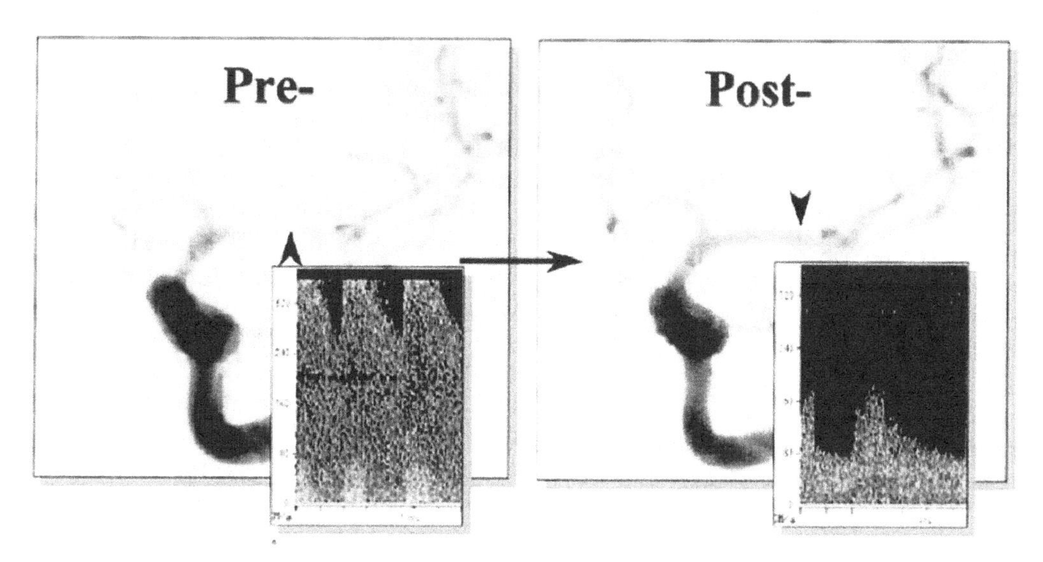

FIGURE 6–7. Angioplasty for severe vasospasm and the velocity changes on transcranial Doppler. A 51-year-old woman with subarachnoid hemorrhage developed severe MCA vasospasm detected by transcranial Doppler as an MFV/PI of 302/0.3 and an MCA/ICA MFV ratio >10. After angioplasty with papaverine the velocity decreased to 106/1.0 with an MCA/ICA MFV ratio of 3.

Hyperemia often results in elevated MFVs in intracranial and feeding extracranial vasculature (Table 6–2). Hyperemia is common in patients with SAH receiving HHH therapy, and early in the postoperative period after CEA or CABG. Hyperperfusion syndrome after CEA includes headache and seizures and usually produces a >30% increase in MCA MFV unilateral to the reconstructed carotid artery.

Collateral Patterns and Flow Direction

The intracranial collateral channels are dormant under normal circulatory conditions. A collateral channel opens when a pressure gradient develops between the two arterial systems that have anastomoses. TCD can detect some of these collateral pathways: reversed OA, anterior crossfilling via AComA, and PComA flow either to or from the anterior circulation. Flow direction will depend on the direction of collateralization. When present, a collateral flow rarely implies an anatomic variant, but most often implies the presence of a flow-limiting lesion proximal to the recipient arterial system and the origin of the collateral channel detected.

The direction of flow determines which arterial system is the donor (the source of flow) and which is the recipient (the collateral flow destination). TCD can therefore provide information on whether any collateral channel is functioning and in which direction it is working. This information should be used to estimate the level of the arterial obstruction and to refine the extracranial duplex ultrasound or MRA findings. For example, a severe extracranial ICA stenosis with >70% diameter reduction is hemodynamically significant and is almost always accompanied by abnormal TCD findings.[17] A battery of TCD parameters may be used to decide on the severity of ICA lesions, particularly when the applicability of other tests is limited.

Reversed Ophthalmic Artery

A low pulsatility flow is primarily directed away from the probe with transorbital insonation at 50–62 mm. The differential diagnosis includes siphon flow and/or low velocity OA flow signals. Additional findings may include no substantial difference in MFVs detected in OA and siphon, high velocities in the ICA siphon suggesting either a high grade proximal ICA and/or siphon stenosis, and no flow signals at depths ≥60 mm suggesting ICA occlusion.

Interpretation

If the reversed OA is the only abnormal finding, this indicates possible proximal ICA stenosis. Occasionally, this may be the only sign of ICA dissection or occlusion. If the reversed OA is found with a blunted MCA signal, there is a probable proximal ICA and/or siphon stenosis or occlusion. If the reversed OA is found with at least one other collateral channel (anterior crossfilling, or PComA) there is a definite proximal ICA high-grade stenosis or occlusion.

Common sources of error include ICA dissection, terminal ICA occlusion distal to the OA origin, and retrograde filling of the ICA siphon with a normal OA direction. Furthermore, a normal OA direction does not rule out proximal ICA stenosis.

Anterior Communicating Artery

The collateral flow through AComA cannot be distinguished from the neighboring ACAs due to the smaller AComA length and diameter and a large gate of insonation. Therefore, we report anterior crossfilling via AComA as opposed to the velocity and direction of flow in AComA itself.

Anterior Crossfilling

Elevated A1-ACA MFVs on the donor side present as ACA > MCA and/or donor ACA MFVs more than 1.2 times greater than contralateral ACA, possible stenotic-like flow at depths 72–78 mm directed away from the donor side, and a normal or low MFV in A1-ACA of the recipient side with or without A1 flow reversal. The differential diagnosis includes distal A1-ACA stenosis and compensatory flow increase if one A1 segment is atretic. The finding of a reversed A1 segment and vessel identification is operator dependent.

Interpretation

If only elevated donor ACA velocities are found, the differential diagnosis includes A1-ACA stenosis and atresia of the contralateral A1 segment. With the latter, the donor A1 segment supplies both A2 segments (may be present in normal individuals as well as in patients with ICA or MCA stenoses). If an elevated donor ACA velocity is found with a stenotic flow at midline depths, the differential includes the distal A1 stenosis, ICA siphon stenosis, and crossfilling via AComA. If an elevated donor ACA MFV is found with a reversed contralateral A1, this indicates probable proximal ICA stenosis. If an elevated donor ACA MFV is found with the stenotic-like flow at midline depths and a reversed contralateral A1 ACA, there is a definite proximal ICA stenosis or occlusion.

Posterior Communicating Artery

PComA connects the posterior and anterior cerebral arterial systems and may be detected by TCD since it usually has a length >5 mm and a favorable angle of insonation. When functioning, it can be detected as a flow signal consistently present at varying depths from 60 to 75 mm via a transtemporal approach. Under normal conditions, this area has no detectable flow when the sonographer switches from ICA bifurcation posteriorly to locate PCA. The direction of flow in PComA corresponds to collateralization: the anterior-to-posterior collateral flow is directed away from the probe, whereas the posterior-to-anterior collateral flow is directed toward the probe. The vessel identification is difficult since the PComA is prone to anatomic variations.

Collateralization via PComA

The flow signals directed either away from or toward the probe with posterior angulation of the transducer over the temporal window are consistently found at 60–75 mm. The velocity range is similar to or higher then those detected in M1-MCA and ICA bifurcation (anterior-to-posterior collateral flow) or basilar artery (posterior-to-anterior collateral flow). A possible stenotic-like flow may be found at depths of 60–75 mm with a similar probe direction. The differential diagnosis includes terminal ICA or PCA stenoses.

Interpretation

PComA identification is operator dependent. If found, PComA implies arterial obstruction in one of the following arteries. If a posterior-to-anterior collateral flow is found, a probable proximal ICA stenosis is present. If an anterior-to-posterior collateral flow is found, a probable BA or dominant VA stenosis is present.

Reversed Flow in the Basilar Artery

If an occlusion develops in the proximal basilar artery, a pressure gradient develops between the carotid circulation and posterior cerebral arteries, superior cerebellar arteries, and perforating vessels. If a thrombus or embolus in the proximal basilar artery does not completely occlude the vessel immediately, the patient may be able to recruit posterior communicating arteries and deliver blood from the carotids via the reversed basilar stem to parts of the cerebellum and smaller distal basilar branches. This collateral flow reaches the low-resistance system of cerebellar anastomoses and the brainstem parenchyma. This is why patients may have neurological dysfunction of variable clinical severity and good diastolic velocities on Doppler. Identification of low-resistance flow moving toward the probe, i.e., reversed basilar flow at 80–100 mm, may indicate continuing perfusion of vital brain structures and often explains the good level of consciousness and partial neurological deficits despite the presence of a proximal basilar obstruction.[49]

Cerebral Embolization

TCD can detect microembolization of cerebral vessels in real time. As an investigational tool, TCD is used to monitor CEA, CABG, angioplasty/stenting, as well as stroke patients with presumed cardiac or arterial sources for brain embolization. All microembolic signals (MES) detected by TCD are asymptomatic since the size of the particles producing them is comparable to or even smaller then the diameter of the brain capillaries. However, the MES cumulative count is related to the incidence of the neuropsychological deficit after CABG, and its significance as a risk factor for stroke is under investigation.[50,51] During surgery or intraarterial procedures microembolic signals can be of different composition, either solid or gaseous. Identification of embolic material is important since air bubbles have a lower pathogenic impact. Recently, multifrequency TCD had shown promising results in differentiating the nature of the embolus.[52]

Nevertheless, it is important to know how to detect and identify MES because occasionally the TCD examiner may be the only witness to cerebral microembolization and this finding may suggest a vascular origin of the neurological event and allow clinicians to investigate potential sources of embolism (heart chambers and septum, aortic arch, arterial stenosis or dissection).

The gold standard for MES identification is an on-line interpretation of video- or digitally taped flow signals. The spectral recording should be obtained with minimal gain at a fixed angle of insonation. The probe should be maintained with a fixation device for at least 0.5–1 h monitoring. The use of two-channel simultaneous registration and a prolonged time of monitoring may improve the yield of the procedure. Multigated or multiranged registration at different insonation depths may improve differentiation of embolic signals from artifacts.[51]

According to the International Cerebral Hemodynamics Society definition,[53] MES have the following:

1. Random occurrence during the cardiac cycle.
2. Brief duration (usually <0.1 s).
3. High intensity (>3 dB over background).
4. Primarily unidirectional signals (if fast Fourier transformation is used).
5. Audible component (chirp, pop).

To avoid discrediting this promising method, the research studies should report the following 14 parameters: ultrasound device, transducer type and size, insonated artery, insonation depth, algorithms for signal intensity measurement, scale settings, detection threshold, axial extension of sample volume, fast Fourier transform (FFT) size (number of points used), FFT length (time), FFT overlap, transmitted ultrasound frequency, high-pass filter settings, and the recording time.[54] No current system of automated embolus detection seems to have the required sensitivity and specificity for clinical use.[54]

In 2004 Mackinnon *et al.* presented the first ambulatory TCD system (like a "Holter" monitor for MCA flow velocity) able to offer good-quality recordings of >5 h. In view of the demonstrated temporal variability in embolization, this technique is likely to improve the predictive value of recording for asymptomatic embolic signals and may be particularly useful in patients in whom embolic signals are relatively infrequent, such as those with asymptomatic carotid stenosis and atrial fibrillation.[55]

Increased Intracranial Pressure

A normal intracranial waveform is detected by TCD when the brain acts as a low-resistance vascular system at normal or low ICP values (Figure 6–3). When ICP increases up to the diastolic pressure of the resistance vessels, the EDV decreases and flow deceleration occurs more rapidly. If ICP is greater than diastolic but less than systolic pressures, the result is either a triphasic waveform as in the peripheral arteries or a sharp-peak systolic flow with an absent end-diastolic component. A further increase in ICP may lead to cerebral circulatory arrest.

Increased ICP may result in high resistance waveforms: PI ≥ 1.2, decreased or absent EDV, or triphasic or reverberating flow. The following algorithm may help to differentiate the mechanisms of increased resistance to flow.

If PI ≥ 1.2 and a positive end-diastolic flow is present in

1. All arteries: hyperventilation; hypertension; increased ICP.
2. Unilateral: compartmental ICP increase; stenoses distal to the site of insonation; intracranial hemorrhage with mass effect or hydrocephalus.[56]
3. One artery: distal obstruction (spasm, stenosis, edema).

If PI ≥ 2.0 and end-diastolic flow is absent in

1. All arteries: extremely high ICP; possible arrest of cerebral circulation.
2. Unilateral: compartmental ICP increase, occlusion distal to the insonation site.
3. One artery: distal obstruction (occlusion, severe spasm, edema).

Cerebral Circulatory Arrest

A progressive elevation of ICP to extreme levels due to brain edema and mass effect can lead to stepwise compression of small to large intracranial arteries causing cerebral circulatory arrest. A prolonged absence of brain perfusion will eventually lead to brain death.

If cerebral circulatory arrest is suspected, use the following algorithm:

1. Positive MCA or BA end-diastolic flow = no cerebral circulatory arrest.
2. Absent end-diastolic flow = uncertain cerebral circulatory arrest (too early or too late).
3. Reversed minimal end-diastolic flow = possible cerebral circulatory arrest (continue monitoring).
4. Reverberating flow = probable cerebral circulatory arrest (confirm in both MCAs at depths of 50–58 mm and BA at 80–90 mm, then monitor arrest for 30 min).

TCD cannot be used to diagnose brain death since this is a clinical diagnosis. It can be used to confirm cerebral circulatory arrest except in infants less than 6 months old.[57] TCD can be used to monitor the progression to cerebral circulatory arrest. Once the reverberating flow is found it should be monitored for at least 30 min in the three major intracranial arteries to avoid false-positive findings. For example, a transient cerebral circulatory arrest can occur in patients with SAH and head trauma due to A-waves of ICP.[58] TCD can also be used to determine the appropriate time for other confirmatory tests (i.e., to minimize studies with residual CBF), and to discuss the upcoming issues with the patient's family.

The criteria and accuracy for TCD testing for cerebral circulatory arrest were addressed in an International Consensus statement.[59]

Steal Syndrome

Subclavian "steal" is a hemodynamic condition of a reversed flow in one vertebral artery to compensate for a proximal hemodynamic lesion in the unilateral subclavian artery. Thus blood flow is diverted or "stolen" from the brain to feed the arm (Figure 6–8). The subclavian steal usually represents an accidental finding since it rarely produces neurological symptoms. If asymptomatic it is called a "subclavian steal phenomenon." If symptoms of vertebrobasilar ischemia are present, it is called a "subclavian steal syndrome."[60]

The main findings include a difference in BP between arms >20 mm Hg and usually systolic flow reversal with PI ≥ 1.2 in one vertebral artery (Figures 6–3 and 6–8) as well as a low resistance flow in the donor artery. Right to left subclavian steal is found in 85% of cases.[60]

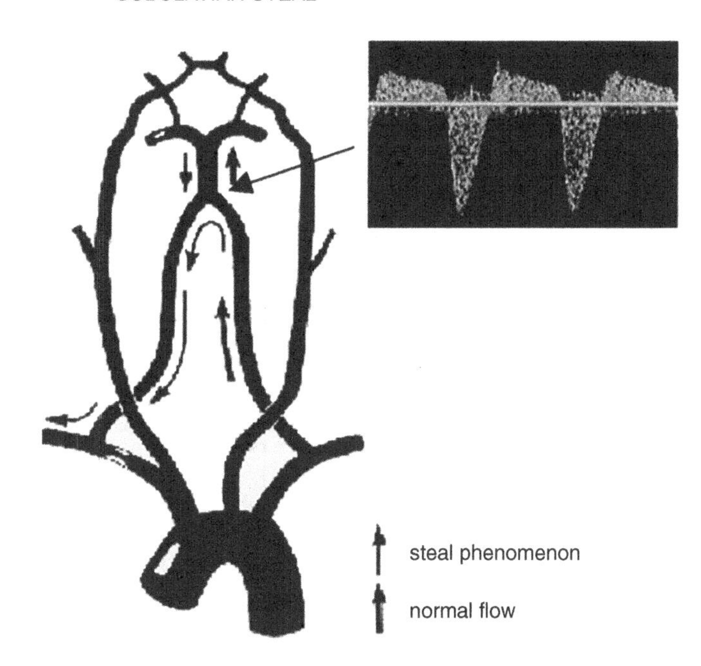

FIGURE 6–8. Subclavian steal. Subclavian steal results in a reversed flow direction in one of the vertebral arteries *(scheme)*, an alternating flow pattern on transcranial Doppler, and retrograde filling of the reversed vertebral artery.

If the difference in BP between the arms is 10–20 mm Hg and the steal waveforms are not present at rest, or flow reversal is incomplete, the hyperemia test should be performed either to provoke the steal or to augment flow reversal. The cuff should be inflated to oversystolic BP values and flow reduction to the arm should be maintained for at least 0.5–1 min. The cuff should be quickly released and any augmentation of flow should be monitored by TCD.

Transcranial Doppler in Acute Stroke

TCD may facilitate the diagnosis of cerebral arterial occlusion and can improve outcomes. First, it can be used to identify the presence and location of an obstructive intracranial thrombus confirming the vascular origin of the patient's neurological symptoms.[61] Second, it provides valuable information about the collateral flow to the vascular territory distal to the artery occlusion, and helps in selecting patients for intraarterial interventions.[62] Third, it provides real-time bedside monitoring of thrombolysis. And finally, it augments residual flow and speeds up thrombolysis, allowing patients to recover from stroke more rapidly and completely.

Arterial Occlusion

The diagnosis of an intracranial arterial occlusion with TCD is difficult. The operator must be experienced and the best results are usually obtained for M1-MCA, ICA siphon, and BA. The main prerequisite is a good window of insonation and to prove this, other arteries should be identified through the same approach. The main finding is no detectable signals from the location where the artery is expected to be.

The specific findings for **MCA** include no signal at any depth of 40–65 mm via a transtemporal approach. Secondary findings are a flow diversion/compensatory increase in ACA and/or PCA, no signals from ACA and ICA with PCA flow identified, and proximal M1-MCA high-resistance flow. The findings need to be confirmed by insonation across the midline from the contralateral temporal window.

The specific findings for **ICA siphon** include no signals at 62–70 mm via a transorbital approach. Secondary findings include a collateral flow in PComA and/or crossfilling via AComA, a blunted MCA flow signal, and a contralateral ICA compensatory flow/velocity increase.

The specific findings for **BA** include no signals at any depth of 80–100+ mm via a transforaminal approach. Secondary findings include a flow velocity increase in one or both VAs indicating cerebellar collateral flow; a high resistance flow signal in one or both VAs indicating proximal BA occlusion; a high resistance flow signal at the origin of the BA indicating distal BA occlusion; retrograde flow toward the probe at the top of the basilar artery (proximal BA occlusion collateralized via PcomAs); functional PComA(s) with flow directed away from the probe via the temporal window; and low BA velocities with the top-of-the-basilar occlusion.

In 2001 Demchuck *et al.* developed the thrombolysis in brain ischemia (TIBI) classification by using TCD to noninvasively monitor intracranial vessel residual flow signals (Figure 6–9). The TIBI classification correlates with initial stroke severity, clinical recovery, and mortality in IV-tissue plasminogen activator (t-PA)-treated stroke patients. In addition, a flow-grade improvement correlated with clinical improvement. The real advantage of TCD is lost if only flow velocity differences are reported and other hemodynamic findings are ignored. TIBI flow grades show information that can be obtained through waveform analysis providing qualitative and quantitative information of the flow status.[63]

Patient Management Optimization

Although TCD does not provide estimates of brain parenchymal perfusion[64,65] or transcortical collateralization of flow, it offers information about collateral flow

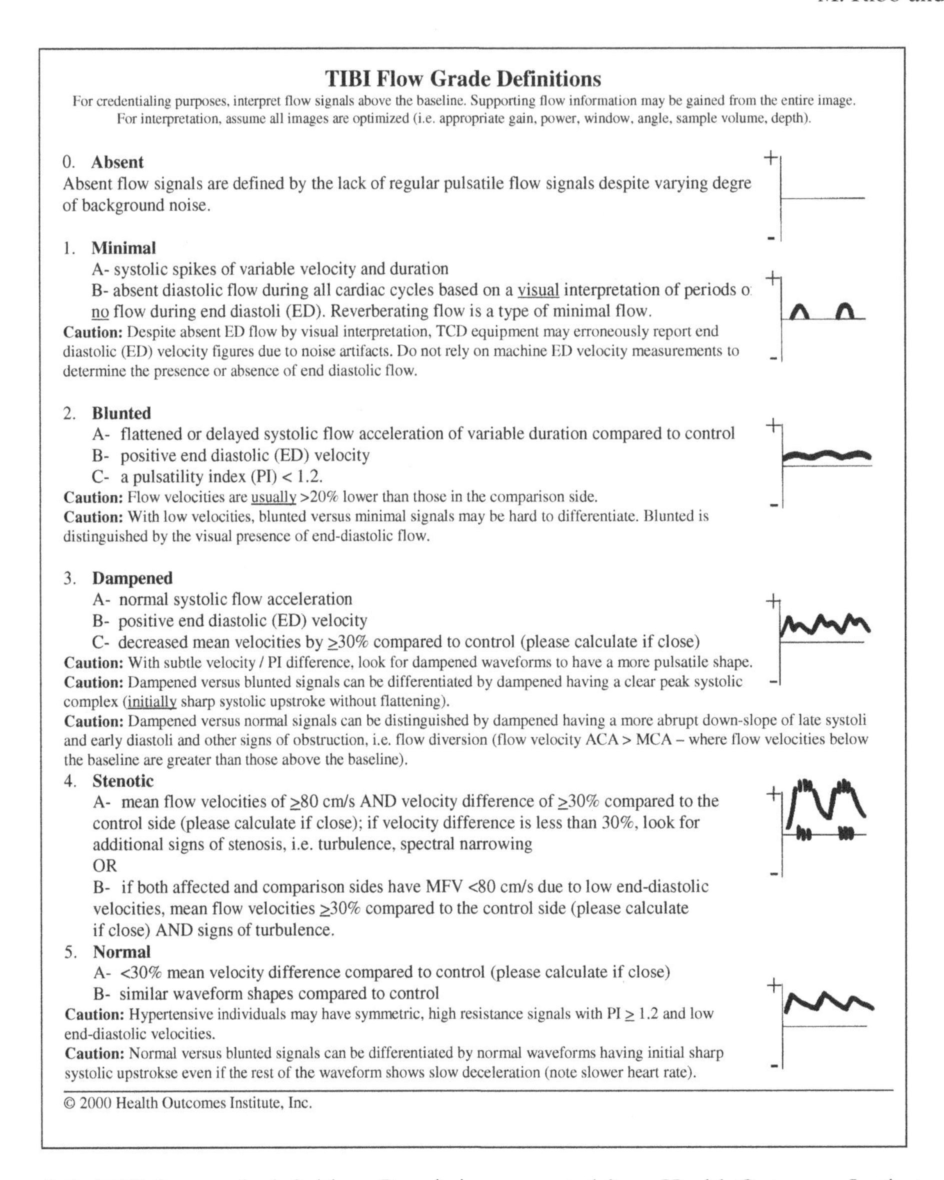

TIBI Flow Grade Definitions

For credentialing purposes, interpret flow signals above the baseline. Supporting flow information may be gained from the entire image. For interpretation, assume all images are optimized (i.e. appropriate gain, power, window, angle, sample volume, depth).

0. **Absent**
Absent flow signals are defined by the lack of regular pulsatile flow signals despite varying degre of background noise.

1. **Minimal**
A- systolic spikes of variable velocity and duration
B- absent diastolic flow during all cardiac cycles based on a visual interpretation of periods o no flow during end diastoli (ED). Reverberating flow is a type of minimal flow.
Caution: Despite absent ED flow by visual interpretation, TCD equipment may erroneously report end diastolic (ED) velocity figures due to noise artifacts. Do not rely on machine ED velocity measurements to determine the presence or absence of end diastolic flow.

2. **Blunted**
A- flattened or delayed systolic flow acceleration of variable duration compared to control
B- positive end diastolic (ED) velocity
C- a pulsatility index (PI) < 1.2.
Caution: Flow velocities are usually >20% lower than those in the comparison side.
Caution: With low velocities, blunted versus minimal signals may be hard to differentiate. Blunted is distinguished by the visual presence of end-diastolic flow.

3. **Dampened**
A- normal systolic flow acceleration
B- positive end diastolic (ED) velocity
C- decreased mean velocities by ≥30% compared to control (please calculate if close)
Caution: With subtle velocity / PI difference, look for dampened waveforms to have a more pulsatile shape.
Caution: Dampened versus blunted signals can be differentiated by dampened having a clear peak systolic complex (initially sharp systolic upstroke without flattening).
Caution: Dampened versus normal signals can be distinguished by dampened having a more abrupt down-slope of late systoli and early diastoli and other signs of obstruction, i.e. flow diversion (flow velocity ACA > MCA – where flow velocities below the baseline are greater than those above the baseline).

4. **Stenotic**
A- mean flow velocities of ≥80 cm/s AND velocity difference of ≥30% compared to the control side (please calculate if close); if velocity difference is less than 30%, look for additional signs of stenosis, i.e. turbulence, spectral narrowing
OR
B- if both affected and comparison sides have MFV <80 cm/s due to low end-diastolic velocities, mean flow velocities ≥30% compared to the control side (please calculate if close) AND signs of turbulence.

5. **Normal**
A- <30% mean velocity difference compared to control (please calculate if close)
B- similar waveform shapes compared to control
Caution: Hypertensive individuals may have symmetric, high resistance signals with PI ≥ 1.2 and low end-diastolic velocities.
Caution: Normal versus blunted signals can be differentiated by normal waveforms having initial sharp systolic upstrokse even if the rest of the waveform shows slow deceleration (note slower heart rate).

FIGURE 6–9. TIBI flow grade definitions. Permission requested from Health Outcomes Institute, Inc.

supply at the level of the Circle of Willis and major proximal branches[66,67] as described above. Information about the perfusion status of the affected brain tissue may help optimize and individualize patient management. For example, in the setting of an acute vertebrobasilar occlusion, identification of the reversed basilar artery flow indicates good collaterals through the posterior communicating arteries, associated with favorable outcomes.[49] In the last year, the development of new software for TCCD able to detect perfusion defects after echocontrast administration is very promising.[50] Finally information obtained from an acute neurovascular ultrasound examination has shown significant potential as a screening tool for intravenous/intraarterial lysis protocols.[62]

Monitoring Thrombolytic Therapy with Ultrasound

Once the arterial occlusion is located, the ultrasound probe can be fixated with a head frame allowing monitoring of the blood flow in the affected artery during t-PA infusion. The first noticeable improvement of flow to the brain occurs at a median time of 17 min after t-PA bolus. Median time to completion of recanalization is 35 min after bolus,[68] and those patients who complete recanalization before the end of 1 h t-PA infusion are 3.5 times more likely to achieve favorable outcome at 3 months. An average rate of spontaneous complete recanalization of the MCA occlusion appears to be about 6% per hour during the first 6 h after symptom onset.[69–71]

Systemic t-PA increases the complete recanalization rate to 12.7%/h. Early complete recanalization is closely associated with dramatic clinical recovery.[72]

However, one-third of early complete recanalizations do not result in immediate clinical improvement. Despite this, one-third of patients with silent recanalizations recover completely at 3 months, indicating the existence of a stunned brain syndrome.[73]

Continuous TCD monitoring of the affected artery shows persistence of the occlusion, thrombus migration, partial or complete recanalization, and reocclusion. Also, visualization of microembolic signals during thrombolysis may indicate thrombus degradation or imminent recanalization. After recanalization, early arterial reocclusion affects up to 25% of t-PA-treated patients, more commonly those with partial or incomplete initial recanalization. Arterial reocclusion accounts for two-thirds of patients who experience deterioration following improvement with t-PA therapy.[74] TCD demonstration of frequent arterial reocclusion with intravenous t-PA has fostered interest in combination therapies, i.e., a thrombolytic drug with anticoagulants, GP IIb IIIa antagonists, or a direct thrombin inhibitor.[75–77]

Ultrasound Enhanced Thrombolysis

In the past 30 years numerous scientists showed in experimental models that ultrasound facilitates the activity of fibrinolytic agents within minutes of its exposure to thrombus and blood-containing drugs.[78–84] The mechanisms of ultrasound-enhanced thrombolysis include improved drug transport, reversible alteration of fibrin structure, and increased t-PA binding to fibrin[78–86] for frequencies ranging from kHz to those used in diagnostic ultrasound.[83,84] Although kHz frequencies penetrate better with less heating, a combination of t-PA with an experimental kHz delivery system resulted in excessive risk of intracerebral hemorrhage (ICH) in stroke patients.[87–89] We used diagnostic 2 MHz transcranial Doppler to evaluate acute stroke patients and reported an unexpectedly high rate of complete recanalization and dramatic clinical recovery when t-PA infusion was continuously monitored with TCD for diagnostic purposes. The CLOTBUST trial (Combined Lysis of Thrombus in Brain ischemia using transcranial Ultrasound and Systemic t-PA) was a phase II multicenter randomized clinical trial (Houston, Barcelona, Edmonton, Calgary).[90] The CLOTBUST trial demonstrated that in stroke patients treated with intravenous t-PA, continuous TCD monitoring of intracranial occlusion safely augments t-PA-induced arterial recanalization (38% vs. 13% of sustained complete MCA recanalization at 2 h after TPA bolus). This early boost in recanalization resulted in a trend toward clinical recovery at 3 months (42% vs. 29%), the subject of a properly powered phase III trial. TCD has a positive biological activity that aids systemic thrombolytic therapy in patients with acute ischemic stroke. The phase II CLOTBUST trial provides clinical evidence for the existence of ultrasound-enhanced thrombolysis in humans that can amplify the existing therapy for ischemic stroke. Early brain perfusion augmentation, complete recanalization, and dramatic clinical recovery are feasible goals for ultrasound-enhanced thrombolysis. A further increase of this effect is being tested with eco-contrast agents that seem to multiply the energy delivered to the clot by ultrasound and by enhancing the lytic effects.[91]

Other Clinical Applications

There are several established clinical applications of TCD that were recently evaluated by an international group of experts (Table 6–4).[92,93] TCD provides a bedside tool for detection of intracranial stenosis, occlusion, collateral channels, and microembolic activity,[49] including testing for the right-to-left shunts, like patent foramen ovale or pulmonary fistulas.[95]

TCD has a pivotal role in predicting the risk of ischemic stroke in children with sickle cell disease. In a prospective study by Adams *et al.*, mean velocities greater than 170–200 cm/s were associated with a 44% increase in relative risk of ischemic stroke over 5 years.[12,96–98] A subsequent randomized trial showed a 90% relative stroke risk reduction when blood transfusion was administered in children with TCD findings of MFV ≥ 200 cm/s.[99]

TCD has an established role in detecting and monitoring arterial vasospasm in patients with SAH.[20,46–48] TCD helps to decide when to start, enforce, and continue HHH therapy, when to perform DSA with angioplasty and papaverine to combat severe vasospasm, and when to transfer patients from the intensive care unit after vasospasm has subsided.[46,48]

TCD offers a quick bedside test to detect markedly elevated ICP, thus providing an opportunity for decompression or hyperventilation to be performed before clinical deterioration.[57,58] TCD also allows detection of a combination of vasospasm and hydrocephalus as well as progression of ICP to cerebral circulatory arrest.

The capacity of TCD to monitor both brain perfusion and embolization in real time has led to numerous applications of TCD during surgical and interventional procedures. Stump *et al.* showed that 58% of microembolic signals during cardiopulmonary bypass are associated with surgical maneuvers or time intervals while the cumulative embolic count was predictive of postoperative neuropsychological deficit.[100] Spencer reported that when surgeons responded to TCD information during CEA monitoring, the incidence of permanent deficits

TABLE 6–4. Accuracy of TCD ultrasonography by indication.[a]

Indication	Sensitivity, %	Specificity, %	Reference standard	Evidence/class
Sickle cell disease	86	91	Conventional angiography	A/I
Right-to-left cardiac shunts	70–100	≥95	Transesophageal echocardiography	A/II
Intracranial stenoocclusive disease			Conventional angiography	
Anterior circulation	70–90	90–95		B/II–III
Posterior circulation	50–80	80–96		B/III
Occlusion				
MCA	85–95	90–98		B/III
ICA, VA, BA	55–81	96		B/III
Extracranial ICA stenosis			Conventional angiography	
Single TCD variable	3–78	60–100		C/II–III
TCD battery	49–95	42–100		C/II–III
TCD battery + carotid duplex	89	100		C/II–III
Vasomotor reactivity testing				
≥70% extracranial ICA stenosis/occlusion			Conventional angiography, clinical outcomes	B/II–III
Carotid endarterectomy			EEG, MRI, clinical outcomes	B/II
Cerebral microembolization			Experimental model, pathology, MRI, neuropsychological tests	
General				B/II–IV
Coronary artery bypass graft surgery microembolization				B/II–III
Prosthetic heart valves				C/III
Cerebral thrombolysis			Conventional angiography, MR angiography, clinical outcome	B/II–III
Complete occlusion	50	100		
Partial occlusion	100	76		
Recanalization	91	93		
Vasospasm after spontaneous subarachnoid hemorrhage			Conventional angiography	I–II
Intracranial ICA	25–30	83–91		
MCA	39–94	70–100		
ACA	13–71	65–100		
VA	44–100	82–88		
BA	77–100	42–79		
PCA	48–60	78–87		
Vasospasm after traumatic subarachnoid hemorrhage			Conventional angiography	I–III
Cerebral circulatory arrest and brain death	91–100	97–100	Conventional angiography, EEG, clinical outcome	II

[a]Permission requested from the Therapeutics and Technology Assessment Subcommittee of the American Academy of Neurology (Neurology 2004;62:1468–1481).
[b]TCD, transcranial Doppler; MCA, middle cerebral artery; ICA, internal carotid artery; VA, vertebral artery; BA, basilar artery; ACA, anterior cerebral artery; PCA, posterior cerebral artery.

decreased from 7% to 2% for 500 operations.[101] As shown by TCD, cerebral embolization was present in 54%, hypoperfusion in 29%, and combined embolism plus hypoperfusion in 17% of these complications.[100] During CEA TCD can provide useful information.[100] It can show microembolization during skin preparation suggesting fragile plaque structure. If MCA MFV does not recover from <30% of precrossclamping values, a shunt may be needed. TCD detection of flow changes through ECA collaterals can help avoid embolization/hypoperfusion with ECA manipulations. An MCA MFV drop during plaque removal indicates a drop in BP or a kink in a shunt. TCD shows microembolism during release of carotid crossclamps. Finally, a prolonged >30s MCA MFV increase to greater than 1.5 times precrossclamp values after the CEA indicates hyperperfusion syndrome, which can be treated with TCD monitoring.[94,101]

Conclusions

Transcranial Doppler is a portable and inexpensive tool that is widely used. However, TCD requires intense and in-depth training as well as experience in both performing the test and interpreting the results. The absence of temporal windows is present in 5–15% of all patients when the ultrasound beam cannot penetrate the skull.[1,3] Due to these limitations and the failure to change the management plan in patients screened for carotid artery disease, Comerota *et al.* advised not incorporating TCD as part of the routine noninvasive cerebrovascular examination.[102,103] However, the technology has improved rapidly. The contrast agents, such as stabilized gaseous microbubbles, overcome the absent windows.[97] Detection of multigated bilateral emboli and compatibility of TCD with other monitoring modalities are realities. Very portable and sensitive units are available to serve as a "neurological stethoscope" to the brain vasculature at the bedside. At the same time, clinicians need to identify the best responders for acute stroke therapies, patients at high risk of stroke with asymptomatic and moderate carotid stenoses, and decide on surgical procedure selection (i.e., CABG+CEA) and stenting. A neurovascular ultrasound examination that combines urgent bedside carotid duplex and TCD is becoming a valuable source of diagnostic information in acute stroke patients, helping in decision making [61] and even enhancing the effects of fibrinolytic drugs.[90]

References

1. Aaslid R, Markwalder TM, Nornes H. Noninvasive transcranial Doppler ultrasound recording of flow velocity in basal cerebral arteries. J Neurosurg 1982;57:769–774.
2. Moehring MA, Spencer MP. Power M-mode transcranial Doppler ultrasound and simultaneous single gate spectrogram. Ultrasound Med Biol 2002;28:49–57.
3. Otis SM, Ringelstein EB. The transcranial Doppler examination: Principles and applications of transcranial Doppler sonography. In: Tegeler CH, Babikian VL, Gomez CR (eds). *Neurosonology*, pp. 140–155. St. Louis: Mosby, 1996.
4. Postert T, Braun B, Meves S, Koster O, Przuntek H, Weber S, Buttner T. Contrast-enhanced transcranial color-coded sonography in acute hemispheric brain infarction. Stroke 1999;30:1819–1826.
5. Bartels E, Flugel KA. Quantitative measurements of blood flow velocity in basal cerebral arteries with transcranial duplex colorflow imaging. A comparative study with conventional transcranial Doppler sonography. J Neuroimag 1994;4:77–81.
6. Gerriets T, Seidel G, Fiss I, Modrau B, Kaps M. Contrast enhanced transcranial color-coded duplex sonography: Efficiency and validity. Neurology 1999;52:1133–1137.
7. Hennerici MMS. *Cerebrovascular Ultrasound: Theory, Practice and Future Developments.* Cambridge: Cambridge University Press, 2001.
8. Gerriets T, Stolz E, Modrau B, Fiss I, Seidel G, Kaps M. Sonographic monitoring of midline shift in hemispheric infarctions. Neurology 1999;52:45–49.
9. Kontos HA. Validity of cerebral arterial blood flow calculations from velocity measurements. Stroke 1989;20: 1–3.
10. Giller CA, Bowman G, Dyer H, Mootz L, Krippner W. Cerebral arterial diameters during changes in blood pressure and carbon dioxide during craniotomy. Neurosurgery 1993;32:737–742.
11. Aaslid R, Lindegaard KF, Sorteberg W, Nornes H. Cerebral autoregulation dynamics in humans. Stroke 1989;20: 45.
12. Adams RJ, McKie V, Nichols F, *et al.* The use of transcranial ultrasonography to predict stroke in sickle cell disease. N Engl J Med 1992;326:605–610.
13. Babikian V, Sloan MA, Tegeler CH, DeWitt LD, Fayad PB, Feldmann E, Gomez CR. Transcranial Doppler validation pilot study. J Neuroimag 1993;3:242–249.
14. Bragoni M, Feldmann E. Transcranial Doppler indicies of intracranial hemodynamics. In: Tegeler CH, Babikian VL, Gomez CR (eds). *Neurosonology*, pp. 129–139. St. Louis: Mosby, 1996.
15. Lindegaard KF, Gromilund P, Aaslid R, *et al.* Evaluation of cerebral AVMs using transcranial Doppler ultrasound. J Neurosurg 1986;65:335–344.
16. Lindegaard KF, Bakke SJ, Gromilund P, *et al.* Assessment of intracranial hemodynamics in carotid artery disease by transcranial Doppler ultrasound. J Neurosurg 1985;63: 890–898.
17. Wilterdink JL, *et al.* Transcranial Doppler ultrasound battery reliably identifies severe internal carotid artery stenosis. Stroke 1997;28:133–136.
18. Kelley RE, *et al.* Transcranial Doppler ultrasonography of the middle cerebral artery in the hemodynamic assessment of internal carotid artery stenosis. Arch Neurol 1990;49:960–964.
19. Canthelmo NL, *et al.* Correlation of transcranial Doppler and noninvasive tests with angiography in the evaluation of extracranial carotid disease. J Vasc Surg 1990;11: 786–792.
20. Lindegaard KF, Nornes H, Bakke SJ, *et al.* Cerebral vasospasm diagnosis by means of angiography and blood velocity measurements. Acta Neurochir (Wien) 1987;100: 12–24.
21. Hennerici M, Neuerburg-Heusler D. *Vascular Diagnosis with Ultrasound: Clinical References with Case Studies*, p. 96. Stuttgart: Thieme, 1998.
22. North American Symptomatic Carotid Endarterectomy Trial Collaborators. Beneficial effect of carotid endarterectomy in symptomatic patients with high grade carotid stenosis. N Engl J Med 1991;325:445–453.
23. European Carotid Surgery Trialists' Collaborative Group. MRC European carotid surgery trial: Interim results for symptomatic patients with severe (70–99%) stenosis and with mild (0–29%) stenosis. Lancet 1991;337:1235–1244.
24. Executive Committee for the Asymptomatic Carotid Atherosclerosis Study. Endarterectomy for asymptomatic carotic artery stenosis. JAMA 1995;273:1421–1428.
25. Fischer M. Carotid plaque morphology in symptomatic and asymptomatic patients. In: Caplan LR, Shifrin EG, Nicolaides AN, Moore WS (eds). *Cerebrovascular Ischemia: Investigation and Management*, pp. 19–24. London: Med-Orion, 1996.
26. Thomas DJ. The Asymptomatic Carotid Surgery Trial: a neurologist's view. In: Caplan LR, Shifrin EG, Nicolaides

AN, Moore WS (eds). *Cerebrovascular Ischemia: Investigation and Management*, pp. 411–421. London: Med-Orion, 1996.
27. Bornstein NM, Gur AY, Shifrin EG, Morag BA. The value of a combined transcranial Doppler and Diamox test in assessing intracerebral hemodynamics. In: Caplan LR, Shifrin EG, Nicolaides AN, Moore WS (eds). *Cerebrovascular Ischemia: Investigation and Management*, pp. 143–148. London: Med-Orion, 1996.
28. Bishop CCR, Insall M, Powell S, Rutt D, Browse NL. Effect of internal carotid artery occlusion on middle cerebral artery blood flow at rest and in response to hypercapnia. Lancet 1986;29:710.
29. Silvestrini M, Vernieri F, Pasqualetti P, Matteis M, Passarelli F, Troisi E, Caltagirone C. Impaired cerebral vasoreactivity and risk of stroke in patients with asymptomatic carotid artery stenosis. JAMA 2000;283:2122–2127.
30. Ringelstein EB. CO_2-reactivity: dependence from collateral circulation and significance in symptomatic and asymptomatic patients. In: Caplan LR, Shifrin EG, Nicolaides AN, Moore WS (eds). *Cerebrovascular Ischemia: Investigation and Management*, pp. 149–154. London: Med-Orion, 1996.
31. Babikian VL, Schwarze JJ. Cerebral blood flow and cerebral physiology. In: Tegeler CH, Babikian VL, Gomez CR (eds). *Neurosonology*, pp. 140–155. St. Louis: Mosby, 1996.
32. Markus HS, Harrson MJG. Estimation of cerebrovascular reactivity using transcranial Doppler, including the use of breath-holding as the vasodilatory stimulus. Stroke 1992;23:668–673.
33. Silvestrini M, Troisi E, Matteis M, Cupini LM, Caltagirone C. Transcranial Doppler assessment of cerebrovascular reactivity in symptomatic and asymptomatic carotid stenosis. Stroke 1996;27:1970–1973.
34. Kleiser B, Scholl D, Widder B. Assessment of cerebrovascular reactivity by Doppler CO_2 and Diamox testing: Which is the appropriate method? Cerebrovasc Dis 1994;4:134.
35. Burt RW, Witt RM, Cikrit DF, Carter J. Increased retention of HMPAO following acetazolamide administration. Clin Nucl Med 1991;16:568.
36. Hojer-Pedersen E. Effect of acetazolamide on cerebral blood flow in subacute and chronic cerebrovascular disease. Stroke 1987;18:887.
37. Dahl A, Lindegaard KF, Russel D, Nyberg-Hansen, Rootwelt K, Sorteberg W, Nornes H. A comparison of transcranial Doppler and cerebral blood flow studies to assess cerebrovascular reactivity. Stroke 1992;23:15.
38. Dahl A, Russel D, Nyberg-Hansen R, Rootwelt K, Bakke SJ. Cerebral vasoreactivity in unilateral carotid artery disease. Stroke 1994;25:621.
39. De Chiara S, *et al.* Cerebrovascular reactivity by transcranial Doppler ultrasonography in insulin-dependent diabetic patients. Cerebrovasc Dis 1993;3:11:111–115.
40. Sugimori H, *et al.* Cerebral hemodynamics in hypertensive patients compared with normotensive volunteers. Stroke 1994;25:1384–1389.
41. Rubba P, *et al.* Cerebral blood flow velocity and systemic vascular resistance after acute reduction of low-density lipoprotein in familial hypercholesterolemia. Stroke 1993;24:1154–1161.
42. Kleiser B, Widder B. Course of carotid artery occlusions with impaired cerebrovascular reactivity. Stroke 1992;23:171–174.
43. Shinoda J, *et al.* Acetazolamide reactivity on cerebral blood flow in patients with subarachnoid hemorrhage. Acta Neurochir (Wien) 1991;109:102–108.
44. Hassler W, Chioffi F. CO_2 reactivity of cerebral vasospasm after aneurysmal subarachnoid hemorrhage. Acta Neurochir (Wien) 1989;98:167–175.
45. Seiler RW, Nirkko A. Effect of nimodipine on cerebrovascular response to CO_2 in asymptomatic individuals and patients with subarachnoid hemorrhage: A transcranial Doppler ultrasound study. Neurosurgery 1990;27:247–251.
46. Sloan MA. Transcranial Doppler monitoring of vasospasm after subarachnoid hemorrhage. In: Tegeler CH, Babikian VL, Gomez CR (eds). *Neurosonology*, pp. 156–171. St. Louis: Mosby, 1996.
47. Newell DW, *et al.* Distribution of angiographic vasospasm after subarachnoid hemorrhage: Implications for diagnosis by TCD. Neurosurgery 1990;27:574–577.
48. Piepgras A, *et al.* Reliable prediction of grade of angiographic vasospasm by transcranial Doppler sonography. Stroke 1994;25:260.
49. Ribo M, Garami Z, Uchino K, Song J, Molina CA, Alexandrov AV. Detection of reversed basilar flow with power-motion doppler after acute occlusion predicts favorable outcome. Stroke 2004;35:79–82.
50. Wiesmann M, Meyer K, Albers T, Seidel G. Parametric perfusion imaging with contrast-enhanced ultrasound in acute ischemic stroke. Stroke 2004;35:508–513.
51. Markus H. Doppler embolus detection: stroke treatment and prevention. In: Tegeler CH, Babikian VL, Gomez CR (eds). *Neurosonology*, pp. 239–251. St. Louis: Mosby, 1996.
52. Russell D, Brucher R. Online automatic discrimination between solid and gaseous cerebral microemboli with the first multifrequency transcranial doppler. Stroke 2002;33:1975–1980.
53. The International Cerebral Hemodynamics Society Consensus Statement. Stroke 1995;26:1123.
54. Ringlestein EB, *et al.* Consensus on microembolus detection by TCD. Stroke 1998;29:725–729.
55. Mackinnon AD, Aaslid R, Markus HS. Long-term ambulatory monitoring for cerebral emboli using transcranial Doppler ultrasound. Stroke 2004;35:73–78
56. Marti-Fabregas J, Belvis R, Guardia E, Cocho D, Marti-Vilalta JL. Relationship between transcranial Doppler and CT data in acute intracerebral hemorrhage. AJNR Am J Neuroradiol 2005;26:113–118.
57. Hennerici M, Neuerburg-Heusler D. *Vascular Diagnosis with Ultrasound: Clinical References with Case Studies*, p. 120. Stuttgart: Thieme, 1998.
58. Newell D. Trauma and brain death. In: Tegeler CH, Babikian VL, Gomez CR (eds). *Neurosonology*, pp. 189–199. St. Louis: Mosby, 1996.
59. Ducrocq X, Braun M, Debouverie M, Junges C, Hummer M, Vespignani H. Brain death and transcranial doppler:

Experience in 130 cases of brain dead patients. J Neurol Sci 1998;160:41–46.
60. Toole JF. *Cerebrovascular Disorders*, 4th ed., pp. 199–123. New York: Raven Press, 1990.
61. Chernyshev OY, Garami Z, Calleja S, Song J, Campbell MS, Noser EA, Shaltoni H, Chen CI, Iguchi Y, Grotta JC, Alexandrov AV. Yield and accuracy of urgent combined carotid/transcranial ultrasound testing in acute cerebral ischemia. Stroke 2005;36:32–37.
62. Saqqur M, Shuaib A, Alexandrov AV, Hill MD, Calleja S, Tomsick T, Broderick J, Demchuk AM. Derivation of transcranial Doppler criteria for rescue intra-arterial thrombolysis. Multicenter experience from the interventional management of stroke study. Stroke 2005;36: 865.
63. Demchuk AM, Burgin WS, Christou I, Felberg RA, Barber PA, Hill MD, Alexandrov AV. Thrombolysis in brain ischemia (TIBI) transcranial Doppler flow grades predict clinical severity, early recovery, and mortality in patients treated with intravenous tissue plasminogen activator. Stroke 2001;32:89–93.
64. Wiesmann M, Meyer K, Albers T, Seidel G. Parametric perfusion imaging with contrast-enhanced ultrasound in acute ischemic stroke. Stroke 2004;35:508–513.
65. Wilterdink JL, Feldmann E, Furie KL, Bragoni M, Benavides JG. Transcranial Doppler ultrasound battery reliably identifies severe internal carotid artery stenosis. Stroke 1997;28:133–136.
66. Christou I, Felberg RA, Demchuk AM, Grotta JC, Burgin WS, Malkoff M, Alexandrov AV. A broad diagnostic battery for bedside transcranial Doppler to detect flow changes with internal carotid artery stenosis or occlusion. J Neuroimag 2001;11:236–242.
67. von Reutern GM. *Ultrasound Diagnosis of Cerebrovascular Disease: Doppler Sonography of the Extra- and Intracranial Arteries Duplex Scanning.* Stuttgart: Thieme, 1993.
68. Alexandrov AV, Burgin WS, Demchuk AM, El-Mitwalli A, Grotta JC. Speed of intracranial clot lysis with intravenous tissue plasminogen activator therapy: Sonographic classification and short-term improvement. Circulation 2001; 103:2897–2902.
69. Molina CA, Montaner J, Abilleira S, Ibarra B, Romero F, Arenilla JF, Alvarez-Sabin J. Timing of spontaneous recanalization and risk of hemorrhagic transformation in acute cardioembolic stroke. Stroke 2001;32:1079–1084.
70. Furlan A, Higashida R, Wechsler L, Gent M, Rowley H, Kase C, Pessin M, Ahuja A, Callahan F, Clark WM, Silver F, Rivera F. Intra-arterial prourokinase for acute ischemic stroke. The proact II study: A randomized controlled trial. Prolyse in acute cerebral thromboembolism. JAMA 1999;282:2003–2011.
71. Uchino KMC, Saqqur M, Demchuk AM, Felberg RA, Calleja S, Wojner AW, Alexandrov AV. Likelihood of early arterial recanalization with intravenous tpa and its predictors: A multicenter transcranial doppler study. Stroke 2003;34:347(abstract).
72. Molina CA RM, Rubiera M, Montaner J, Arenillas JF, Santamarina E, Alvarez-Sabin J. Predictors of early arterial reocclusion after tpa-induced recanalization. Stroke 2004;35:250(abstract).
73. Alexandrov AV, Hall CE, Labiche LA, Wojner AW, Grotta JC. Ischemic stunning of the brain: Early recanalization without immediate clinical improvement in acute ischemic stroke. Stroke 2004;35:449–452.
74. Alexandrov AV, Grotta JC. Arterial reocclusion in stroke patients treated with intravenous tissue plasminogen activator. Neurology 2002;59:862–867.
75. Schmulling S, Rudolf J, Strotmann-Tack T, Grond M, Schneweis S, Sobesky J, Thiel A, Heiss WD. Acetylsalicylic acid pretreatment, concomitant heparin therapy and the risk of early intracranial hemorrhage following systemic thrombolysis for acute ischemic stroke. Cerebrovasc Dis 2003;16:183–190.
76. Straub S, Junghans U, Jovanovic V, Wittsack HJ, Seitz RJ, Siebler M. Systemic thrombolysis with recombinant tissue plasminogen activator and tirofiban in acute middle cerebral artery occlusion. Stroke 2004;35:705–709.
77. Sugg R, Pary JK, Uchino K, Shaltoni HM, Gonzales NR, Alexandrov AV, Ford SR, Shaw SG, Mathern DE, Grotta JC. Tpa argatroban stroke study (tarts). International Stroke Conference 2005 (abstract).
78. Trubestein G, Engel C, Etzel F, Sobbe A, Cremer H, Stumpff U. Thrombolysis by ultrasound. Clin Sci Mol Med Suppl 1976;3:697s–698s.
79. Lauer CG, Burge R, Tang DB, Bass BG, Gomez ER, Alving BM. Effect of ultrasound on tissue-type plasminogen activator-induced thrombolysis. Circulation 1992;86(4):1257–1264.
80. Blinc A, Francis CW, Trudnowski JL, Carstensen EL. Characterization of ultrasound-potentiated fibrinolysis *in vitro*. Blood 1993;81(10):2636–2643.
81. Kimura M, Iijima S, Kobayashi K, Furuhata H. Evaluation of the thrombolytic effect of tissue-type plasminogen activator with ultrasonic irradiation: *In vitro* experiment involving assay of the fibrin degradation products from the clot. Biol Pharm Bull 1994;17(1):126–130.
82. Akiyama M, Ishibashi T, Yamada T, Furuhata H. Low-frequency ultrasound penetrates the cranium and enhances thrombolysis *in vitro*. Neurosurgery 1998;43(4): 828–832; discussion 832–833.
83. Suchkova V, Siddiqi FN, Carstensen EL, Dalecki D, Child S, Francis CW. Enhancement of fibrinolysis with 40-kHz ultrasound. Circulation 1998;98(10):1030–1035.
84. Behrens S, Daffertshofer M, Spiegel D, Hennerici M. Low-frequency, low-intensity ultrasound accelerates thrombolysis through the skull. Ultrasound Med Biol 1999;25(2):269–273.
85. Behrens S, Spengos K, Daffertshofer M, Schroeck H, Dempfle CE, Hennerici M. Transcranial ultrasound-improved thrombolysis: Diagnostic vs. therapeutic ultrasound. Ultrasound Med Biol 2001;27(12):1683–1689.
86. Spengos K, Behrens S, Daffertshofer M, Dempfle CE, Hennerici M. Acceleration of thrombolysis with ultrasound through the cranium in a flow model. Ultrasound Med Biol 2000;26(5):889–895.
87. Daffertshofer M, Hennerici M. Ultrasound in the treatment of ischaemic stroke. Lancet Neurol 2003;2(5): 283–290.

88. Alexandrov AV, Demchuk AM, Burgin WS, Robinson DJ, Grotta JC. Ultrasound-enhanced thrombolysis for acute ischemic stroke: Phase I. Findings of the CLOTBUST trial. J Neuroimag 2004;14(2):113–117.
89. Alexandrov AV, Wojner AW, Grotta JC. CLOTBUST: Design of a randomized trial of ultrasound-enhanced thrombolysis for acute ischemic stroke. J Neuroimag 2004;14(2):108–112.
90. Alexandrov AM, Grotta JC, Ford SR, Garami Z, Montaner J, Alvarez-Sabin J, Saqqur M, Demchuk AM, Chernyshev OY, Moye LA, Hill MD, Wojner AW, for the CLOTBUST Investigators. A multi-center randomized trial of ultrasound-enhanced systemic thrombolysis for acute ischemic stroke. N Engl J Med 2004;351:2170–2178.
91. Cintas P, Nguyen F, Boneu B, Larrue V. Enhancement of enzymatic fibrinolysis with 2-MHz ultrasound and microbubbles. J Thromb Haemost 2004;2(7):1163–1166.
92. Babikian VL, Feldmann E, Wechsler LR, Newell DW, Gomez CR, Bogdahn U, Caplan LR, Spencer MP, Tegeler CH, Ringelstein EB, Alexandrov AV. Transcranial Doppler ultrasonography: 1997 update. Neurology 1998;50(Suppl. 4).
93. Sloan MA, Alexandrov AV, Tegeler CH, Spencer MP, Caplan LR, Feldmann E, Wechsler LR, Newell DW, Gomez CR, Babikian VL, Lefkowitz D, Goldman RS, Armon C, Hsu CY, Goodin DS. Assessment: Transcranial Doppler ultrasonography: Report of the therapeutics and technology assessment subcommittee of the American Academy of Neurology. Neurology 2004;62: 1468–1481.
94. Alexandrov AV, Babikian VL, Adams RJ, Tegeler CH, Caplan LR, Spencer MP. The evolving role of transcranial Doppler in stroke prevention and treatment. J Stroke Cerebrovasc Dis 1998;7:101–104.
95. Jauss M, Zanette E. Detection of right-to-left shunt with ultrasound contrast agent and transcranial Doppler sonography. Cerebrovasc Dis 2000;10:490–496.
96. Bendixen BH, Adams HP, Leira EC, Change KC, Hanson MD, Woolson RF, Clarke WR. Responses to treatment with a low molecular weight heparinoid or placebo among persons with acute ischemic stroke secondary to large atherosclerosis. Neurology 1998;50:A345 (abstract).
97. Nabavi DG, Droste DW, Kemeny V, Schulte-Altendorneburg G, Weber S, Ringelstein EB. Potential and limitations of echocontrast-enhanced ultrasonography in acute stroke patients: A pilot study. Stroke 1998;29;949–954.
98. Adams RJ, McKie VC, Carl EM, *et al.* Long-term stroke risk in children with sickle cell disease screened with transcranial Doppler. Ann Neurol 1997;42:699–704.
99. The STOP Trial. NIH Alert. October, 1997.
100. Stump DA, Newman SP. Embolus detection during cardiopulmonary bypass. In: Tegeler CH, Babikian VL, Gomez CR (eds). *Neurosonology*, pp. 252–255. St. Louis: Mosby, 1996.
101. Spencer MP. Transcranial Doppler monitoring and causes of stroke from carotid endarterectomy. Stroke 1997; 28:685–691.
102. Comerota AJ, Katz ML, Hosking JD, Hashemi HA, Kerr RP, Carter AP. Is transcranial Doppler a worthwhile addition to screening tests for cerebrovascular disease? J Vasc Surg 1995;21:90–97.
103. Ries F. Echocontrast agents in transcranial Doppler sonography. In: Tegeler CH, Babikian VL, Gomez CR (eds). *Neurosonology*, pp. 221–228. St. Louis: Mosby, 1996.

7 Ultrasonic Characterization of Carotid Plaques

Andrew N. Nicolaides, Maura Griffin, Stavros K. Kakkos, George Geroulakos, Efthyvoulos Kyriacou, and Niki Georgiou

Introduction

The multidisciplinary approach combining angiography, high-resolution ultrasound, thrombolytic therapy, plaque pathology, histochemistry, coagulation studies, and more recently molecular biology has led to the realization that carotid plaque rupture is a key mechanism underlying the development of cerebrovascular events.[1–3]

Plaques with a large extracellular lipid-rich core, thin fibrous cap, reduced smooth muscle density, and increased numbers of activated macrophages and mast cells appear to be most vulnerable to rupture.[3,4] Fibrous caps may rupture because of reduced collagen synthesis as well as increased matrix degradation or in response to extrinsic mechanical or hemodynamic stresses.[5] Plaques at the carotid bifurcation coincide with points at which stresses produced by biomechanical and hemodynamic forces are maximal.[6]

Histological studies on the vascular biology of symptomatic and asymptomatic carotid plaques have recently been reviewed by Golledge *et al.*[7] They showed that the features of unstable plaques removed from symptomatic patients were surface ulceration and plaque rupture (48% of symptomatic versus 31% of asymptomatic, $p < 0.001$), thinning of the fibrous cap, and infiltration of the cap by a greater number of macrophages and T-lymphocytes.

The identification of unstable plaques *in vivo* and subsequent plaque stabilization may prove to be an important modality for a reduction in the lethal consequences of atherosclerosis.[8,9] This putative concept of plaque stabilization, although attractive, has not yet been rigorously validated in humans. Indirect data from clinical trials involving lipid lowering/modification and lifestyle/risk factor modification provide strong support for this new approach.[10]

Conventional angiography has been used for several decades to investigate the presence and severity of internal carotid artery stenosis, but its invasive nature means that it cannot be repeated frequently and carries a risk of stroke of 1.2%. In addition, angiography provides little information on plaque structure. In contrast, high-resolution ultrasound has enabled us to study the presence, rate of progression or regression of plaques, and most importantly their consistency.

Ultrasonic characteristics of unstable (vulnerable) plaques have been determined[11–13] and populations or individuals at increased risk for cardiovascular events can now be identified.[14] In addition, high-resolution ultrasound has enabled us to identify the different ultrasonic characteristics of unstable carotid plaques associated with amaurosis fugax, transient ischemic attacks (TIAs), stroke, and different patterns of computed tomography (CT) brain infarction.[12,13] This information has provided new insight into the pathophysiology of the different clinical manifestations of extracranial atherosclerotic cerebrovascular disease using noninvasive methods.

The aim of this chapter is to highlight the advances in ultrasonic plaque characterization and their potential applications in clinical practice.

Ultrasonic Plaque Classification

High-resolution ultrasound provides information not only on the degree of carotid artery stenosis but also on the characteristics of the arterial wall including the size and consistency of atherosclerotic plaques. Several studies have indicated that "complicated" carotid plaques are often associated with ipsilateral neurological symptoms and share common ultrasonic characteristics, being more echolucent (weak reflection of ultrasound and therefore containing echo-poor structures) and heterogeneous (having both echolucent and echogenic areas). In contrast, "uncomplicated" plaques, which are often asymptomatic, tend to be of uniform consistency (uniformly hypoechoic or uniformly hyperechoic) without evidence of ulceration.[11,15,16]

A.F. Aburahma, J.J. Bergan (eds.), *Noninvasive Cerebrovascular Diagnosis*, DOI 10.1007/978-1-84882-957-2_7,

Table 7–1. Design of published studies on carotid plaque characterization in relation to risk for neurologic events.

Reference	Carotid bifurcations *n*	Follow-up in years	Type of patients A = asymptomatic S = symptomatic	Plaque characteristics studied
O'Holleran *et al.*, 1987[18]	296	3.8	A	Calcified, dense, soft
Sterpetti *et al.*, 1988[25]	238	2.8	A and S	Homogeneous, heterogeneous
Langsfeld *et al.*, 1989[26]	419	1.8	A	Plaque types 1 to 4
Bock *et al.*, 1993[27]	242	2.3	A	Echolucent, echogenic
Polak *et al.*, 1998[22]	270	3.3	A	Hypo-, iso-, hyperechoic
Mathiesen *et al.*, 2001[28]	223	3.0	A	Plaque types 1 to 4
Grønholdt *et al.*, 2001[29]	111	4.4	A	Grayscale median
	135	4.4	S	Grayscale median
Liapis *et al.*, 2001[30]	442	3.7	A and S	Plaque types 1 to 4
AbuRahma *et al.*, 1998[31]	391	3.1	A	Homogeneous, heterogeneous
Carra *et al.*, 2003[32]	291	2.7	A	Homogeneous, heterogeneous

Different classifications of plaque ultrasonic appearance have been proposed. Reilly classified[15] carotid plaques as homogeneous and heterogeneous, defining as homogeneous plaques those with "uniformly bright echoes" that are now known as uniformly hyperechoic (type 4) (see below). Johnson classified plaques as dense and soft,[17,18] Widder as echolucent and echogenic based on the their overall level of echo patterns,[19] while Gray-Weale described four types: type 1, predominantly echolucent lesions, type 2, echogenic lesions with substantial (>75%) components of echolucency, type 3, predominately echogenic with small area(s) of echolucency occupying less than a quarter of the plaque, and type 4, uniformly dense echogenic lesions.[20] Geroulakos subsequently modified the Gray-Weale classification by using a 50% area cut-off point instead of 75% and by adding a fifth type, which as a result of heavy calcification on its surface cannot be correctly classified.[11]

In an effort to improve the reproducibility of visual (subjective) classification, a consensus conference has suggested that echodensity should reflect the overall brightness of the plaque with the term hyperechoic referring to echogenic (white) and the term hypoechoic referring to echolucent (black) plaques.[21] The reference structure, to which plaque echodensity should be compared, should be blood for hypoechoic, the sternomastoid muscle for isoechoic, and bone for hyperechoic plaques. More recently, a similar method has been used by Polak.[22]

In the past a number of workers had confused echogenicity with homogeneity.[15] It is now realized that measurements of texture are different from measurements of echogenicity. The observation that two different atherosclerotic plaques may have the same overall echogenicity but frequently have variations of texture within different regions of the plaque was made as early as 1983.[23] The term homogeneous should therefore refer to plaques of uniform consistency irrespective of whether they are predominantly hypoechoic or hyperechoic. The term heterogeneous should be used for plaques of nonuniform consistency, i.e., having both hypoechoic and hyperechoic components (Gray-Weale[20] types 2 and 3). Although O'Donnnell had proposed this otherwise simple classification in 1985[16] and Aldoori in 1987,[24] there has been considerable diversity in terminology used by others, as shown in Table 7–1.[18,22,25–32] Because of this confusion, frequently plaques having intermediate echogenicity or being complex are inadequately described. For example, echolucent plaques have been considered as heterogeneous.[26] A reflection of this confusion is a report from the committee on standards for noninvasive vascular testing of the Joint Council of the Society for Vascular Surgery and the North American Chapter of the International Society for Cardiovascular Surgery proposing that carotid plaques should be classified as homogeneous or heterogeneous.[33]

Regarding the clinical significance of carotid plaque heterogeneity, it seems that the heterogeneous plaques described in the three studies published in the 1980s (Table 7–1) include hypoechoic plaques. Also heterogeneous plaques in all studies listed in Table 7–1 contain hypoechoic areas (large or small) and appear to be the plaques that are associated with symptoms or if found in asymptomatic individuals they are the plaques that subsequently tend to become symptomatic.

Correlation with Histology

Reilly has shown for the first time that carotid plaque characteristics on B-mode ultrasound performed before operation correlate with carotid plaque histology.[15] As indicated above, by evaluating visually the sonographic characteristics of carotid plaques, two patterns were identified: a homogeneous pattern containing uniform hyperechoic echoes corresponding to dense fibrous tissue and a heterogeneous pattern containing a mixture of hyperechoic areas representing fibrous tissue and anechoic areas that represent intraplaque hemorrhage or lipid.[33] Thus, it was realized early that ultrasound could not distinguish between hemorrhage and lipid. Because most heterogeneous lesions contained intraplaque hemorrhage and ulcerated lesions, it was thought at the time that the presence of a plaque hemorrhage reflected the potential for plaque rupture and development of symptoms. However, it was subsequently realized that plaque hemorrhage was very common and was found in equal frequency in both symptomatic and asymptomatic plaques[34] and that ultrasound was highly sensitive in demonstrating plaque hemorrhage (27/29, 93%), as well as specific (84%).[16,31,35] It was both sensitive and specific in demonstrating calcification in carotid endarterectomy specimens.[36]

Aldoori reported that plaque hemorrhage was seen histologically in 21 patients, 19 (78%) of whom were diagnosed preoperatively as having echolucent heterogeneous plaques on ultrasound imaging.[24] Gray-Weale[20] also validated his plaque classification by demonstrating a statistically significant relationship ($p < 0.001$) between ultrasound appearance of type 1 and 2 plaques (echolucent appearance) and the presence of either intraplaque hemorrhage or ulceration in the endarterectomy specimen. It is now apparent from those ultrasound-histology correlations that Reilly's heterogeneous plaques correspond closely to Gray-Weale's echolucent (types 1 and 2) plaques.

The above findings were confirmed by studies performed in the 1990s using the new generation of ultrasound scanners with their improved resolution. Van Damme[37] reported that fibrous plaques (dense homogeneous hyperechoic lesions) were detected with a specificity of 87% and a sensitivity of 56%. Recent intraplaque hemorrhage was echographically apparent as a hypoechoic area in 88% of cases, corresponding to a specificity of 79% and a sensitivity of 75%. Kardoulas,[38] in another study, confirmed Van Damme's results on fibrous plaques, with fibrous tissue being significantly greater (73%) in plaques with an echogenic character compared with those with an echolucent morphology (63%; $p = 0.04$).

More recently the European carotid plaque study group that performed a multicenter study confirmed that plaque echogenicity was inversely related to hemorrhage and lipid ($p = 0.005$) and directly related to collagen content and calcification ($p < 0.0001$).[39]

Plaque shape (mural vs. nodular) on ultrasound has been shown to be associated with histology features characteristic of unstable plaques. Weinberger[40] demonstrated that mural plaques propagating along the carotid wall had a 72% frequency of recent organizing hemorrhage. In contrast, nodular plaques causing local narrowing of the vessel had only a 23% incidence of organizing hemorrhage ($p < 0.01$).

We now know that stable atherosclerotic plaques have on histological examination a thick fibrous cap, a small lipid core, are rich in smooth muscle cells (SMC) that produce collagen, and have a poor content of macrophages. In contrast, unstable plaques that are prone to rupture and development of symptoms have a thin fibrous cap, a large lipid core, few SMC, and are rich in macrophages.[3] Macrophages are responsible for the production of enzymes, matrix metaloproteinases (stromelysins, gelatinases, collagenases) that play an important role in remodeling the plaque matrix and erosion of the fibrous cap.[41] Recently, Lammie[42] reported a highly significant association between a thin fibrous cap and a large necrotic core ($p < 0.002$) in carotid endarterectomy specimens and a good agreement between ultrasound and pathological measurements of fibrous cap thickness (thick vs. thin fibrous cap, kappa = 0.53).

There is considerable debate on the question of whether thrombosis on the surface of the plaque, being an otherwise significant feature of complicated plaques, can discriminate between symptomatic and asymptomatic plaques. Acute thrombosis on ultrasound appears as a completely echolucent defect adjacent to the lumen[43] and it is almost certain that by the time the operation is performed (usually several weeks after the event) the thrombus has undergone remodeling.

Natural History Studies

Johnson did the first study, which has shown the value of ultrasonic characterization of carotid bifurcation plaques in asymptomatic patients, in the early 1980s.[17,18] In that study, hypoechoic carotid plaques in comparison to hyperechoic or calcified ones increased the risk of stroke during a follow-up period of 3 years; this effect was prominent in patients with carotid stenosis more than 75% (as estimated by cross-sectional area calculations and spectral analysis), as stroke occurred in 19% of them. None of the patients with calcified plaques developed a stroke.

A second study performed in the 1980s by Sterpetti[25] has shown that the severity of stenosis (lumen diameter reduction greater than 50%) and the presence of a heterogeneous plaque were both independent risk factors for the development of new neurological deficits (TIA and stroke). Twenty-seven percent of the patients with heterogeneous plaques and hemodynamically significant stenosis developed new symptoms. Unfortunately, their study had mixed cases as 37% of the patients had a history of previous neurologic symptoms, mainly hemispheric ones. History of these neurological symptoms was a risk factor for the development of new neurological symptoms during the follow-up period, although this was found only in the univariate analysis. Because no subgroup analysis was performed, no conclusion can be drawn regarding asymptomatic or symptomatic patients.

In a similar study of patients with asymptomatic carotid stenosis AbuRahma[31] reported that the incidence of ipsilateral strokes during follow-up was significantly higher in patients having heterogeneous plaques than in those having homogeneous ones: 13.6% versus 3.1% ($p = 0.0001$; odds ratio: 5). Similarly, the incidence rate of all neurological events (stroke or TIA) was higher in patients with heterogeneous than in those with homogeneous plaques: 27.8% versus 6.6% ($p = 0.001$; odds ratio, 5.5). Heterogeneous plaques were defined as those composed of a mixture of hypoechoic, isoechoic, and hyperechoic lesions, and homogeneous plaques as those that consisted of only one of the three components. Similar results indicating an increased risk in patients with heterogeneous plaques were reported by Carra[32] (Table 7–2).

The study published in the 1980s by Langsfeld[26] confirmed that patients with *hypoechoic plaques* (type 1, predominantly echolucent raised lesion, with a thin "eggshell" cap of echogenicity and type 2, echogenic lesions with substantial areas of echolucency) had a twofold risk of stroke: 15% in comparison to 7% in those having *hyperechoic plaques* [type 3, predominately echogenic with small area(s) of echolucency deeply localized and occupying less than a quarter of the plaque and type 4, uniformly dense echogenic lesions]. A confounding factor was that patients with greater than 75% stenosis were also at increased risk. However, the overall incidence of new symptoms was low, in contrast with the previous studies, perhaps because only asymptomatic patients were included in that study. Based on their results, the authors proposed an aggressive approach in those patients with greater than 75% stenosis and heterogeneous plaques. There is some confusion regarding the interchangeable use of the terms heterogeneous and hypoechoic in that article. The authors raised the point that it is important for each laboratory to verify its ability to classify plaque types. The same group in another study published 4 years later reported a 5.7% annual vessel event rate (TIA and stroke) for echolucent carotid plaques versus 2.4% for the echogenic ones ($p = 0.03$).[27]

Given the fair interobserver reproducibility for type 1 plaques, the use of reference points was proposed: anechogenicity to be standardized against circulating blood, isoechogenicity against sternomastoid muscle, and hyperechogenicity against bone (cervical vertebrae). This method was used in the late 1990s by Polak,[22] who investigated the association between stroke and internal carotid artery plaque echodensity in 4886 asymptomatic individuals aged 65 years or older, who were followed up prospectively for 48 months. Some 68% of those had carotid artery stenosis, which exceeded 50% in 270 patients. In this study plaques were subjectively characterized as hypoechoic, isoechoic, or hyperechoic in relation to the surrounding soft tissues. Hypoechoic plaques causing 50–100% stenoses were associated with a significantly higher incidence of ipsilateral, nonfatal stroke than iso- or hyperechoic plaques of the same degree of stenosis (relative risk 2.78 and 3.08, respectively). The authors of this study suggested that quantitative methods of grading carotid plaque echomorphology such as computer-assisted plaque characterization might be more precise in determining the association between hypoechoic (echolucent) plaques and the incidence of stroke. Subsequent studies[28–30] have supported the finding that

TABLE 7–2. Results of prospective studies of plaque characterization in relation to risk for neurologic events.

Reference	Endpoint	Stenosis	Findings
O'Holleran *et al.*, 1987[18]	Stroke, transient ischemic attack (TIA)	>75%	Cumulative 5 year stroke risk was 80% for soft (echolucent plaques) 10% for dense (echogenic and calcified plaques)
Sterpetti *et al.*, 1988[25]	Stroke, TIA	>50%	Events: 27% for heterogeneous plaques 9% for homogeneous plaques
Langsfeld *et al.*, 1989[26]	Neurological symptoms	>75%	Events: 15% for echolucent plaques 9% for echogenic plaques
Bock *et al.*, 1993[27]	Stroke, TIA	—	Annual event rate: 5.7% for echolucent plaques 2.4% for echogenic plaques
Polak *et al.*, 1998[22]	Stroke	>50%	RR for ipsilateral stroke was 2.78 in hypoechoic plaques
Mathiesen *et al.*, 2001[28]	Neurological	>35%	RR for cerebrovascular events was 4.6 in subjects with echolucent plaques
Grønholdt *et al.*, 2001[29]	Ipsilateral stroke	>80%	RR for ischemic stroke was 7.9 in subjects with echolucent plaques
Liapis *et al.*, 2001[30]	Stroke, TIA	>70%	RR was 2.96 for stroke and 2.02 for TIA in echolucent plaques
AbuRahma *et al.*, 1998[31]	Stroke, TIA	—	Ipsilateral stroke occurred in 13.6% of heterogeneous plaques 3.1% of homogeneous plaques
Carra *et al.*, 2003[32]	Stroke, TIA	>70%	Ipsilateral event occurred in 5% of heterogeneous plaques 1.3% of homogeneous plaques

hypoechoic plaques are associated with an increased risk when compared with hyperechoic plaques (see below). We now know that echolucent and heterogeneous plaques are not mutually exclusive and the risk is increased in both. Type 2 plaques, which are associated with the highest incidence of neurological events, are by definition included in both echolucent and heterogeneous groups (see the section on plaque types below).

The Need for B-Mode Image Normalization

Ultrasound examination and plaque characterization have been until now highly subjective. When the examination is performed in a dimly lit room the gain is usually reduced by the operator; when it is performed in a brightly lit room the gain is increased. Although the human eye can adjust to the image brightness to a certain extent, reproducible measurements of echodensity are not possible. Ultrasonic image normalization, which was introduced in the late 1990s, has enabled us to overcome this problem.

Computer-assisted plaque measurements of echodensity were initially made from digitized B-mode images of plaques taken from a duplex scanner with fixed instrument settings including gain and time control. The median of the frequency distribution of gray values of the pixels within the plaque (grayscale median—GSM, scale 0–255, 0 = black, 255 = white) was used as the measurement of echodensity. Early work had demonstrated that plaques with a GSM of less than 32, i.e., echolucent plaques had a 5-fold increase in the prevalence of silent brain infarcts on CT brain scans.[44] Other teams found similar results but the cut-off point was different from 32.[45] Soon it became apparent that ultrasonic image normalization was necessary, so that images captured under different instrument settings, from different scanners, by different operators, and through different peripherals such as video or magnetooptical disk could be comparable.

As a result a method has been developed to normalize images by means of digital image processing using blood and adventitia as the two reference points.[46] With the use of commercially available software (Adobe Photoshop version 3.0 or later, Adobe Systems Inc.) and the "histogram" facility, the GSM of the two reference points (blood and adventitia) in the original B-mode image was determined. Algebraic (linear) scaling of the image was performed with the "curves" option of the software so that in the resultant image the GSM of blood was equal to 0 and that of the adventitia to 190. Thus brightness of all pixels in the image including those of the plaque became adjusted according to the two reference points. This resulted in a significant improvement in the comparability of the ultrasonic tissue characteristics.

Appropriate areas of blood and adventitia for image normalization and the avoidance of areas of acoustic shadow in the selection of the plaque area are imperative. The duplex settings recommended are as follows: maximum dynamic range, low persistence, and high frame rate. A high-frequency linear array transducer ideally 7–10 MHz should be used. A high dynamic range ensures a greater range of grayscale values. High frame rate ensures good temporal resolution. In addition to these presets the time gain compensation curve should be positioned vertically through the lumen of the vessel, as there is little attenuation of the beam at this point. This ensures that the adventitia of the anterior wall has the same brightness as the adventitia of the posterior wall. The overall gain should be adjusted to give optimum image quality (bright echoes with minimum noise in the blood). A linear postprocessing curve should also be used and finally where possible the ultrasound beam should be at 90° to the arterial wall (Figure 7–1).

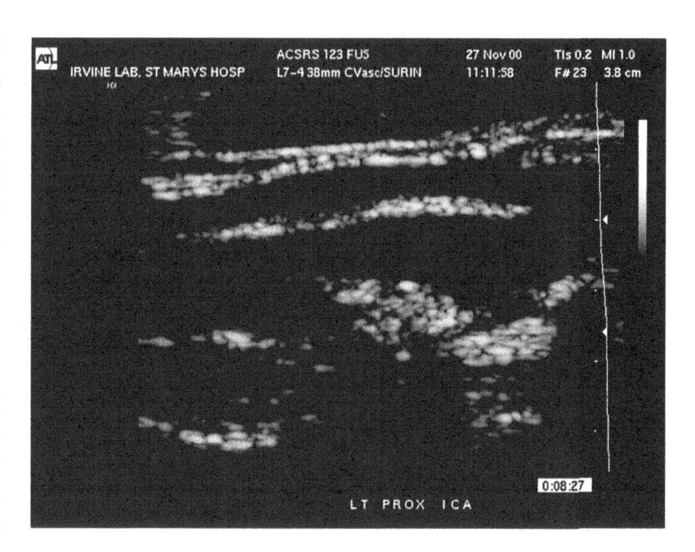

FIGURE 7–1. Image obtained for plaque analysis. The ultrasound beam is at right angles to the adventitia; the time gain compensation curve (TGC) is vertical through the vessel lumen; a bright segment of adventitia is visible adjacent to the plaque.

The previously discussed guidelines should result in the following: an area of noiseless blood, an echodense piece of adventitia in the vicinity of the plaque, and visualization of the extent and borders of the plaque. It is here that color images can provide further information about plaque outline.

Two major reproducibility studies have been performed in order to establish the validity of the method of image normalization and the value of GSM measurements.[47,48] These studies have demonstrated that GSM after image normalization is a highly reproducible measurement that could be used in natural history studies of asymptomatic carotid atherosclerotic disease, aiming to identify patients at higher risk of stroke. A key issue for the successful reproducibility of normalized images is that only the inner half of the

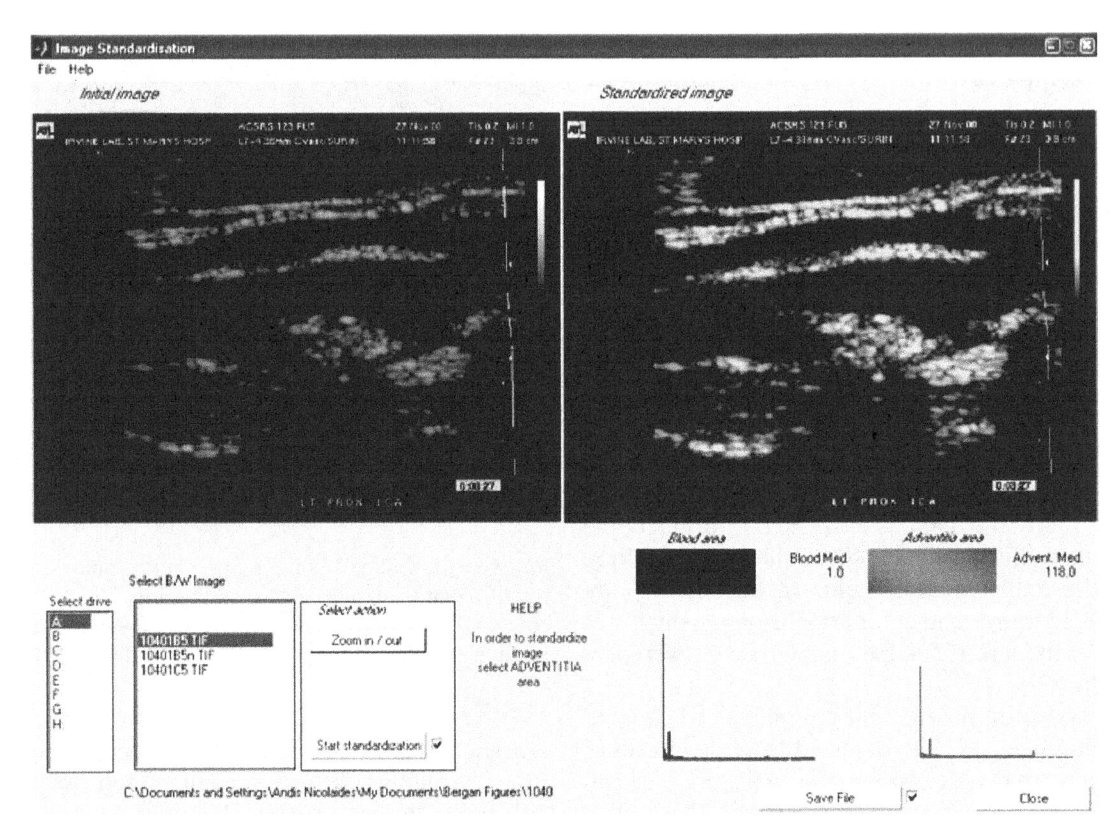

FIGURE 7–2. A user-friendly method of image normalization. Original image is on the left. By sampling pixels representing blood and pixels of center of adventitia after magnification, the normalized image is produced on the right. This image can be saved in a database.

brightest section of adventitia should be sampled for normalization.

Adequate training is essential if the level of reproducibility reported above is to be achieved. It is necessary not only in the use of the software but also in the appropriate scanning technique.

The authors have developed a research software package, now commercially available, that can be used to analyze ultrasonic images of plaques. This package has five main modules. The first provides a user-friendly way to normalize images (Figure 7–2). A zooming facility allows enlargement of the image so that the middle half of the adventitia can be selected accurately. The second provides a means of calibration and of making measurements of distance or area in mm and mm^2, respectively. The third provides a method of normalizing images to a standard pixel density (20 pixels per mm). This is because a number of texture features are pixel density dependent and various degrees of image magnification even on the same scanner do alter the pixel density (see section on "Texture Features"). The fourth provides the user with a means of selecting the area of interest (plaque) and saving it as a separate file (Figure 7–3). An image enhancement facility allows clearer visualization of the edges of the plaque. The fifth classifies plaques according to the Geroulakos classification[11] and extracts a number of texture features and saves them on a file for subsequent statistical analysis. In addition, images are color contoured. Pixels with a grayscale value in the range of 0–25 are colored black. Pixels with values 26–50, 51–75, 76–100, 101–125, and greater than 125 are colored blue, green, yellow, orange, and red, respectively (Figure 7–4). In addition, this module allows printing of the plaque images and selected features or saving the latter in a file (Figure 7–5). For the purpose of automatic classification by computer, the Geroulakos classification has been redefined in terms of pixels and gray levels. Examples of plaque types 1–4 are shown in Figure 7–6. For plaque type 5 only the calcified or visible bright areas of the plaque should be selected ignoring the areas of acoustic shadows where information on plaque texture is lacking.

Type 1. Uniformly echolucent (black): (less than 15% of the plaque area is occupied by colored areas, i.e., with pixels having a grayscale value greater than 25). If the fibrous cap is not visible, the plaque can be detected as a black filling defect only by using color flow or power Doppler.

Type 2. Mainly echolucent: (colored areas occupy 15–50% of the plaque area).

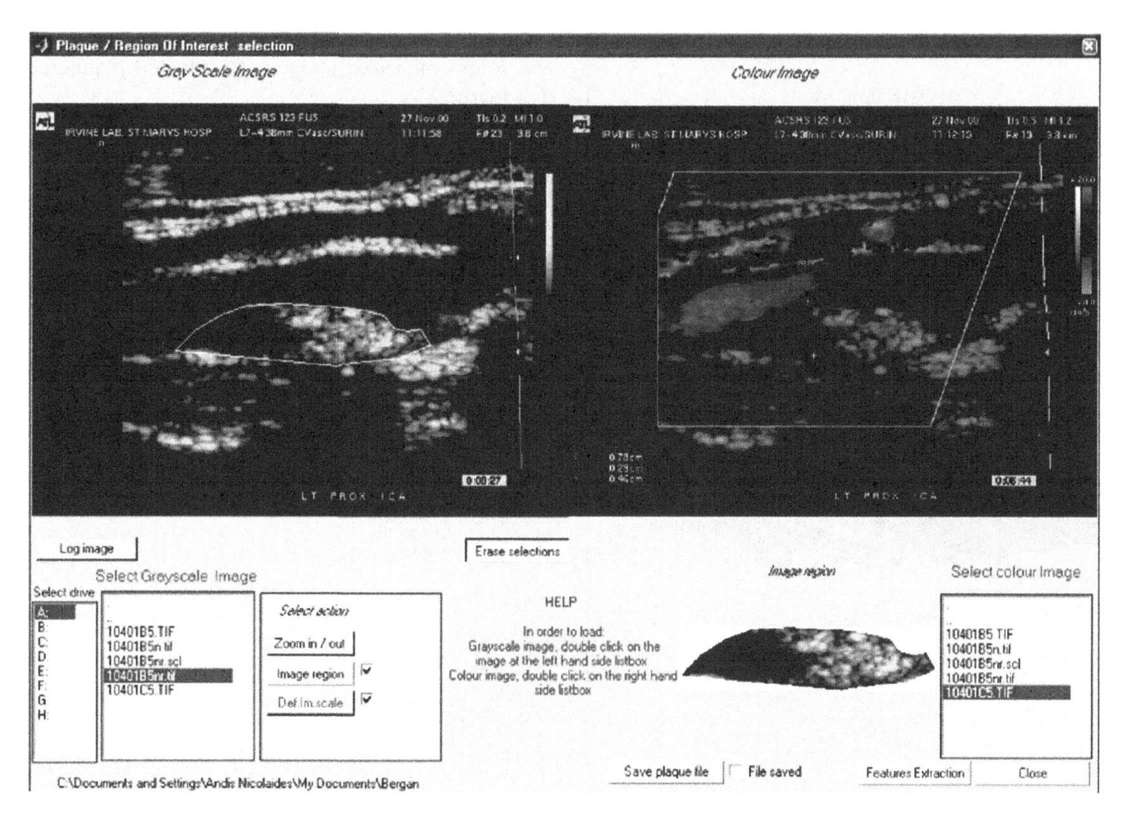

FIGURE 7–3. This module provides the facility for outlining the plaque and saving it as a separate file in the database. The color image on the right provides some indication of the extent of hypoechoic areas near the lumen.

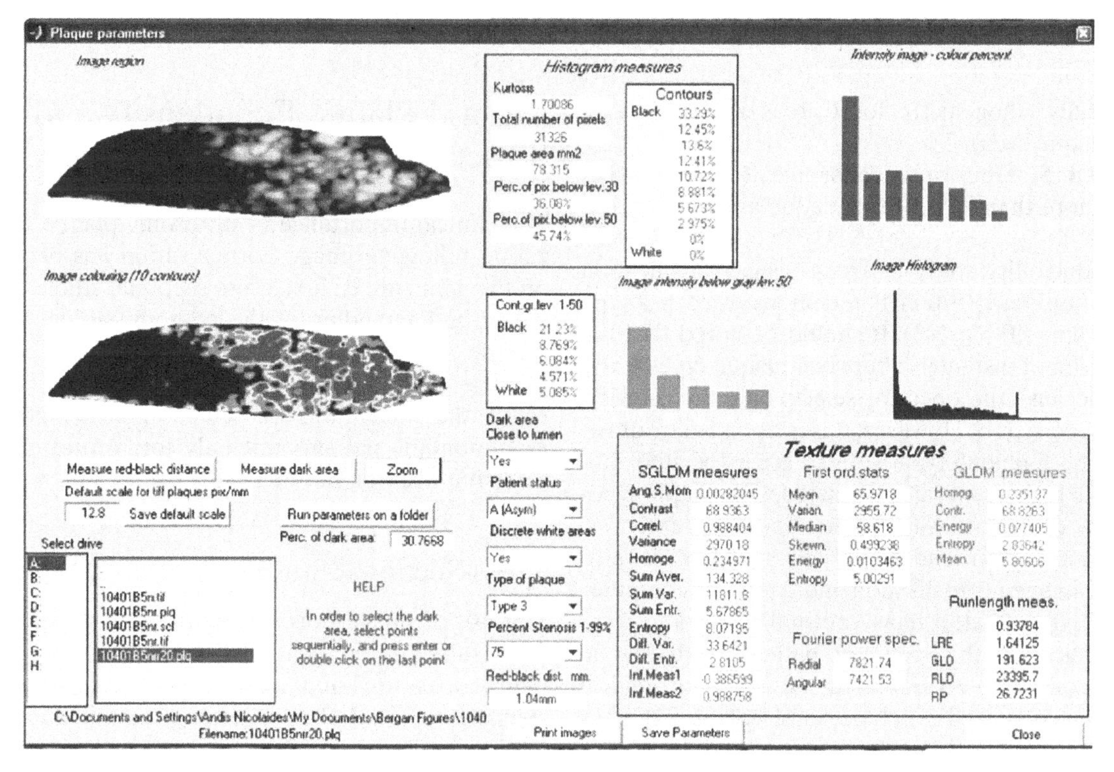

FIGURE 7–4. This module extracts a large number of well-established standard first-order and second-order statistical features used in image analysis. The program determines the type of plaque automatically and allows input from the operator about the presence of a dark area adjacent to the lumen, presenting symptoms and percent carotid stenosis.

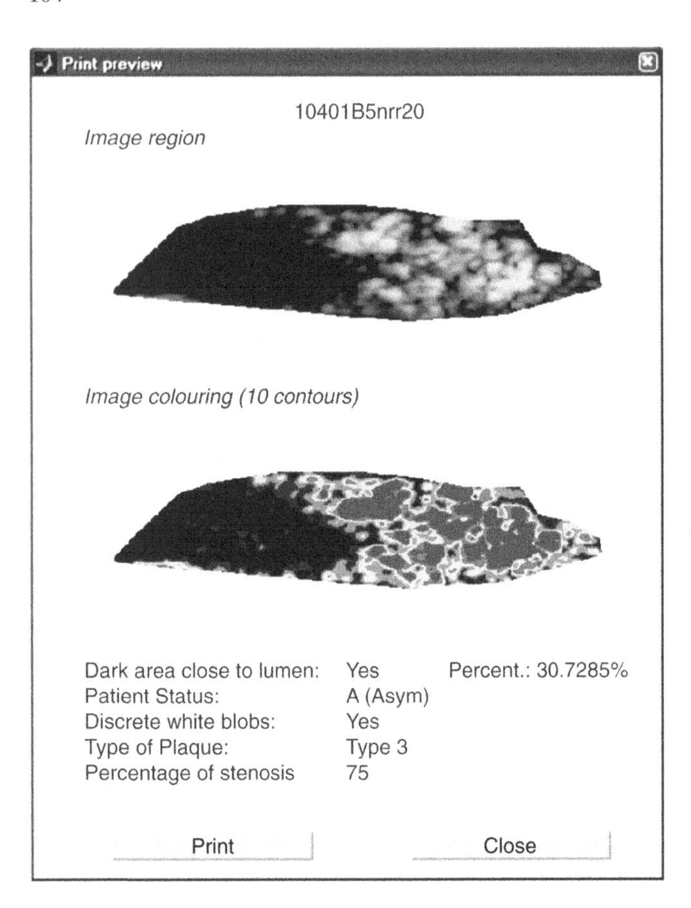

FIGURE 7–5. Printout of normalized grayscale image of plaque and color contoured image with selected plaque characterization features.

Type 3. Mainly echogenic: (colored areas occupy 50–85% of the plaque area).

Type 4 and 5. Uniformly echogenic: (colored areas occupy more than 85% of the plaque area).

A reproducibility study between visual classification and computer classification has demonstrated a kappa statistic of 0.61 (Table 7–3). It should be noted that the computer cannot distinguish between plaque types 4 and 5. This is because the operator selects only the calcified area of plaque type 5. However, this is not a major drawback since both plaque types 4 and 5 are associated with low risk. The high event rate associated with plaque types 1–3 and low event rate with plaques 4 and 5 found after image normalization and visual classification is also found after image normalization and typing by computer (Table 7–4). In fact, after image normalization and computer classification the group of patients with plaque types 1–3 contains 99 (93.5%) of all 106 neurological events. When compared with type 4 and 5 plaques the relative risk is 3.3 (95% CI 1.56–7.00). Also, after image normalization and computer classification plaque types 1–3 contain 44 (93.6%) of all 46 strokes (RR 3.4 with 95% CI 1.07–10.9).

Carotid Plaque Echodensity and Structure in Normalized Images

The clinical importance of ultrasonic plaque characterization following image normalization has been focused on two main areas: first, cross-sectional studies aiming at better understanding of the pathophysiology of carotid disease and second, natural history studies seeking to identify high- and low-risk groups for stroke in order to refine the indications on selection of symptomatic or asymptomatic patients not only for carotid endarterectomy but also for stenting.

Cross-Sectional Studies

The use of image normalization and computer analysis has resulted in the identification of differences in carotid plaque structure—in terms of echodensity and degree of stenosis—not only between symptomatic and asymptomatic plaques in general but also between plaques associated with retinal or hemispheric symptoms.[49] In a series of asymptomatic and symptomatic patients presenting with amaurosis fugax, TIAs, and stroke with good

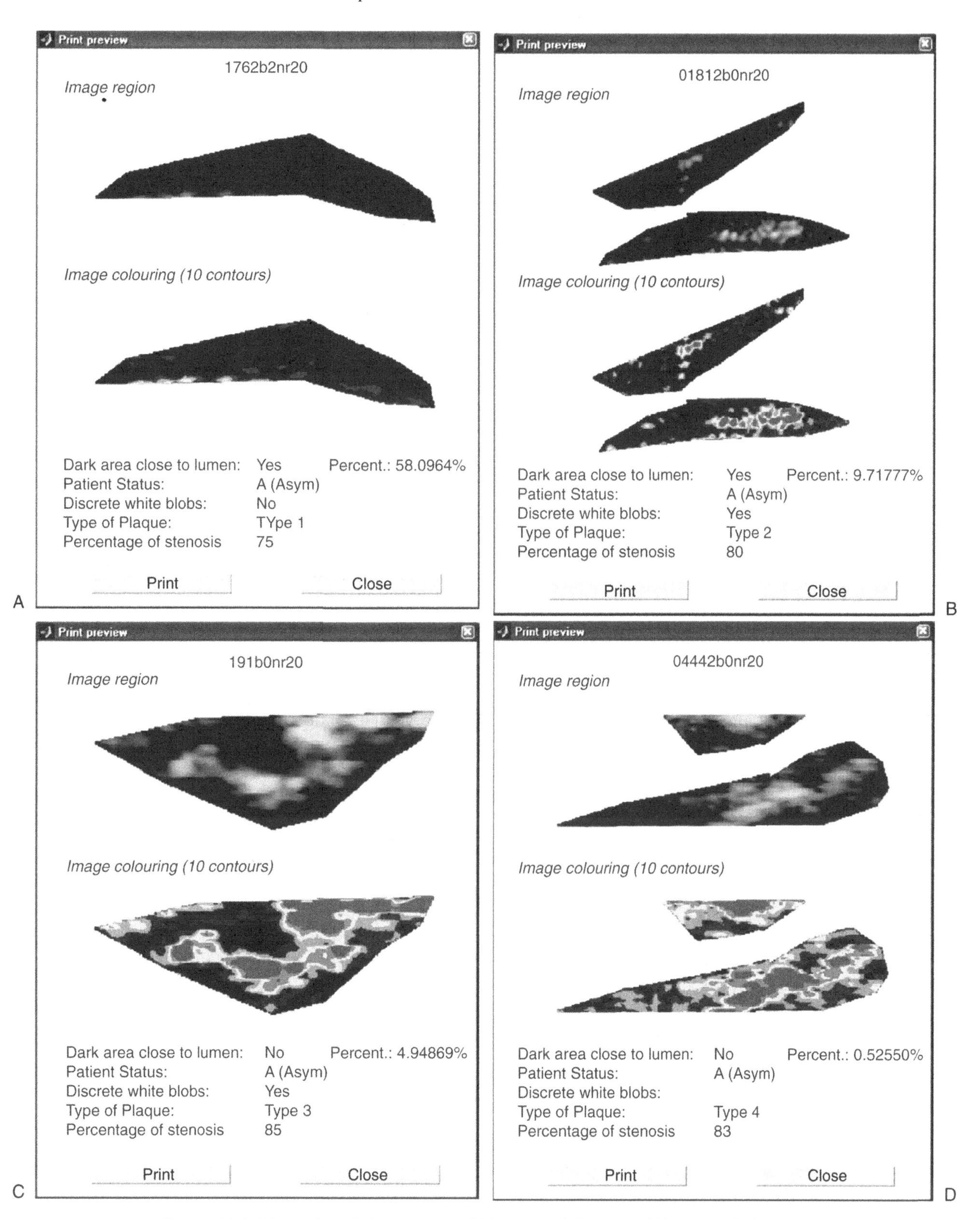

FIGURE 7–6. Examples of plaque types: (A) type 1, (B) type 2, (C) type 3, (D) type 4.

Table 7–3. Relationship between plaque visual classification after image normalization and plaque classification by computer (kappa = 0.61).[a]

Plaque type: visual classification after image normalization	Plaque type classification by computer after image normalization				
	1	2	3	4/5	Total
1	57 (51%)	53 (47%)	2 (1.8%)	0	112 (100%)
2	6 (1.6%)	251 (68%)	110 (30%)	3 (0.8%)	370 (100%)
3	0	9 (3%)	281 (91%)	20 (6.5%)	310 (100%)
4/5	0	0	92 (34%)	178 (66%)	270 (100%)
Total	63 (6%)	313 (29%)	486 (46%)	201 (19%)	1062 (100%)

[a]Because of the low event rate in plaque types 4 and 5 and because the computer cannot distinguish between them these plaques have been grouped together.

recovery having 50–99% stenosis on carotid duplex scan, plaques associated with symptoms were significantly more hypoechoic, with higher degrees of stenosis than those not associated with symptoms (mean GSM = 13.3 versus 30.5 and mean degree of stenosis = 80.5% versus 72.2%). Furthermore, plaques associated with amaurosis fugax were hypoechoic (mean GSM = 7.4) and severely stenotic (mean stenosis 85.6%). Plaques associated with TIAs and stroke had a similar echodensity and a similar degree of stenosis (mean GSM = 14.9 versus 15.8 and degree of stenosis = 79.3% versus 78.1%).[50] These findings confirm previous reports, which have shown that hypoechoic plaques are more likely to be associated with symptoms. In addition, they support the hypothesis that amaurosis fugax has a pathophysiological mechanism different from that of TIAs and stroke.

Our group has found that GSM separates echomorphologically the carotid plaques associated with silent nonlacunar CT-demonstrated brain infarcts from plaques that are not so associated. The median GSM of plaques associated with ipsilateral nonlacunar silent CT-demonstrated brain infarcts was 14, and that of plaques that were not so associated was 30 ($p = 0.003$).[48] Additionally, emboli counted on transcranial Doppler (TCD) in the ipsilateral middle cerebral artery were more frequent in the presence of low-plaque echodensity (low GSM), but not in the presence of a high degree of stenosis. These data support the embolic nature of cerebrovascular symptomatology.[49]

There are several biological findings that can explain the association of hypoechoic plaques with symptoms. Our group has found that hypoechoic plaques with a low GSM have a large necrotic core volume.[51] In addition, hypoechoic plaques have increased macrophage infiltration on histological examination of the specimen after endarterectomy.[52]

The role of biomechanical forces in the induction of plaque fatigue and rupture has been emphasized.[53–55] In our group of patients, carotid plaques associated with amaurosis fugax were hypoechoic and were associated with very high-grade stenoses. It may well be that the plaques that are hypoechoic and homogeneous undergo low internal stresses and therefore do not rupture but progress to tighter stenosis with poststenotic dilatation, turbulance, and platelet adhesion in the poststenotic area resulting in the eventual production of showers of small platelet emboli. Such small platelet emboli may be too small to produce hemispheric symptoms but are detected by the retina. In contrast, plaques associated with TIAs and stroke were less hypoechoic and less stenotic than those associated with amaurosis fugax. These plaques are hypoechoic but more heterogeneous and may undergo stronger internal stresses. Therefore, they may tend to

Table 7–4. The ipsilateral AF, TIAs, and strokes that occurred during follow-up in patients with different types of plaque after image normalization and classification by computer.[a]

Plaque type classified by computer	Events absent	AF	TIAs	Stroke	All events	Total
1	56 (88.9%)	2 (3.2%)	1 (1.6%)	4 (6.3%)	7 (11.1%)	63 (100%)
2	271 (86.6%)	6 (1.9%)	17 (5.4%)	19 (6.1%)	42 (13.4%)	313 (100%)
3	435 (89.7%)	10 (2.1%)	19 (3.9%)	21 (4.3%)	50 (10.3%)	485 (100%)
4/5	194 (97.1%)	0	5 (2.5%)	2 (1.5%)	7 (3.5%)	201 (100%)
Total	956 (90.0%)	18 (1.7%)	42 (3.8%)	46 (4.4%)	106 (10.0%)	1062 (100%)

[a]AF, amaurosis fugax; TIAs, transient ischemic attacks.

rupture at an earlier stage (lower degrees of stenosis), producing larger particle debris (plaque constituents or thrombi) that deprive large areas of the brain of adequate perfusion.

Prospective Studies

The Tromsø study conducted in Norway involving 223 subjects with carotid stenosis > 35% has found that subjects with echolucent atherosclerotic plaques have increased risk of ischemic cerebrovascular events independent of degree of stenosis.[28] The authors give no details on the patient's neurological history. The adjusted relative risk for all cerebrovascular events in subjects with echolucent plaques was 4.6 (95% CI 1.1–18.9), and there was a significant linear trend ($p = 0.015$) for higher risk with increasing plaque echolucency. Ipsilateral neurological events were also more frequent in patient's with echolucent or predominantly echolucent plaques (17.4% and 14.7%, respectively). The authors concluded that evaluation of plaque morphology in addition to the grade of stenosis might improve clinical decision making and differentiate treatment for individual patients and that computer-quantified plaque morphology assessment, being a more objective method of ultrasonic plaque characterization, may further improve this.

This method has been recently used by Grønholdt,[29] who found that echolucent plaques causing >50% diameter stenosis were associated with increased risk of future stroke in symptomatic ($n = 135$) but not asymptomatic ($n = 111$) individuals. Echogenicity of carotid plaques was evaluated with high-resolution B-mode ultrasound and computer-assisted image processing. The mean of the standardized median grayscale values of the plaque was used to divide plaques into echolucent and echorich. Relative to symptomatic patients with echorich 50–79% stenotic plaques, those with echorich 80–99% stenotic plaques, echolucent 50–79% stenotic plaques, and echolucent 80–99% stenotic plaques had relative risks of ipsilateral ischemic stroke of 3.1 (95% CI, 0.7–14), 4.2 (95% CI, 1.2–15), and 7.9 (95% CI, 2.1–30), equivalent to absolute risk increase of 11%, 18%, and 28%, respectively. The authors suggested that measurement of echolucency, together with the degree of stenosis, might improve selection of patients for carotid endarterectomy. The relatively small number of asymptomatic individuals was probably the reason why plaque characterization was not helpful in predicting risk in the asymptomatic group.

Ultrasonic Plaque Ulceration

Several studies have indicated a strong association between macroscopic plaque ulceration and the development of embolic symptoms (amaurosis fugax, TIAs, stroke) and signs such as silent infarcts on CT brain scans.[56–60] However, the ability of ultrasound to identify plaque ulceration is poor.[15,19,61–67] The sensitivity is low (41%) when the stenosis is greater than 50% and moderately high (77%) when the stenosis is less than 50%. This is because ulceration is much easier to detect in the presence of mild stenosis, when the residual lumen and plaque surface are more easily seen, than with severe stenosis, when the residual lumen and the surface of the plaque are not easily defined because they are not always in the plane of the ultrasound beam.

Two studies have investigated plaque surface characteristics and the type of plaque in relation to symptoms. The first one was a retrospective analysis of 578 symptomatic patients (242 with stroke and 336 with TIAs) recruited for the B-scan Ultrasound Imaging Assessment Program. A matched case-control study design was used to compare brain hemispheres with ischemic lesions to unaffected contralateral hemispheres with regard to the presence and characteristics of carotid artery plaques. Plaques were classified as smooth when the surface had a continuous boundary, irregular when there was an uneven or pitted boundary, and pocketed when there was a crater-like defect with sharp margins. The results demonstrated an odds ratio of 2.1 for the presence of an irregular surface and of 3.0 for hypoechoic plaques in carotids associated with TIAs and stroke.[68]

The second study included 258 symptomatic and 65 asymptomatic patients. Carotid plaque morphology was classified according to Gray-Weale,[20] and plaque surface features were assessed. The results demonstrated that plaque types 1 and 2 were more common in symptomatic patients. The incidence of ulceration was 23% in the symptomatic and 14% in the asymptomatic group ($p = 0.04$).[69]

In the absence of any prospective natural history studies in which ultrasound has been used for identifying plaque ulceration, the finding of plaque ulceration cannot be used for making clinical decisions.

Stenosis: A Confounding Factor

Natural history studies have demonstrated that the risk of developing ipsilateral symptoms including stroke increases with increasing severity of internal carotid artery stenosis (Table 7–5). In addition, a number of important messages have emerged recently. One is that the different methods used on either side of the Atlantic to express the degree of stenosis have a different relationship to risk. Another is the realization that a considerable number of events occur in patients with low grade asymptomatic carotid stenosis. Also, the relationship between risk and degree of internal carotid stenosis depends on the methodology used. Finally, both the

TABLE 7–5. Natural history studies of patients with asymptomatic internal carotid artery stenosis in which grades of stenosis up to 99% have been included.[a]

Publication	Grading of stenosis				Mean follow-up (years)	Events			Event rate (annual)		
	Area	N%	E%	*n*		TIAs +AF[b]	Stroke	TIAs+ stroke	TIAs +AF	Stroke	TIAs+ Stroke
Johnson *et al.*, 1985[6]	**<75**	<50%	<70%	176	3	12	3	15	2.3%	0.6%	1.7%
	>75	>50%	>70%	121		57	12	69	15.7%	3.3%	19%
Chambers and Norris,	**<75**	<50%	<70%	387	2	8	6	14	1.0%	0.1%	1.8%
1986[8]	**>75**	>50%	>70%	113		16	6	22	7.0%	2.6%	9.7%
Hennerici *et al.*, 1987[9]		**<80%**	<88%	119	2.5	15	4	19	5.0%	1.3%	6.4%
		>80%	>88%	36		2	3	5	2.2%	3.3%	5.5%
Norris *et al.*, 1991[10]		**<50%**	<70%	303	3.4	11	13	24	1.1%	1.3%	2.3%
		50–75%	72–85%	216		28	5	33	3.8%	0.6%	4.5%
		75–99%	85–99%	177		36	11	47	6.0%	1.8%	7.8%
Zhu and Norris, 1991[11]		**<50%**	<72%	734[c]	4	12	10	22	0.4%	0.3%	0.7%
		50–74%	72–85%	172[c]		12	2	14	1.7%	0.3%	2.0%
		75–99%	85–99%	94[c]		23	6	29	6.1%	1.6%	7.7%
MacKey *et al.*, 1997[12]		<12%	**<50%**	358	3.6	5	5	10	0.4%	0.4%	0.8%
		12–65%	**50–79%**	207		3	6	9	0.4%	0.8%	1.2%
		65–99%	**79–99%**	113		12	7	19	2.9%	1.7%	4.7%
Nadareishvili *et al.*,		**<50%**	<72%	108	10	—	—	10	—	—	0.9%
2002[13]		**50–99%**	72–99%	73		—	—	12	—	—	7.7%
ECST (asymptomatic		<47%	**0–69%**	2113	4.5	—	54		—	0.5%	—
side) 1995[14]		47–99%	**70–99%**	127		—	13		—	2.3%	—
NASCET (asymptomatic		**<50%**	<72%	1496	5	—	116	—	—	1.5%	—
side)		**50–74%**	72–85%	172		—	31	—	—	2.8%	—
Inzitary *et al.*, 2000[15]		**75–99%**	85–99%	73		—	12	—	—	3.3%	—
		<60%	<77%	1604		—	128	—	—	1.6%	—
		60–99%	77–99%	73		—	34	—	—	3.1%	—
ACSRS		12–49%	**50–69%**	194	3.5	7	3	10	0.4%	0.4%	1.5%
Nicolaides *et al.*, 2005[84]		50–82%	**70–89%**	593		31	23	54	1.5%	1.1%	2.6%
		82–99%	**90–99%**	328		24	20	44	2.1%	1.7%	3.8%

[a]The method used to grade the stenosis in each study (area, N% = NASCET or E% = ECST) is shown in bold.
[b]AF, amaurosis fugax; TIAs, transient ischemic attacks.
[c]Indicates carotid arteries rather than patients.

severity of internal carotid stenosis and plaque characterization texture features are independent predictors of risk and can complement each other. Thus, plaque characterization cannot be considered independent of stenosis.

Two main methods are currently used to express percent diameter stenosis. The first one defines the residual lumen as a percentage of the normal distal internal carotid artery (ICA). It has been used in North America since the late 1960s and more recently the North American Symptomatic Carotid Endarterectomy Trial (NASCET)[70] and the Asymptomatic Carotid Atherosclerosis Study (ACAS).[71] It has become known as the North American, "NASCET," or "N" method.[72] The second method expresses the residual lumen as a percentage of the diameter of the carotid bulb and has been used in the European Carotid Surgery Trial (ECST).[73] It has become known as the European or "ECST" or "E" method.[74] The relationship between both methods is shown in Figure 7–7.

Several natural history studies[17,27,75–82] indicate that the risk of stroke in asymptomatic patients is low (0.1–1.6% per year) for NASCET stenosis less than 75–80% and higher (2.0–3.3% per year) with greater degrees of stenosis (Table 7–5). Different cut-off points, ranges, and methods of grading stenosis have been used in these natural history studies[17,27,75–82] and randomized controlled trials.[70,71,73,83] Universal agreement as to the best method for grading ICA stenosis and optimum cut-off points in relation to risk have not yet been established.

The NASCET randomized controlled study has used angiography and a cut-off point of 70% stenosis in relation to the distal internal carotid, which is equivalent to 83% stenosis in relation to the bulb (Figure 7–7). The ECST randomized controlled study has used angiography also, but a cut-off point of 70% stenosis in relation to the bulb, which is equivalent to 47% stenosis in relation to the distal ICA. Many vascular surgeons are under the impression that these cut-off points are similar! The only similarity is the value of 70%. In reality the difference in terms of plaque size or residual lumen is considerable. However, with increasing degrees of stenosis the values of the two methods converge and the discrepancy decreases (Figure 7–7).

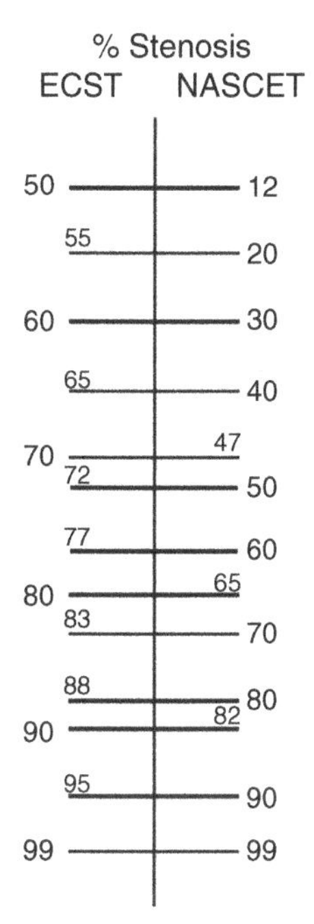

FIGURE 7–7. The relationship between ECST and NASCET percentage stenosis. The conversion scale is based on the following equations: NASCET stenosis = (ECST stenosi − 43) × (100/57) and ECST stenosis = [NASCET stenosis × (57/100) + 43]. Note: a 43% stenosis of the bulb reduces the lumen to the diameter of the lumen of the normal distal internal carotid artery. (Reproduced from Nicolaides *et al.*, 2005. Eur J Vasc Endovasc Surg 30, 275–284, with permission.)

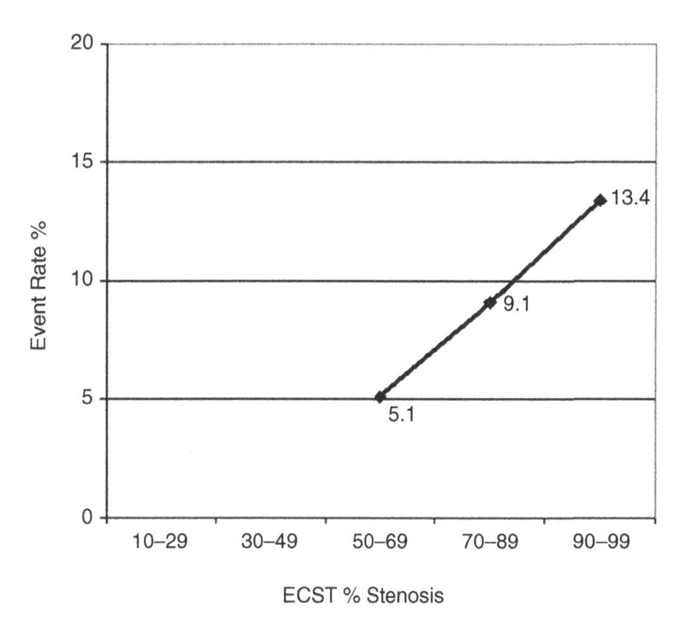

FIGURE 7–8. The incidence of ipsilateral ischemic hemispheric events in relation to the ECST percentage stenosis of the internal carotid artery in the ACSRS study. (Reproduced from Nicolaides *et al.*, 2005. Eur J Vasc Endovasc Surg 30, 275–284, with permission.)

The results of the Asymptomatic Carotid Stenosis and Risk of Stroke (ACSRS) prospective natural history study have demonstrated that the risk of ipsilateral ischemic hemispheric events has a linear relationship with ECST stenosis (Figure 7–8) but not with NASCET stenosis (Figure 7–9).[84]

Natural history studies including the ACSRS that have included patients with asymptomatic carotid stenosis up to 99% (Table 7–5) have demonstrated that a considerable number of events occur at low grades of stenosis. In fact, in the ACSRS study 37 (34%) of 108 ipsilateral ischemic hemispheric events including 16 (35%) of the 46 strokes (Table 7–6) occurred in patients with stenosis less than 60% NASCET (<77% ECST), the selection criterion for carotid endarterectomy in asymptomatic patients as indicated from the findings of the ACAS trial. Only 10 (9%) of the events including 3 (3%) strokes occurred in patients with stenosis less than 70% ECST, equivalent to approximately 50% NASCET. The question that has been posed is whether plaque characterization can improve the selection of patients at increased risk in the range of 50–70% NASCET (equivalent to 72–83% ECST).

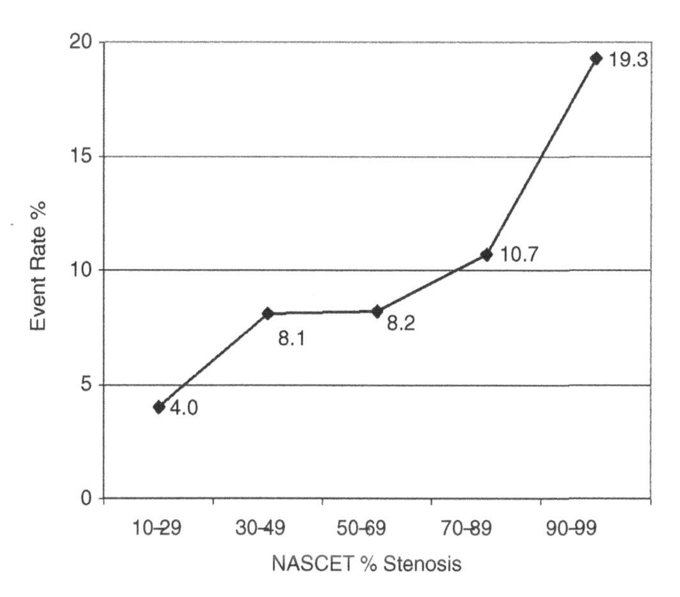

FIGURE 7–9. The incidence of ipsilateral ischemic hemispheric events in relation to the NASCET percentage stenosis of the internal carotid artery in the ACSRS study. (Reproduced from Nicolaides *et al.*, 2005. Eur J Vasc Endovasc Surg 30, 275–284, with permission.)

TABLE 7–6. The number of different ipsilateral ischemic hemispheric neurological events in relation to less than 60% and 60–99% NASCET internal carotid artery stenosis (chi square 4.6; $p = 0.21$).[a]

% NASCET stenosis	AF	TIA	Stroke	All events	All patients
<60	6 (1.2%)	15 (3.0%)	16 (3.2%)	37 (7.4%)	499
60–99	12 (1.9%)	29 (4.6%)	30 (4.7%)	71 (11.2%)	636
Total	18 (1.6%)	44 (3.9%)	46 (4.1%)	108 (9.7%)	1115

[a]AF, amaurosis fugax; TIAs, transient ischemic attacks.

Plaque Type and Risk

As pointed out above, most natural history studies performed in the past have used different methods of plaque classification without prior image normalization. It is now realized that image normalization results in marked change in the appearance of plaques with reclassification of a large number. The relationship between plaque classification before image normalization and after image normalization in patients admitted to the ACSRS study is shown in Table 7–7.[85] Before image normalization 131 plaques were classified as type 1, 288 as type 2, 319 as type 3, 166 as type 4, and 188 as type 5. It can be seen that after image normalization 66% of type 1, 49% of type 2, 46% of type 3, 66% of type 4, and 82% of type 5 were reclassified as a different plaque type (kappa statistic 0.22) demonstrating that there was a poor agreement between plaque classification before and after image normalization. After image normalization 652 (60%) of the plaques changed category. This marked change in plaque category is found in all plaque types including type 5. Before image normalization plaques with a calcified cap that had more than 15% of the plaque obscured by an acoustic shadow were classified as type 5. After image normalization the area of plaque adjacent to the calcification and acoustic shadow could be seen and outlined more easily in relation to blood. This area changed considerably in many plaques and explains why a large number of plaques initially classified as type 5 changed to type 4, 3, and even 2 after image normalization (Table 7–7).

The ipsilateral neurological events (amaurosis fugax, TIAs, and stroke) that occurred in the ACSRS study during follow-up in patients with different types of plaque before and after image normalization are shown in Tables 7–8 and 7–9, respectively. It can be seen that after image normalization the incidence of events in relation to different plaque types has changed. After image normalization there was a decreased incidence in patients with plaque types 4 and 5 with the vast majority of events occurring in plaque types 1, 2, and 3. Before image normalization only 82 (71%) of the 116 neurological events occurred in plaque types 1–3, but after image normalization the number increased to 109 (94%).

When plaque types 1–3 are compared with plaque types 4 and 5 before image normalization the relative risk of having an event is 1.12 (95% CI 0.76 to 1.66) (chi square, $p = 0.45$). Also, 37 (73%) of the 51 ischemic strokes have occurred in patients with plaque types 1–3 (Table 7–8). When plaque types 1–3 are compared with plaque types 4 and 5 after image normalization the relative risk of having an event is 4.8 (95% CI 2.27–10.28) (chi square, $p = 0.0001$). Also, 49 (96%) of the 51 ischemic strokes have occurred in patients with plaque types 1–3 (Table 7–9).

When echolucent plaques (types 1 and 2) are compared with echogenic (types 3 and 4) plaques the incidence of ipsilateral neurological events is 61 (14.9%) out of 409 in the former and 53 (8.3%) out of 635 in the latter (Table 7–9) (RR 1.6 95% CI 1.16–2.32) (chi square, $p = 0.003$).

TABLE 7–7. The relationship between plaque classification before and after image normalization (kappa = 0.22).

Plaque type before image normalization	Plaque type after image normalization					
	1	2	3	4	5	Total
1	44 (34%)	54 (41%)	22 (17%)	11 (7%)	0	131 (100%)
2	23 (8%)	148 (51%)	97 (34%)	16 (6%)	4 (1.4%)	288 (100%)
3	10 (3%)	68 (21%)	173 (54%)	54 (17%)	14 (4%)	319 (100%)
4	0	35 (21%)	62 (37%)	57 (34%)	12 (7%)	166 (100%)
5	0	27 (19%)	96 (51%)	47 (25%)	18 (10%)	188 (100%)
Total	77 (7%)	332 (31%)	450 (41%)	185 (17%)	48 (6%)	1092 (100%)

TABLE 7–8. The ipsilateral AF, TIAs, and strokes that occurred during follow-up in patients with different types of plaque before image normalization.[a]

Plaque type	Events absent	AF	TIAs	Stroke	All events	Total
1	125 (95.4%)	1 (0.8%)	4 (3.1%)	1 (0.8%)	6 (4.6%)	131 (100%)
2	243 (84.4%)	3 (1.0%)	19 (6.6%)	23 (8.0%)	45 (15.6%)	288 (100%)
3	288 (90.3%)	5 (1.6%)	13 (4.0%)	13 (4.0%)	31 (9.7%)	319 (100%)
4	146 (88.0%)	6 (3.6%)	4 (2.4%)	10 (6.0%)	20 (12%)	166 (100%)
5	174 (92.5%)	4 (2.1%)	6 (3.2%)	4 (2.6%)	14 (7.5%)	188 (100%)
Total	976 (89.4%)	19 (1.7%)	46 (4.2%)	51 (4.7%)	116 (10.6%)	1092 (100%)

[a]AF, amaurosis fugax; TIAs, transient ischemic attacks.

When heterogeneous plaques (types 2 and 3) are compared with homogeneous plaques (types 1 and 4) the incidence of ipsilateral neurological events is 102 (13%) out of 782 in the former and 12 (4.6%) out of 262 in the latter (Table 7–5) (RR 2.8 95% CI 1.59–5.10) (chi square, $p = 0.0001$).

Before image normalization the ipsilateral neurological event rate was high in all plaque types (Table 7–8). After image normalization the event rate was high in plaque types 1–3 and low in types 4 and 5 (Table 7–9). This justifies grouping plaques 1–3 as high risk and 4 and 5 as low risk (see below).

Several research teams have indicated that the risk for stroke is higher with echolucent plaques (types 1 and 2) when compared with echogenic plaques (types 3 and 4) (Table 7–2). Others have claimed that heterogeneous plaques are associated with a higher risk for stroke than homogeneous plaques (Table 7–2). As pointed out earlier the results of the ACSRS study are compatible with both findings. This is because type 2 plaques that are associated with the highest stroke risk (Table 7–9) are included by most authors in both the echolucent and heterogeneous groups. The low risk associated with type 4 plaques can be explained by the fact that these plaques contain a large amount of collagen that is uniformly distributed, giving them stability. With decreasing amounts of collagen that is not uniformly distributed, the plaques may become increasingly unstable reaching a maximum risk in type 2 plaques that have a large lipid core and relatively little unevenly distributed collagen. It is now believed that type 2 and 3 plaques are unstable and tend to rupture because they are of nonuniform consistency and have nonuniform stresses within them during each pulsation. This is in contrast to type 1 plaques that have a uniform consistency and tend to progress without early rupture presenting with symptoms only when the stenosis becomes severe.[48]

Plaque Type, Stenosis, and Risk

The relationship between plaque type, stroke, and ipsilateral internal carotid stenosis (mild, moderate, and severe) has been explored in the ACSRS natural history study.[85] In this study the relationship between stenosis expressed as percentage stenosis of the bulb (ECST method) and stroke is shown in Figure 7–10. As in all other natural history studies the stroke rate increases with increasing degrees of internal carotid stenosis.

Table 7–10 shows the incidence of ipsilateral ischemic stroke in relation to both plaque type and severity of stenosis. For stenosis in the 50–69% range the incidence of stroke is low irrespective of plaque type (Table 7–10: cells a and e). For stenosis in the 70–89% range the stroke rate was 5.7% in patients with plaque types 1–3 and 0.8% in patients with plaque types 4 and 5 (Table 7–10: cells b and f). For stenosis in the 90–99% range the stroke rate is 7.7% in patients with plaque types 1–3 and zero in patients with plaque types 4 and 5 (Table 7–10: cells c and g).

TABLE 7–9. The ipsilateral AF, TIAs, and strokes that occurred during follow-up in patients with different types of plaque after image normalization.[a]

Plaque type	Events absent	AF	TIAs	Stroke	All events	Total
1	70 (91.0%)	2 (2.6%)	1 (1.3%)	4 (5.2%)	7 (9.1%)	77 (100%)
2	278 (84.1%)	7 (2.1%)	23 (6.7%)	24 (7.1%)	54 (15.9%)	332 (100%)
3	419 (93.1%)	10 (2.2%)	17 (3.8%)	21 (4.7%)	48 (10.7%)	450 (100%)
4	180 (97.3%)	0	3 (1.6%)	2 (1.1%)	5 (2.7%)	185 (100%)
5	46 (95.8%)	0	2 (4.2%)	0	2 (4.2%)	48 (100%)
Total	976 (89.4%)	19 (1.7%)	46 (4.2%)	51 (4.7%)	116 (10.6%)	1092 (100%)

[a]AF, amaurosis fugax; TIAs, transient ischemic attacks.

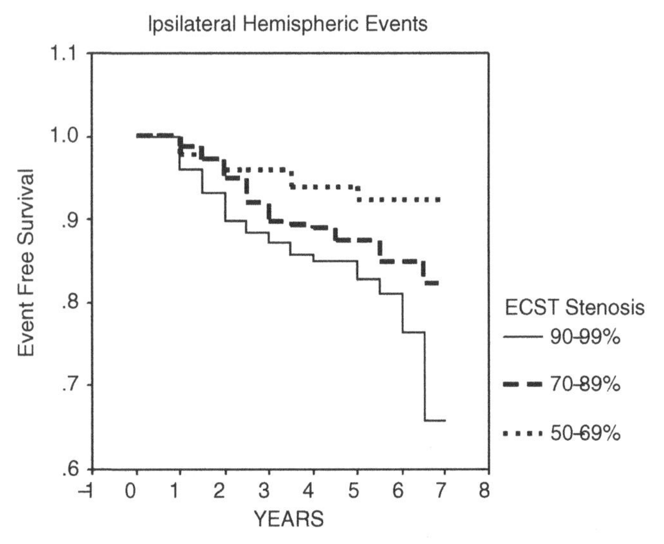

FIGURE 7–10. The ipsilateral hemispheric event-free cumulative survival rate in relation to the ECST percentage stenosis of the internal carotid artery (50–69% group: n = 101; 70–89% group: n = 593; 90–99% group: n = 328). Overall log rank: 11.7, p = 0.0026; 50–69 vs. 70–89%, p = 0.045; 70–89 vs. 90–99%, p = 0.020; 50–69 vs. 90–99%, p = 0.0014. (Reproduced from Nicolaides *et al.,* 2005. Eur J Vasc Endovasc Surg 30, 275–284, with permission.)

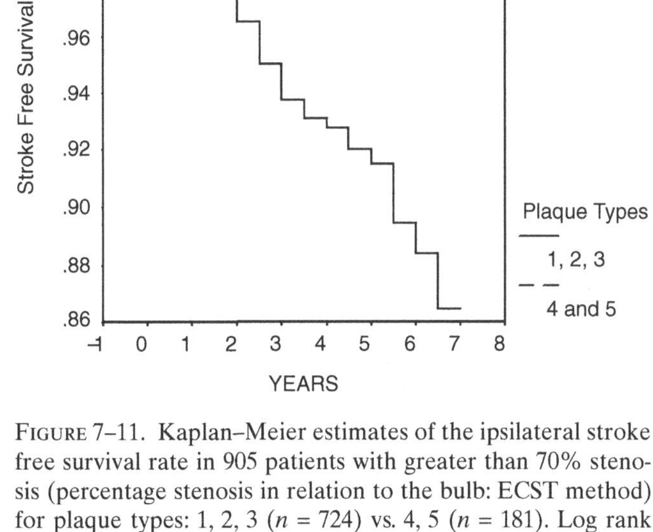

FIGURE 7–11. Kaplan–Meier estimates of the ipsilateral stroke free survival rate in 905 patients with greater than 70% stenosis (percentage stenosis in relation to the bulb: ECST method) for plaque types: 1, 2, 3 (n = 724) vs. 4, 5 (n = 181). Log rank p = 0.0028. (Reproduced from Nicolaides *et al.,* 2005. Vascular 13, 211–221, with permission.)

Thus, for the 905 patients with stenosis in the range of 70–99% (cells b, c, f, and g in Table 7–10) the incidence of stroke was (47/724) 6.5% (cells b and c) in plaque types 1, 2, and 3 and only (1/181) 0.55% (cells f and g) in plaque types 4 and 5 (RR 11.7 with 95% CI 1.63–84.5) (chi square with Yates correction 9.0; p = 0.003). The cumulative stroke-free survival rate in these 905 patients with greater than 70% stenosis for plaque types 1–3 and 4 and 5 is shown in Figure 7–11. For patients with plaque types 1–3 the cumulative stroke rate is 14% at 7 years (2% per year) and for patients with plaque types 4 and 5 the cumulative event rate is 1% at 7 years (0.14% per year).

The results of the ACSRS study indicate that for asymptomatic patients with internal carotid stenosis less than 70%, the annual risk of stroke is low (1.6%) irrespective of plaque type (Table 7–10). It is 4.6% for grades of stenoses 70–89% and 6.5% for 90–99%. The incidence of stroke in the ACSRS study is also very low (0.9%) for plaque types 4 and 5 irrespective of the degree of stenosis and increases to 5.7% with plaque types 1–3. Thus, it appears that the lesions that are associated with greater than 70% stenosis that are types 1–3 (cells b and c in Table 7–6) (RR 11.7 with 95% CI 1.63–84.5) identify a higher risk group. This higher risk group has a cumulative annual stroke rate of 2% per year in contrast to plaques types 4 and 5 producing greater than 70% stenosis that have a cumulative annual stroke rate of 0.14% per year (Figure 7–11).

The results of the ACAS randomized controlled trial[71] have suggested that surgery is beneficial in those patients who have an asymptomatic greater than 60% internal

TABLE 7–10. The incidence of ipsilateral ischemic stroke in relation to plaque type after image normalization and severity of stenosis.

Plaque type after image normalization	Grade of stenosis (ECST)			
	50–69%	70–89%	90–99%	Total
1, 2 and 3	2/135 (1.5%) a	26/453 (5.7%) b	21/271 (7.7%) c	**49/859 (5.7%) d**
4 and 5	1/52 (1.9%) e	1/129 (0.8%) f	0/52 g	**2/235 (0.9%) h**
Total	**3/187 (1.6%) i**	**27/582 (4.6%) j**	**21/323 (6.5%) k**	**51/1092 (4.7%) l**

carotid stenosis as measured by the NASCET method, which is equivalent to 77% ECST stenosis (Table 7–7). Similar results have been produced by the ACST randomized controlled study,[83] but in the publication of the latter study it has not been stated whether the cut-off point of 70% stenosis based on duplex is meant to be in relation to the distal internal carotid (NASCET method) or the bulb (ECST method). Plaque characterization was not performed in the ACAS study. Plaque classification into echolucent or echogenic plaques was attempted in the ACST study but no significant difference was found. In the ACST study plaque classification was performed locally without image normalization and without recording of images for assessment at the coordinating center and for enhanced quality control.

The results of the ACSRS study suggest that asymptomatic patients with plaque types 4 and 5 classified as such after image normalization and taking into consideration not only the calcified area but also the area of the plaque adjacent to the calcification not affected by acoustic shadow are at low risk even when they produce a severe stenosis. In the ACSRS study 181 (20%) of the 905 plaques with greater than 70% ECST stenosis fell into this category (Table 7–10). Also, patients with plaque types 1–3 with ECST stenosis in the range of 70–83%, which is approximately equivalent to 50–70% NASCET, are at increased risk and may need prophylactic carotid endarterectomy.

Texture Features Other Than Grayscale Median

With the exception of GSM, very few studies have investigated the association between textural features of carotid plaque ultrasonic images and patient symptoms.[86–88] The use of a GSM cut-off point of 40, by demonstrating an odds ratio of approximately four, has achieved only partial separation of symptomatic from asymptomatic carotid plaques.[89] Thus, it has been suggested that the additional use of textural features might improve the identification of high-risk plaques.[90,91] Ultrasonic texture characterization using computer algorithms has been successfully applied to liver images.[92,93]

Several of the texture features offered by the fifth module of the image analysis software have been found to be associated with plaques of different symptomatology. Many of these features measure similar parameters and good results have been obtained with several combinations. One example is given below. The value of these texture features was tested in a cross-sectional study of 409 patients referred to the vascular laboratory for diagnostic duplex scanning. Of these 242 were asymptomatic, 40 presented with amaurosis fugax, 72 with TIAs, and 55 with stroke. Plaques were classified into three main groups (Figure 7–12) on the basis of image normalization and six features, two (homogeneity and angular second movement) based on the spatial gray level dependence matrix method (SGLDM), Runlength-SRE, plaque type (1–5), GSM, and black area close to the lumen using discriminant function analysis. Black area close to the lumen was defined as an area with gray scale pixels in the range of 0–25 that is greater than 15% of the total plaque area. The discriminant function classified plaques into three groups (Figure 7–12). The group on the left in Figure 7–12 consisted of asymptomatic plaques, the group at the top of plaques that were asymptomatic or were associated with TIAs or stroke, and the group at the bottom right of plaques that were asymptomatic or associated with amaurosis fugax. It can be argued that because all plaques start by being asymptomatic, it is very likely that the group at the top of the figure is that of unstable plaques that tend to produce TIAs or stroke. Similar arguments can be produced for the other groups. This methodology is being tested in the ACSRS natural history study and features shown to be associated with symptomatic plaques in the cross-sectional study above are proving to be good predictors of stroke.

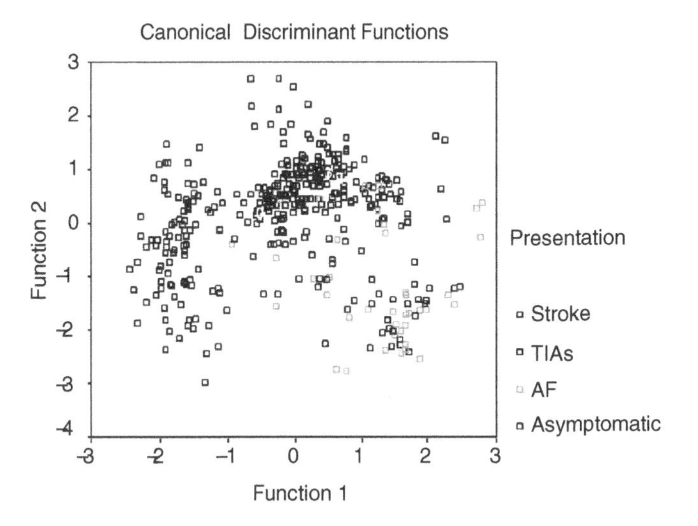

FIGURE 7–12. Discriminant function analysis of 409 plaques after image normalization (242 asymptomatic, 40 presenting with AF, 72 with TIAs, and 55 with stroke and good recovery). Three main groups of plaques are displayed.

Schulte-Altedorneburg reported that thrombosis at the plaque surface was often seen in "completely echolucent" plaques ($p < 0.001$).[94] It is likely that the echolucent plaque component represents the thrombus or its combination with the lipid core. A recent study has demonstrated a strong association between symptomatic plaques and intraluminal thrombus attached to the plaque.[95] It may well be that the presence of a black area adjacent to the lumen identifies many plaques associated with thrombus formation. This needs to be tested in future studies.

Table 7–11. The incidence of ipsilateral ischemic hemispheric events in relation to black area near the lumen after image normalization and severity of stenosis in the first 1098 patients admitted to the ACSRS.

		Black area adjacent to lumen				
		Absent		Present		
Stenosis	Number	Events	No events	Events	No events	OR (95% CI)
50–69%	304	5 (3.4%)	140	18 (11%)	141	3.57 (1.29 to 9.89)
70–89%	655	6 (2.2%)	260	61 (16%)	328	8.10 (3.43 to 18.93)
90–99%	139	2 (4.6%)	41	25 (26%)	71	7.21 (1.62 to 32.05)

Future Perspectives—The Asymptomatic Carotid Stenosis and Risk of Stroke Study

The methodology of computer-assisted carotid plaque characterization after image normalization is now being applied in a prospective multicenter international natural history study of asymptomatic carotid stenosis with stroke as the primary end-point. The aim of the ACSRS study[84,85,95] is to identify a high-risk subgroup that has an ipsilateral stroke rate greater than 4% (ideally greater than 7%), based on clinical risk factors and the findings of the non-invasive investigations, mainly ultrasonic carotid plaque characterization (echodensity and texture) in addition to degree of stenosis. In addition, a low-risk subgroup with an ipsilateral stroke rate of less than 1% should be identified.

The ACSRS study is still in progress and the results of texture analysis of plaques have not yet been published. Only preliminary analyses with limited resuls are available.

As indicated above a number of texture features can be used in the successful identification of a high-risk group.[96–98] One of the most powerful features is the presence of a black area adjacent to the lumen. This feature has been suggested by Pedro *et al.*[99] and has also been shown to be associated with symptomatic plaques in the author's cross-sectional study (Figure 7–12). When applied to the ACSRS study this feature alone can identify a high-risk group for symptoms (Table 7–11). The increased risk is present across all grades of stenosis (Figures 7–13–7–15).

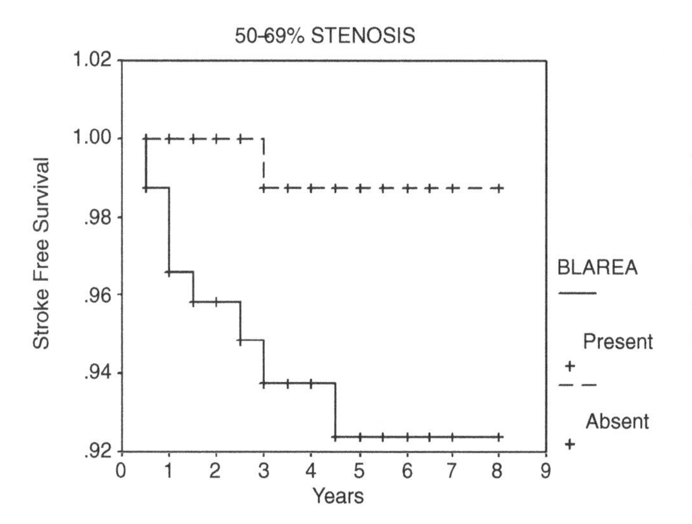

Figure 7–13. Kaplan–Meier estimates of the ipsilateral stroke free survival rate in patients admitted to the ACSRS study with 50–69 ECST percentage stenosis for plaques with ($n = 159$) and without ($n = 145$) a black area adjacent to the lumen after image normalization. Log rank $p = 0.018$.

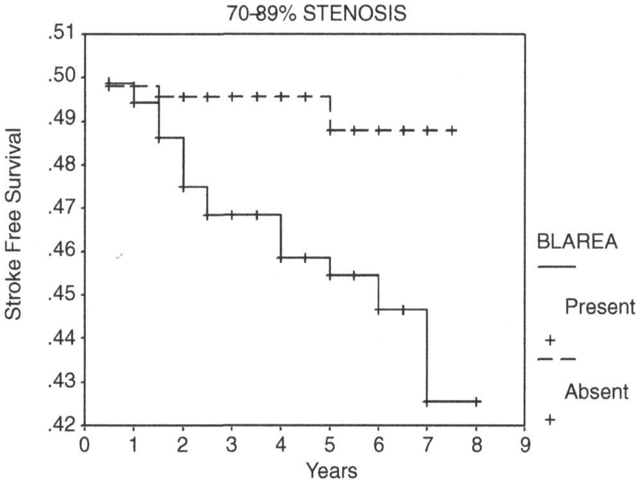

Figure 7–14. Kaplan–Meier estimates of the ipsilateral stroke free survival rate in patients admitted to the ACSRS study with 70–89 ECST percentage stenosis for plaques with ($n = 389$) and without ($n = 266$) a black area adjacent to the lumen after image normalization. Log rank $p = 0.002$.

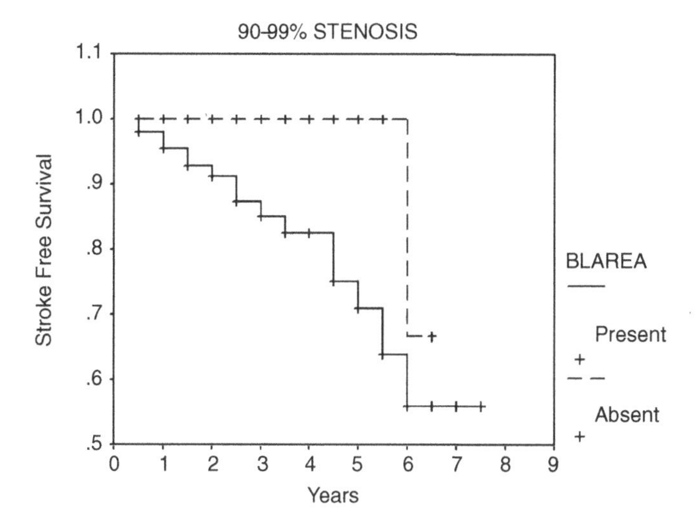

FIGURE 7-15. Kaplan–Meier estimates of the ipsilateral stroke free survival rate in patients admitted to the ACSRS study with 90–99 ECST percentage stenosis for plaques with ($n = 112$) and without ($n = 43$) a black area adjacent to the lumen after image normalization. Log rank $p = 0.02$.

Conclusions

Ultrasound, apart from being a valuable diagnostic tool, provides useful information on the natural history of carotid artery atherosclerosis. The high resolution of modern equipment and our ability to normalize images have provided the basis for reproducible plaque characterization features that can identify unstable plaques. The identification of a high-risk group of patients based on ultrasound features other than stenosis is becoming a reality. It should lead to a better selection of patients for carotid endarterectomy. Innovations such as algorithms and software identifying patients at high risk for stroke are expected to become available on duplex scanners in the near future.

References

1. Libby P. Molecular basis of acute coronary syndromes. Circulation 1995;91:2844–2850.
2. Clinton S, Underwood R, Hayes L, *et al.* Macrophage-colony stimulating factor gene expression in vascular cells and human atherosclerosis. Am J Pathol 1992;140:301–316.
3. Davies MJ, Richardson PD, Woolf N, Katz DR, Mahn J. Risk of thrombosis in human atherosclerotic plaques: Role of extracellular lipid, macrophage and smooth muscle cell content. Br Heart J 1993;69:377–381.
4. Falk E. Why do plaques rupture. Circulation 1992;86(6): 30–42.
5. Glagov S, Bassiouny HS, Sakaguchi Y, Goudet CA, Vito RP. Mechanical determinants of plaque modeling, remodeling and disruption. Atherosclerosis 1997;131:3–4.
6. Shah PK. Role of inflammation and metalloproteinases in plaque disruption and thrombosis. Vasc Med 1998;3: 199–206.
7. Golledge J, Greenhalgh RM, Davies AH. The symptomatic carotid plaque. Stroke 2000;31(3):774–781.
8. Shah PK. Pathophysiology of plaque rupture and the concept of plaque stabilization. Cardiol Clin 1996;14(1): 17–29.
9. Muller WD, Faust M, Kotzka J, Krone W. Mechanisms of plaque stabilization. Herz 1999;24:26–31.
10. Rabbani R, Topol EJ. Strategies to achieve coronary arterial plaque stabilization. Cardiovasc Res 1999;41:402–417.
11. Geroulakos G, Ramaswami G, Nicolaides A, James K, Labropoulos N, Belcaro G, Holloway M. Characterisation of symptomatic and asymptomatic carotid plaques using high-resolution real time ultrasonography. Br J Surg 1993; 80:1274–1277.
12. Sabetai MM, Tegos TJ, Nicolaides AN, *et al.* Hemispheric symptoms and carotid plaque echomorphology. J Vasc Surg 2000;31:39–49.
13. Tegos TJ, Sabetai MM, Nicolaides AN, El-Atrozy TS, Dhanjil S, Stevens JM. Patterns of brain computed tomography infarction and carotid plaque echogenicity. J Vasc Surg 2001;33:334–339.
14. Belcaro G, Nicolaides AN, Laurora G, *et al.* Ultrasound morphology classification of the arterial wall and cardiovascular events in a 6-year follow-up study. Arterioscler Thromb Vasc Biol 1996;16:851–856.
15. Reilly LM, Lusby RJ, Hughes L, Ferrell LD, Stoney RJ, Ehrenfeld WK. Carotid plaque histology using real-time ultrasonography: Clinical and therapeutic implications. Am J Surg 1983;146:188–193.
16. O'Donnell TF Jr, Erdoes L, Mackey WC, Mc Cullough J, Shepard A, Heggerick P, Isner J, Callow AD. Correlation of B-mode ultrasound imaging and arteriography with pathologic findings at carotid endarterectomy. Arch Surg 1985; 120:443–449.
17. Johnson JM, Kennelly MM, Decesare D, Morgan S, Sparrow A. Natural history of asymptomatic carotid plaque. Arch Surg 1985;120:1010–1012.
18. O'Holleran LW, Kennelly MM, Decesare D, McClurken M, Johnson JM. Natural history of asymptomatic carotid plaque. Five year follow-up study. Am J Surg 1987;154: 659–662.
19. Widder B, Paulat K, Hachspacher J, *et al.* Morphological characterization of carotid artery stenoses by ultrasound duplex scanning. Ultrasound Med Biol 1990;16:349–354.
20. Gray-Weale AC, Graham JC, Burnett JR, Burne K, Lusby RJ. Carotid artery atheroma: Comparison of preoperative B-mode ultrasound appearance with carotid endarterectomy specimen pathology. J Cardiovasc Surg 1988;29: 676–681.
21. deBray JM, Baud JM, Dauzat M for the Consensus Conference. Concensus on the morphology of carotid plaques. Cerebrovasc Dis 1997;7:289–296.
22. Polak JF, Shemanski L, O'Leary DH, *et al.* for the Cardiovascular Health Study. Hypoechoic plaque at US of the carotid artery: An independent risk factor for incident stroke in adults aged 65 years or older. Radiology 1998; 208:649–654.

23. Wolverson MK, Bashiti HM, Peterson GJ. Ultrasonic tissue characterization of atheromatous plaques using a high resolution real time scanner. Ultrasound Med Biol 1983; 9:599–609.
24. Aldoori MI, Baird RN, Al-Sam SZ, *et al.* Duplex scanning and plaque histology in cerebral ischaemia. Eur J Vasc Surg 1987;1:159–164.
25. Sterpetti AV, Schultz RD, Feldhaus RJ, *et al.* Ultrasonographic features of carotid plaque and the risk of subsequent neurologic deficits. Surgery 1988;104:652–660.
26. Langsfeld M, Gray-Weale AC, Lusby RJ. The role of plaque morphology and diameter reduction in the development of new symptoms in asymptomatic carotid arteries. J Vasc Surg 1989;9:548–557.
27. Bock RW, Gray-Weale AC, Mock PA, Robinson DA, Irwig L, Lusby RJ. The natural history of asymptomatic carotid artery disease. J Vasc Surg 1993;17:160–171.
28. Mathiesen EB, Bønaa KH, Joakimsen O. Echolucent plaques are associated with high risk of ischemic cerebrovascular events in carotid stenosis. The Tromsø Study. Circulation 2001;103:2171–2175.
29. Grønholdt M-LM, Nordestgaard BG, Schroeder TV, Vorstrup S, Sillesen H. Ultrasonic echolucent carotid plaques predict future strokes. Circulation 2001;104:68–73.
30. Liapis CD, Kakisis JD, Kostakis AG. Carotid stenosis. Factors affecting symptomatology. Stroke 2001;32:2782–2786.
31. AbuRahma AF, Kyer PD III, Robinson PA, Hannay RS. The correlation of ultrasonic carotid plaque morphology and carotid plaque hemmorhage: Clinical implications. Surgery 1998;124:721–728.
32. Carra G, Visona A, Bonanome A, Lusiani L, Pesavento R, Bortolon M, Pagnan A. Carotid plaque morphology and cerebrovascular events. Int Angiol 2003;22:284–289.
33. Thiele BL, Jones AM, Hobson RW, Bandyk DF, Baker WH, Sumner DS, Rutherford RB. Standards in non-invasive cerebrovascular testing. Report from the committee on standards for non-invasive vascular testing of the Joint Council of the Society for Vascular Surgery and the North American Chapter of the International Society for Cardiovascular Surgery. J Vasc Surg 1992;15:995–1003.
34. Fisher CM, Ojemann RG. A clinicopathologic study of carotid endarterectomy plaques. Rev Neurol (Paris) 1986; 142:573–576.
35. Bluth EI, Kay D, Merritt CR, *et al.* Sonographic characterization of carotid plaque: detection of hemorrhage. Am J Roentgenol 1986;146:1061–1065.
36. Bendick PJ, Glover JL, Hankin R, *et al.* Carotid plaque morphology: Correlation of duplex sonography with histology. Ann Vasc Surg 1988;2:6–13.
37. Van Damme H, Trotteur G, Vivario M, *et al.* Echographic characterization of carotid plaques. Acta Chir Belg 1993; 93:233–238.
38. Kardoulas DG, Katsamouris AN, Gallis PT, *et al.* Ultrasonographic and histologic characteristics of symptom-free and symptomatic carotid plaque. Cardiovasc Surg 1996;4: 580–590.
39. European Carotid Plaque Study Group. Carotid artery plaque composition—Relationship to clinical presentation and ultrasound B-mode imaging. Eur J Vasc Endovasc Surg 1995;10:23–30.
40. Weinberger J, Marks SJ, Gaul JJ, *et al.* Atherosclerotic plaque at the carotid artery bifurcation. Correlation of ultrasonographic imaging with morphology. J Ultrasound Med 1987;6:363–366.
41. Shah PK, Falk E, Badimon JJ, *et al.* Human monocyte-derived macrophages induce collagen breakdown in fibrous caps of atherosclerotic plaques. Potential role of matrix degrting metaloproteinases and implications for plaque rapture. Circulation 1995;92:1565–1569.
42. Lammie GA, Wardlaw J, Allan P, *et al.* What pathological components indicate carotid atheroma activity and can these be identified reliably using ultrasound? Eur J Ultrasound 2000;11:77–86.
43. Urbano LA, Perren F, Rossetti AO, *et al.* Thrombus in the internal carotid artery complicating an "unstable" atheromatous plaque. Circulation 2003;107:e19–20.
44. El-Barghouty NM, Nicolaides A, Bahal V, Geroulakos G, Androulakis A. The identification of high risk carotid plaque. Eur J Vasc Surg 1996;11:470–478.
45. Biasi GM, Sampaolo A, Mingazzini P, de Amicis P, El-Barghouti N, Nicolaides AN. Computer analysis of ultrasonic plaque echolucency in identifying high risk carotid bifurcation lesions. Eur J Vasc Endovasc Surg 1999;17:476–479.
46. El-Atrozy T, Nicolaides A, Tegos T, Zarka AZ, Griffin M, Sabetai M. The effect of B-mode image standardisation on the echodensity of symptomatic and asymptomatic carotid bifurcation plaques. Int Angiol 1998;17:179–186.
47. Tegos TJ, Sabetai MM, Nicolaides AN, *et al.* Comparability of the ultrasonic tissue characteristics of carotid plaques. J Ultrasound Med 2000;14:399–407.
48. Sabetai MM, Tegos TJ, Nicolaides AN, Dhanjil S, Pare GJ, Stevens JM. Reproducibility of computer-quantified carotid plaque echogenicity. Stroke 2000;31:2189–2196.
49. Tegos TJ, Sabetai MM, Nicolaides AN, *et al.* Correlates of embolic events detected by means of transcranial Doppler in patients with carotid atheroma. J Vasc Surg 2001;33:131–138.
50. Sabetai MM, Tegos TJ, Nicolaides AN, El-Atrozy TS, Dhanjil S, Griffin M, Belcaro G, Geroulakos G. Hemispheric symptoms and carotid plaque echomorphology. J Vasc Surg 2000;31:39–49.
51. Sabetai MS, Coker J, Sheppard M, Tegos T, Belcaro G, Stansby G, Nicolaides AN. The association of carotid plaque necrotic core volume and echogenicity with ipsilateral hemispheric symptoms. Circulation 2001;104(Suppl 2):671 (abst).
52. Gronholdt M-LM, Nordestgaard BG, Bentzon J, Wiebe BM, Zhou J, Falk E, Sillesen H. Macrophages are associated with lipid-rich carotid artery plaques, echolucency on B-mode imaging, and elevated plasma lipid levels. J Vasc Surg 2002;35:137–145.
53. Richardson PD, Davies MJ, Born GVR. Influence of plaque configuration and stress distribution and fissuring of coronary atherosclerotic plaque. Lancet 1989;ii:941–944.
54. Ku DN, McCord BN. Cyclic stress causes rupture of the atherosclerotic plaque cap. Circulation 1993;88(Suppl 1):1362 (abst).

55. Glagov S, Bassiouny HS, Sakaguchi Y, Goudet CA, Vito RP. Mechanical determinants of plaque modeling, remodeling and disruption. Atherosclerosis 1997; 131(Suppl):S13–S14.
56. Zukowski AJ, Nicolaides AN, Lewis RT, Mansfield AO, Williams MA, Helmis E, Malouf GM, Thomas D, Al-Kutoubi A, Kyprianou P, *et al.* The correlation between carotid plaque ulceration and cerebral infarction seen on CT scan. J Vasc Surg 1984;1:782–786.
57. Persson AV, Robichaux WT, Silverman M. The natural history of carotid plaque development. Arch Surg 1983;118:1048–1052.
58. Seager JM, Klingman N. The relationship between carotid plaque composition and neurological symptoms. J Surg Res 1987;43:78–85.
59. Sterpetti AV, Hunter WJ, Schulz RD. Importance of ulceration of carotid plaque. J Cardiovasc Surg 1991;32:154–158.
60. Eliasziw M, Streifler JY, Fox JA. Significance of plaque ulceration in symptomatic patients with high-grade stenosis. Stroke 1994;25:305–308.
61. Fisher GG, Anderson DC, Farber R, Lebow S. Prediction of carotid disease by ultrasound and digital subtraction angiography. Arch Neurol 1985;42:224–227.
62. O'Leary DH, Holen J, Ricotta JJ Roe S, Schenk EA. Carotid bifurcation disease: Prediction of ulceration with B-mode ultrasound. Radiology 1987;162:523–525.
63. Comerota AJ, Katz ML, White JV, Grosh JD. The preoperative diagnosis of the ulcerated carotid atheroma. J Vasc Surg 1990;11:505–510.
64. Farber R, Bromer M, Anderson D, Loewenson R, Yock D, Larson D. B-mode real-time ultrasonic carotid imaging: Impact on decision-making and prediction of surgical findings. Neurology 1984;34:541–544.
65. Ricotta JJ. Plaque characterization by B-mode scan. Surg Clin North Am 1990;70:191–199.
66. Goodson SF, Flanigan DP, Bishara RA, Schuler JJ, Kikta MJ, Meyer JP. Can carotid duplex scanning supplant arteriography in patients with focal carotid territory symptoms? J Vasc Surg 1987;5:551–557.
67. Rubin JR, Bondi JA, Rhodes RS. Duplex scanning versus conventional arteriography for the evaluation of carotid artery plaque morphology. Surgery 1987;102:749–755.
68. Iannuzzi A, Wilcosky T, Mercuri M, Rubba P, Bryan FA, Bond G. Ultrasonographic correlates of carotid atherosclerosis in transient ischemic attack and stroke. Stroke 1995;26:614–619.
69. Golledge J, Cuming R, Ellis M, Davies AH, Greenhalgh RM. Carotid plaque characteristics and presenting symptom. Br J Surg 1997;84:1697–1701.
70. North American Symptomatic Carotid Endarterectomy Trial Collaborators. Beneficial effect of carotid endarterectomy in symptomatic patients with high-grade carotid stenosis. N Engl J Med 1991;325:445–453.
71. Executive Committee for the Asymptomatic Carotid Atherosclerosis Study. Endarterectomy for asymptomatic carotid artery stenosis. J Am Med Assoc 1995;273:1421–1428.
72. Nicolaides AN, Shifrin EG, Bradbury A, Dhanjil S, Griffin M, Belcaro G, Williams M. Angiographic and duplex grading of internal carotid stenosis: Can we overcome the confusion? J Endovasc Surg 1996;3:158–165.
73. European Carotid Surgery Trialists Collaborative Group. MRC European carotid surgery trial: Interim results for symptomatic patients with severe (70–99%) or with mild (0–29%) carotid stenosis. Lancet 1991;337:1235–1243.
74. De Bray JM, Glatt B. Quantification of atheromatous stenosis in the extracranial internal carotid artery. Cerebrovasc Dis 1995;5:414–426.
75. Chambers BR, Norris JW. Outcome in patients with asymptomatic neck bruits. N Engl J Med 1986;315:860–865.
76. Hennericci M, Hulsbomer HB, Hefter H, Lammerts D, Rautenberg W. Natural history of asymptomatic extracranial arterial disease. Results of a long-term prospective study. Brain 1987;110:777–791.
77. Norris JW, Zhu CZ, Bornstein NM, Chambers BR. Vascular risks of asymptomatic carotid stenosis. Stroke 1991;22:1485–1490.
78. Zhu CZ, Norris JW. A therapeutic window for carotid endarterectomy in patients with asymptomatic carotid stenosis. Can J Surg 1991;34:437–440.
79. Mackey AE, Abrahamowicz M, Langlois Y, Battista R, Simard D, Bourque F, *et al.* Outcome of asymptomatic patients with carotid disease. Neurology 1997;48:896–903.
80. Nadareishvili ZG, Rothwell PM, Beletsky V, Pagniello A, Norris JW. Long-term risk of stroke and other vascular events in patients with asymptomatic carotid artery stenosis. Arch Neurol 2002;59:1162–1166.
81. The European Carotid Surgery Trialists Collaborative Group. Risk of stroke in the distribution of an asymptomatic carotid artery. Lancet 1995;345:209–212.
82. Inzitari D, Eliasziw M, Gates P, Sharpe BL, Chan RKT, Meldrum HE, *et al.* The causes and risk of stroke in patients with asymptomatic internal-carotid-artery stenosis. N Engl J Med 2000;342:1693–1700.
83. MRC Asymptomatic Carotid Surgery Trial (ACST) Collaborative Group. Prevention of disabling and fatal strokes by successful carotid endarterectomy in patients without recent neurological symptoms: Randomized controlled trial. Lancet 2004;363:1491–1502.
84. Nicolaides AN, Kakkos SK, Griffin M, Sabetai M, Dhanjil S, Tegos T, Thomas DJ, Giannoukas A, Geroulakos G, Georgiou N, Francis S, Ioannidou E, Dore CJ, and the Asymptomatic Carotid Stenosis and Risk of Stroke (ACSRS) Study Group. Severity of asymptomatic carotid stenosis and risk of ipsilateral hemispheric ischaemic events: Results from the ACSRS Study. Eur J Vasc Endovas Surg 2006;31:336.
85. Nicolaides A, Kakkos SK, Griffin M, Sabetai M, Dhanjil S, Thomas DJ, Geroulakos G, Georgiou N, Francis S, Ioannidou E, Doré CJ. Effect of image normalization on carotid plaque classification and risk of ipsilateral hemispheric events: Results from the ACSRS study. Vascular 2005;13:211–221.
86. Mazzone AM, Urbani MP, Picano E, Paterni M, Borgatti E, De Fabritiis A, *et al.* In vivo ultrasonic parametric imaging of carotid atherosclerotic plaque by video densitometric technique. Angiology 1995;46:663–672.

87. Elatrozy T, Nicolaides A, Tegos T, Griffin M. The objective characterisation of ultrasonic carotid plaque features. Eur J Vasc Endovasc Surg 1998;16:223–230.
88. Tegos TJ, Mavrophoros D, Sabetai MM, Elatrozy TS, Dhanjil S, Karapataki M, *et al.* Types of neurovascular symptoms and carotid plaque ultrasonic textural characteristics. J Ultrasound Med 2001;20:113–121.
89. Elatrozy T. Preoperative characterisation of carotid plaques. Ph.D. thesis. Imperial College, University of London, 2000.
90. Christodoulou CI, Pattichis CS, Pantziaris M, Tegos T, Nicolaides A, Elatrozy T, *et al.* Multi-feature texture analysis for the classification of carotid plaques. In: *IJCNN '99. Proceedings of International Joint Conference on Neural Networks,* 1999 July 10–16, Washington DC. 1999;5:3591–3596.
91. Kyriacou E, Pattichis MS, Christodoulou CI, Pattichis CS, Kakkos S, Griffin M, Nicolaides A. Ultrasound imaging in the analysis of carotid plaque morphology for the assessment of stroke. In: Suri JS, Yyan C, Wilson DL, Laxminarayan S (eds). *Advanced Plaque Imaging: Pixel to Molecular*. Studies in Health Technology and Informatics. IOS Press, 2005;113:241–75 (ISBN:1-58603-516-9).
92. Wu Q. Automatic tumor detection for MRI liver images. Ph.D. thesis. London, England: Imperial College, 1996;48–59.
93. Jirák D, Dezortová M, Tamir P, Hájek M. Texture analysis of human liver. J Magn Reson Imaging 2002;15:68–74.
94. Schulte-Altedorneburg G, Droste DW, Haas N, Kemeny V, Nabavi DG, Fuzesi L, Ringelstein EB. Preoperative B-mode ultrasound plaque appearance compared with carotid endarterectomy specimen histology. Acta Neurol Scand 2000;101:188–194.
95. Fisher M, Paganini-Hill A, Martin A, Cosgrove M, Toole JF, Barnett HJM, Norris J. Carotid plaque pathology. Thrombosis, ulceration and stroke pathogenesis. Stroke 2005;36: 253–257.
96. Nicolaides AN, Griffin M, Kakkos SK, Geroulakos G, Kyriakou E. In: Mansour MA, Labropoulos N (eds). *Evaluation of Carotid Plaque Morphology in Vascular Diagnosis*, pp. 131–148. Philadelphia: Elsevier Saunders, 2005.
97. Nicolaides AN. Asymptomatic carotid stensosis and risk of stroke. Identification of a high risk group (ACSRS). Int Angiol 1995;14:21–23.
98. Nicolaides A, Kakkos S, Sabetai M, Griffin M, Ioannidou E, Francis S, Kyriakou E. Asympomatic carotid stenosis and risk of stroke: Natural history study. Stroke 2005;36:424 (abst).
99. Pedro LM, Fernandes e Fernandes J, Pedro MM, Goncalves I, Dias NV, Fernandes e Fernandes R, Caneiro TF, Balsinha C. Ultrasonographic risk score of carotid plaques. Eur J Vasc Endovasc Surg 2002;24:492–498.

8 Carotid Plaque Echolucency Measured by Grayscale Median Identifies Patients at Increased Risk of Stroke during Carotid Stenting. The Imaging in Carotid Angioplasty and Risk of Stroke Study

A. Froio, G. Deleo, C. Piazzoni, V. Camesasca, A. Liloia, M. Lavitrano, and G. M. Biasi

Stenting of carotid artery disease has emerged as a potential alternative to carotid endarterectomy (CEA), the current gold standard treatment for carotid artery lesions.[1–4] After the initial experience with an unacceptably high rate of neurologic complications, the results have now improved, and, as a consequence, several trials have been planned to compare carotid angioplasty/stenting (CAS) with CEA.[5]

Even though it is generally accepted that the composition and the characteristics of the plaque may influence the outcome of CEA and CAS, especially in the case of CAS in which the plaque is not removed but remodeled, indications for either one of the two procedures are mostly based (both in trial and in clinical practice) on the percentage of stenosis and the presence or absence of preprocedural neurologic symptoms, whereas the features of the plaque are somehow disregarded if not ignored. The reason for this is related to the fact that the percentage of stenosis, as well as the presence or absence of symptoms, is easy to identify and quantify, whereas the plaque is usually defined as soft, lipidic, fibrolipidic, hemorrhagic, colliquated, ulcerated, pretty homogeneous, etc., which makes the parameter rather undetermined and unreliable.[6]

But the advent of high-resolution B-mode scanners and the use of a quantitative, computer-assisted index of echogenicity [such as grayscale median (GSM)] introduced by our team have greatly improved the correlation between plaque characterization and clinical features.[7, 8]

The aim of the Imaging in Carotid Angioplasty and Risk of Stroke (ICAROS) registry was to determine the preprocedural echographic criteria, which can identify the carotid plaque related to a higher risk of stroke during CAS so that a better selection of candidates for CAS may be made.[9,10]

Echographic Evaluation of Carotid Plaque

The study of carotid plaque morphology by ultrasonography, which usually relies on visual characterization based on subjective and qualitative evaluation of the B-mode images, has created controversies concerning the clinical importance of some characteristics of the plaque observed with duplex scan (i.e., ulceration or intraplaque hemorrhage and their correlation with the presence or absence of neurologic symptoms).[11]

Ulceration and hemorrhage are frequently defined according to subjective criteria, which is liable to create some confusion. Carr and colleagues demonstrated this because, in their study, they found both a significant and a nonsignificant correlation between neurologic symptoms and the presence of ulceration and hemorrhage, using different definitions of ulceration (gross ulceration versus microscopic ulceration: correlation only with gross ulceration; $p = 0.02$) and hemorrhage (plaque hemorrhage versus intraplaque hemorrhage: borderline correlation only with intraplaque hemorrhage; $p = 0.06$).[12] As a consequence of this, Greenhalgh wrote: "The fact that it has taken so long for plaque type to be shown to relate to stroke risk in asymptomatic severely stenosed carotid arteries can mean one of two things: it can mean plaque type never has and never will relate to stroke risk or second, that the precise combination of findings has not been clearly recognized."

To overcome the unreliability related to the morphologic characteristics of carotid plaques, we should keep in mind that echography means detection of echoes, that is, detection of echogenicity. Echography can reliably register areas with a lot of echoes (hyperechoic or echogenic) and areas with few echoes (hypoechoic or echolucent).

A.F. Aburahma, J.J. Bergan (eds.), *Noninvasive Cerebrovascular Diagnosis*, DOI 10.1007/978-1-84882-957-2_8,

Echogenicity could be assessed according to the Gray-Weale/Geroulakos classification.[13,14] Only through the advent of high-resolution B-mode scanners did a more reliable analysis of echogenicity became available.

Barnett and colleagues recently wrote: "Modern ultrasound done in well-equipped and closely supervised laboratories can distinguish between echodense (echogenic) and echolucent carotid lesions . . . however, such sophisticated technology did not exist when NASCET was launched in 1987; at that time it was an inadequate method to evaluate both the degree of stenosis and the nature of the carotid lesion causing the symptoms."[15]

The improvement in ultrasonography allowed several authors to assess the relationship between echogenicity and neurologic events. In the Cardiovascular Health Study, 4886 individuals aged 65 years or older without symptoms of cerebrovascular diseases were followed for an average of 3.3 years.[16] Hypoechoic plaques were associated with a risk of stroke. Liapis and colleagues found evidence that in a cohort of patients with carotid stenosis followed for an average of 3.6 years, the presence of echolucent plaques was related to the development of neurologic events.[17] Gronholdt and colleagues and Mathiesen and colleagues performed prospective studies to assess the relationship between plaque morphology and the risk of ischemic stroke.[18,19] In the Tromso Study, subjects with echolucent plaques have an increased risk of ischemic cerebrovascular events, independent of the degree of stenosis and cardiovascular risk factors. Gronholdt and colleagues found evidence that echolucent plaques causing greater than 50% stenosis are associated with a risk of future stroke. Thus, echolucency is now recognized as an important factor in determining future neurologic events.

Further improvement in carotid echographic evaluation has been achieved through the introduction of a computer-assisted *objective* grading of the echogenicity of carotid plaques, namely the GSM.

Grayscale Median Calculation

The GSM is a computer-assisted grading of the echogenicity of carotid plaques. It is a measure of overall plaque echogenicity, which is a quantitative index of the echoes registered from the plaque.

The following conditions are needed to ensure the reliability of the GSM.

Duplex Scanner Setup

Every duplex scanner makes it possible to collect images with the characteristics required for the computer-assisted analysis of echogenicity. For GSM calculation there are no unsuitable duplex scanners.

A 7-MHz linear array single or multifrequency transducer should be used. The dynamic range is the range in acoustic power (in decibels) between the faintest and the strongest signals that can be displayed on the screen. The decrease of the dynamic range increases the apparent contrast in the image. For GSM calculation the maximum dynamic range should be used in order to have the greatest possible display of gray scale values (grayer and flatter image).

The frame rate, which means the number of scannings that the probe does producing the images, must be positioned at the maximum level, ensuring good temporal resolution.

The persistence is the number of frames that are mathematically added to produce each image. Higher persistence tends to suppress noise, but it is always done at the expense of time resolution, and it may blur real targets. The persistence is displayed on the screen device as a series of numbers from 1 to 5 and the right persistence would be 2 or 3 (medium to low level).

A linear postprocessing curve is used because image normalization is achieved with linear scaling.

The overall gain should be increased until the plaque can be easily recognized and noise appears within the lumen. It should then be decreased to obtain a lumen free of noise (black).

The time gain compensation (TGC) curve is adjusted (gently sloping) with the aim of obtaining images where the far and near walls of the artery produce the same echogenicity. At the level of the arterial lumen no gains of the TGC curve must be done. This is essential for normalization of carotid plaques with anterior and posterior components. The consequence of this is that the ultrasound beam should be at 90° to the arterial wall, with a horizontal adventitia.

Image Recording

The patient should be in supine position. The carotid vessels are analyzed using different longitudinal views (anterolateral, lateral, and posterolateral). The minimum depth should be used, so that the plaque occupies a large part of the image. Excessive magnification is not required.

In case of acoustic shadow the image can be analyzed only if >50% of the area depicts acoustic information. The GSM cannot be calculated in plaques without any ultrasound information due to acoustic shadowing. The larger the section of plaque that can be visualized, the more accurate is the information provided by GSM.

Before image recording, the following criteria should be fulfilled:

1. Blood: a noiseless vessel lumen in the vicinity of the plaque.

2. Adventitia: in the proximity of the plaque it should be bright, thick, and horizontal.
3. Plaque: well defined and with the maximum thickness.
4. Anterior and posterior walls of the carotid artery should be visible.

The following images (in longitudinal projections) should be recorded:

1. The B-mode (grayscale) image.
2. The color image: may help in the delineation of the luminal margin of the plaque (especially with hypoechoic dark plaques).

Attention should be paid in order to have B-mode and color image in the same plane.

Digital storage media (magnetooptical disk and compact disk) are preferred to analogic video tape requiring a video grabber card.

Image Normalization and Grayscale Median Calculation

GSM is calculated using Adobe Photoshop (5.0 or higher).

In Adobe Photoshop both the B-mode and the color image should be open. In the B-mode image the color information should be discarded: from the "Image" menu, click on "Mode," then "Grayscale."

Using the "Lasso" tool, drag the pointer to outline the plaque. Then, click on "Histogram" in the "Image" menu. The "median" value shown in the panel is the GSM.

Hypoechoic dark (echolucent) regions are associated with a GSM that tended to approach 0, whereas hyperechoic bright (echogenic) regions are associated with a GSM that tended to approach 255.

The GSM calculated in this manner is not standardized and consequently the GSM is influenced by duplex scanner settings. The lack of reproducibility of nonstandardized GSM has been demonstrated by our group and by others: the GSM cut-off point for the identification of carotid plaques at increased risk of producing stroke was 50 in Milan and 32 in London.[7,20]

Normalization (standardization) allows comparison of images from different scanners by different ultrasonographers. Due to normalization, GSM is a highly reproducible index of echogenicity.

Image normalization is a grayscale transformation using linear scaling: grayscale values of all pixels in an image are adjusted according to two reference points, blood and adventitia. Blood and adventitia were selected (instead of muscles, vertebrae, intima-media complex, etc.) because they are easily and clearly recognizable in the vicinity of the plaque and constitute the two distinct ends of grayscale (blood = dark, adventitia = bright). The process modifies the image such that in the resultant image the GSM of the blood is in the range of 0–5 and the GSM of the adventitia in the range of 185–195.

Several steps are required for image normalization.

Using the "Lasso" tool, drag the pointer to select an area in the blood that should be free of noise. To check this, in the "Image" menu click on "Histogram." The "median" value shown in the panel is the GSM. The GSM of the selected area in the blood should be 0. If not, the gain of duplex scanner is not set properly (see above).

Similarly, using the "Lasso" tool, the brightest part of the adventitia on the same arterial wall of the plaque should be selected. It is important to note the following:

- Image magnification should be performed before adventitia outlining.
- The selected area should not be too small (area, not a point!).
- The selected area should be horizontal.

The GSM of adventitia should then be obtained using the "Histogram" function. Unlike the GSM of blood, every GSM value measured in the adventitia is accepted.

To normalize the image, click on "Image" menu then "Adjustments" and finally "Curves." The straight line shown in the panel represents the relationship between the grayscale of the input (x-axis) image and that of the output (y-axis). Each axis has a black and a white edge: this is the grayscale, ranging from 0 (completely black) to 255 (completely white).

The aim of normalization is to modify the subjectivity related to the echographic examination. This purpose can be achieved using the brightest (adventitia) and the faintest (blood) area of the image: in particular conditions (the duplex scanner settings described above) these areas are independent of the type of duplex scanner and the ultrasonographer. Normalizing the image the faintest point remains unchanged with a GSM value of 0 before and 0 after standardization (a proper gain adjustment is essential for this purpose). On the other hand, the GSM value of the brightest area (adventitia) drives all the normalization process: the adventitial GSM value measured before (input value) is converted arbitrarily to a GSM value of 190 (output value). In the normalized image the GSM value of blood and adventitia is 0 and 190, respectively, independent of the type of duplex scanner and the ultrasonographer.

In Adobe Photoshop, the straight line shown in the panel should be modified so that the new line crosses a new point with the input value corresponding to the measured adventitial GSM value and the output value corresponding to 190.

The image is now standardized. Using the "Lasso" tool the plaque should be outlined. In the "Histogram" panel the following measurements are obtained:

1. GSM, defined as the median of overall gray shades of the pixels in the plaque.

2. Total percentage of echolucent pixels, defined as the percentage of pixels with GSM < 25 (PEP25).

The reproducibility of this method is high.[21,22]

If you need help in measuring the GSM, please feel free to contact us at gsm@unimib.org.

Embolic Burden and Stroke Risk in Carotid Stenting

The embolic risk during CAS is well documented. Markus and colleagues showed that, during angioplasty, multiple embolic signals were detected immediately after balloon inflation in 90% of cases. Embolic signals were common immediately after the procedure (80% of cases) but thereafter became less frequent.[23]

Coggia and colleagues developed an *ex vivo* human model to study the embolic potential of carotid bifurcation angioplasty and stenting. The studies showed that carotid angioplasty and stenting generate embolic particles after each stage of the procedure and that the size of most embolic particles generated was less than 120 µm, with many platelet or cholesterol microthrombi. The maximum size of particles detected in the last phase, i.e., during the balloon angioplasty, was between 1000 and 2100 µm.[24]

Jordan and colleagues showed that CAS, compared with CEA, is accomplished with more than eight times the rate of microemboli when evaluated with transcranial Doppler ultrasonography (8.8 versus 74.0; $p = 0.0001$).[25]

Ohki and colleagues showed that echolucent plaques ($p < 0.05$) and plaques with stenosis of 90% or more ($p < 0.05$) generated a higher number of embolic particles following balloon angioplasty and stenting. Multiple regression analysis revealed that echogenicity and severity of stenosis were significant independent risk factors.[26]

Henry and colleagues showed that the number of particles released during CAS and collected by means of a distal balloon occlusion device was higher in echolucent plaques with a low GSM.[27]

Several studies analyzed the impact of emboli on the brain. Using transcranial Doppler ultrasonography, Ackerstaff and colleagues studied the effect of the total number of particles detected during CEA on perioperative neurologic events. It was demonstrated that microemboli (more than 10) noted during the procedure were related to both intraoperative and postoperative cerebral complications. Isolated microemboli never resulted in new morphologic changes on postoperative cerebral computed tomographic (CT) scans. On the other hand, the detection of more than 10 microemboli was significantly related to new lesions on magnetic resonance imaging (MRI).[28]

Tübler and colleagues analyzed the relationship between particles collected by means of a distal balloon occlusion and the occurrence of neurologic complications during CAS. The maximum area, the maximum diameter, and the number of captured particles were higher in patients with cerebrovascular accidents than in those with uncomplicated procedures.[29]

These studies showed that the incidence of neurologic complications during CAS is related to embolization from carotid plaque: it appears clear that the reduction of embolic particles from the carotid plaque is essential to decrease neurologic deficits.

Based on these assumptions, our group suggested that plaque echogenicity measured by the GSM can be a useful indicator of embolic potential in the carotid arteries.[6,9]

The Imaging in Carotid Angioplasty and Risk of Stroke ICAROS Study

ICAROS was a registry of carotid angioplasty and stenting procedures that reported any cerebral event following the procedure and correlated the risk of cerebral embolization with the echographic characteristics of the carotid plaque. The aim of the ICAROS study was to determine the preprocedural echographic criteria, which can identify the carotid plaque related to a higher risk of stroke during CAS, so that a better selection of candidates for CAS may be performed.

The study was open to all interventionalists performing carotid endovascular procedures. Participants were free to apply their own endovascular techniques and devices, including cerebral protection mechanisms (percutaneous femoral or cervical approach, minimal surgical dissection of the common carotid artery, primary stenting, preliminary and/or postdeployment dilation, etc.), but techniques and instrumentation were precisely documented.

All cerebral ischemic events following the procedure were reported and investigated in detail with physical examination by an independent neurologist and with cerebral CT or MRI. The degree of stenosis was calculated based on the ratio of the peak systolic velocity of the internal carotid artery to that of the common carotid artery. A complete angiographic evaluation of supraaortic trunks, carotid arteries, and intracranial circulation was performed.

Several training courses on how to set up the duplex scanner for the collection of the images were organized worldwide for ultrasonographers from the participating centers. Duplex scanning images were then sent to the coordinating center (Bassini Teaching Hospital), where the optimal color and B-mode images were transferred onto a personal computer. Image normalization and calculation of the GSM were performed by the same operator (who was blinded to clinical data and outcome) by means of Adobe Photoshop 5.0 software, as previously described. The overall rate of neurological complications was 6.7% (28/418), with transient ischemic attack 3.1% (13/418), minor strokes 2.2% (9/418), and major strokes 1.4% (6/418), while no deaths were observed.[10]

The GSM value in complicated patients was significantly lower than in uncomplicated cases, both in the stroke ($p < 0.005$) and in the stroke plus transient ischemic attack (TIA) ($p < 0.005$) subset. A receiver operating characteristic (ROC) curve was used to choose the best GSM cut-off value: the most successful threshold value was 25. The prevalence of a GSM value of less than 25 (echolucent plaques) was high 155/418 (37%) patients. Eleven out of 155 patients with GSM ≤ 25 had a stroke (7.1%) compared to 4 out of 263 patients with GSM > 25 (1.5%, $p = 0.005$). The event rates increased to 12.9% and 3.0%, respectively, when both stroke and TIA were counted ($p = 0.002$).

There were 5/219 (2.3%) strokes in protected and 10/199 (5.0%) in unprotected procedures ($p = 0.18$). However, protection gave different results in the GSM subgroups: in patients with GSM ≤ 25 a brain protection device tended to increase the risk of stroke (12.5% vs. 5.2%, $p = 0.15$), whereas it had a protective value in the echogenic subgroup (0% vs. 4.8%, $p = 0.01$).

The overall neurological complication rate was higher in primary lesions than in restenoses (5.2% vs. 2.2%, p = ns). This difference was observed also in GSM > 25 patients (4.0% vs. 0%, $p < 0.05$) but not in GSM ≤ 25 patients (6.6% vs. 7.8%, p = ns).

The stroke rate was 2.8% for asymptomatic and 5.3% for symptomatic patients (p = ns), with a similar trend in GSM subsets. The neurological complication rate was 1.5% (3/202) in <85% carotid stenosis rate subset and 5.6% (12/216) in ≥85% ($p < 0.05$). The neurological complication rate was significantly higher in patients with positive cerebral CT than in those with negative CT (7.7% vs. 2.4%, $p < 0.05$).

A multivariate regression analysis revealed that GSM (OR = 7.11, $p = 0.0019$) and degree of stenosis (OR = 5.76, $p = 0.010$) are significant independent predictors of stroke alone, while preprocedural symptomatology (OR = 2.92, $p = 0.061$) and preprocedural brain CT (OR = 2.54, $p = 0.099$) are borderline significant. Similar results were found in the analysis of stroke plus TIA as endpoints.

Conclusions

The clinical impact of GSM relies on the ability to identify a vast number of patients at higher risk of stroke during CAS and to distinguish subsets of patients (with restenosis or with the protected procedure) in which the rate of neurological complications is different from the overall population.

A computer-assisted echogenicity evaluation through image normalization and measurement of GSM is a simple method to identify preprocedurally high- risk carotid plaques, in which endovascular treatment could be burdened with a higher risk. GSM is one of the parameters that should be mandatory for indication to treatment in order to quantify the individual risk related to the specific procedure. A low GSM value is not an absolute contraindication to CAS, but an index related to a higher risk for the procedure.

Echographic evaluation of carotid plaque through GSM should therefore always be included in the planning of any clinical trial on the endovascular treatment of carotid lesions.

References

1. Ferguson GG, Eliasziw M, Barr HW, *et al.* The North American Symptomatic Carotid Endarterectomy Trial: Surgical results in 1415 patients. Stroke 1999;30:1751–8.
2. MRC European Carotid Surgery Trial. Interim results for symptomatic patients with severe (70–99%) or with mild (0–29%) carotid stenosis. European Carotid Surgery Trialists' Collaborative Group. Lancet 1991;337:1235–43.
3. Executive Committee for the Asymptomatic Carotid Atherosclerosis Study. Endarterectomy for asymptomatic carotid artery stenosis. JAMA 1995;273:1421–8.
4. Halliday A, Mansfield A, Marro J, *et al.* Prevention of disabling and fatal strokes by successful carotid endarterectomy in patients without recent neurological symptoms: Randomised controlled trial. Lancet 2004;363:1491–502.
5. Roubin GS, New G, Iyer SS, *et al.* Immediate and late clinical outcomes of carotid artery stenting in patients with symptomatic and asymptomatic carotid artery stenosis: A 5-year prospective analysis. Circulation 2001;103:532–7.
6. Biasi GM. Is it time to reconsider the selection criteria for conventional or endovascular repair of carotid artery stenosis in the prevention of cerebral ischemia? J Endovasc Ther 2001;8:339–40.
7. Biasi GM, Mingazzini PM, Baronio L, *et al.* Carotid plaque characterization using digital image processing and its potential in future studies of carotid endarterectomy and angioplasty. J Endovasc Surg 1998;5:240–6.
8. Biasi GM, Sampaolo A, Mingazzini P, De Amicis P, El-Barghouty N, Nicolaides AN. Computer analysis of ultrasonic plaque echolucency in identifying high risk carotid bifurcation lesions. Eur J Vasc Endovasc Surg 1999;17:476–9.
9. Biasi GM, Ferrari SA, Nicolaides AN, Mingazzini PM, Reid D. The ICAROS registry of carotid artery stenting. Imaging in Carotid Angioplasties and Risk of Stroke. J Endovasc Ther 2001;8:46–52.
10. Biasi GM, Froio A, Diethrich EB, *et al.* Carotid plaque echolucency increases the risk of stroke in carotid stenting: The Imaging in Carotid Angioplasty and Risk of Stroke (ICAROS) study. Circulation 2004;110:756–62.

11. European Carotid Plaque Study Group. Carotid artery plaque composition—relationship to clinical presentation and ultrasound B-mode imaging. Eur J Vasc Endovasc Surg 1995;10:23–30.
12. Carr S, Farb A, Pearce WH, Virmani R, Yao JS. Atherosclerotic plaque rupture in symptomatic carotid artery stenosis. J Vasc Surg 1996;23:755–65; discussion 765–6.
13. Geroulakos G, Ramaswami G, Nicolaides A, *et al.* Characterization of symptomatic and asymptomatic carotid plaques using high-resolution real-time ultrasonography. Br J Surg 1993;80:1274–7.
14. Gray-Weale AC, Graham JC, Burnett JR, Byrne K, Lusby RJ. Carotid artery atheroma: Comparison of preoperative B-mode ultrasound appearance with carotid endarterectomy specimen pathology. J Cardiovasc Surg (Torino) 1988; 29:676–81.
15. Barnett HJ, Eliasziw M, Meldrum H. Plaque morphology as a risk factor for stroke. JAMA 2000;284:177.
16. Polak JF, Shemanski L, O'Leary DH, *et al.* Hypoechoic plaque at US of the carotid artery: An independent risk factor for incident stroke in adults aged 65 years or older. Cardiovascular Health Study. Radiology 1998;208: 649–54.
17. Liapis CD, Kakisis JD, Kostakis AG. Carotid stenosis: Factors affecting symptomatology. Stroke 2001;32:2782–6.
18. Mathiesen EB, Bonaa KH, Joakimsen O. Echolucent plaques are associated with high risk of ischemic cerebrovascular events in carotid stenosis: The Tromso study. Circulation 2001;103:2171–5.
19. Gronholdt ML, Nordestgaard BG, Schroeder TV, Vorstrup S, Sillesen H. Ultrasonic echolucent carotid plaques predict future strokes. Circulation 2001;104:68–73.
20. el-Barghouty N, Geroulakos G, Nicolaides A, Androulakis A, Bahal V. Computer-assisted carotid plaque characterisation. Eur J Vasc Endovasc Surg 1995;9:389–93.
21. Elatrozy T, Nicolaides A, Tegos T, Zarka AZ, Griffin M, Sabetai M. The effect of B-mode ultrasonic image standardisation on the echodensity of symptomatic and asymptomatic carotid bifurcation plaques. Int Angiol 1998;17:179–86.
22. Sabetai MM, Tegos TJ, Nicolaides AN, Dhanjil S, Pare GJ, Stevens JM. Reproducibility of computer-quantified carotid plaque echogenicity: Can we overcome the subjectivity? Stroke 2000;31:2189–96.
23. Markus HS, Clifton A, Buckenham T, Brown MM. Carotid angioplasty. Detection of embolic signals during and after the procedure. Stroke 1994;25:2403–6.
24. Coggia M, Goeau-Brissonniere O, Duval JL, Leschi JP, Letort M, Nagel MD. Embolic risk of the different stages of carotid bifurcation balloon angioplasty: An experimental study. J Vasc Surg 2000;31:550–7.
25. Jordan WD Jr, Voellinger DC, Doblar DD, Plyushcheva NP, Fisher WS, McDowell HA. Microemboli detected by transcranial Doppler monitoring in patients during carotid angioplasty versus carotid endarterectomy. Cardiovasc Surg 1999;7:33–8.
26. Ohki T, Marin ML, Lyon RT, *et al.* Ex vivo human carotid artery bifurcation stenting: Correlation of lesion characteristics with embolic potential. J Vasc Surg 1998;27:463–71.
27. Henry M, Henry I, Klonaris C, *et al.* Benefits of cerebral protection during carotid stenting with the PercuSurge GuardWire system: Midterm results. J Endovasc Ther 2002; 9:1–13.
28. Ackerstaff RG, Jansen C, Moll FL, Vermeulen FE, Hamerlijnck RP, Mauser HW. The significance of microemboli detection by means of transcranial Doppler ultrasonography monitoring in carotid endarterectomy. J Vasc Surg 1995;21:963–9.
29. Tubler T, Schluter M, Dirsch O, *et al.* Balloon-protected carotid artery stenting: Relationship of periprocedural neurological complications with the size of particulate debris. Circulation 2001;104:2791–6.

9 Duplex Ultrasound in the Diagnosis of Temporal Arteritis

George H. Meier and Courtney Nelms

Giant cell arteritis is the most common primary arteritis diagnosed, with an average incidence of 15–25 cases per 100,000 population over the age of 50.[1] Giant cell arteritis can be subclassified into at least three main types: cranial, affecting the arteries of the face, head, and posterior cerebral circulation; large vessel, involving the axillary and subclavian arteries; and aortic, leading to aneurysmal degeneration of the ascending aorta or aortic valve insufficiency. Of these, the most common presentation is the cranial form, traditionally referred to as temporal arteritis. In this form, the arteritis involves the superficial temporal arteries as well as the facial artery branches. Involvement of the ophthalmic artery can lead to retinal ischemia and is the second leading cause of acquired blindness in the United States.[2]

In the temporal arteritis form of giant cell arteritis, the diagnosis can often be challenging. The American College of Rheumatology developed clinical criteria for the diagnosis of giant cell arteritis in 1990[3] (Table 9–1). Using these criteria, three of the five criteria must be present to define the diagnosis of temporal arteritis. The presence of a positive biopsy demonstrating giant cell arteritis is only one of the five criteria and is therefore insufficient alone to diagnose giant cell arteritis. Additionally, giant cell arteritis may not involve the artery evenly along its course, resulting in areas of normal artery interspersed with areas of abnormality. In fact, the irregular distribution of arterial involvement is common in temporal arteritis,[4] risking a false negative biopsy if too small a segment of artery is biopsied. Current recommendations suggest that bilateral biopsy should be done even in cases of unilateral symptoms,[5,6] and at least 5 cm of artery should be biopsied on either side. In spite of this approach, a substantial number of temporal artery specimens miss the areas of active disease.[7–10] For these reasons, the absence of histologic evidence of giant cell arteritis is insufficient to rule out the disease and many patients require treatment even in the absence of a positive biopsy.

The pathologic findings resulting in a positive biopsy consist of three dominant findings in temporal arteritis: the presence of a halo of edema around or within the artery wall, usually associated with giant cell formation; stenosis secondary to narrowing after the inflammation abates; or occlusion of the artery due to obliterative arteritis. Therefore, any of these may represent a positive biopsy depending on the stage of the arteritis and the duration of symptoms or treatment. For any diagnostic modality to replace biopsy, these findings must be apparent.

High-resolution duplex ultrasound is a common test for many vascular disorders and the easy access to the superficial temporal artery makes it an obvious modality to consider for the diagnosis of temporal arteritis. Its use in temporal arteritis has two potential utilities. First, the mapping of areas of arterial involvement for biopsy may allow a positive biopsy rate higher than currently seen with blind biopsy. If abnormalities on duplex ultrasound are seen (halo, stenosis, or occlusion), then directed biopsy may produce a higher yield, avoiding the false-negative biopsy discussed above. The second benefit of duplex ultrasound in temporal arteritis may be the benefit of avoiding biopsy completely. If the clinical suspicion is high based on the American College of Radiology (ACR) criteria, then an ultrasound indicating arterial pathology may provide sufficient accuracy to avoid open surgical biopsy altogether. The presence of halo, stenosis, or occlusion on ultrasound evaluation may not need correlation with open biopsy, but in selected patients may warrant treatment without biopsy. While this use of ultrasound has not been established as a standard, the potential is enticing and the avoidance of open biopsy should be the ultimate goal in the diagnosis of temporal arteritis.

A.F. Aburahma, J.J. Bergan (eds.), *Noninvasive Cerebrovascular Diagnosis*, DOI 10.1007/978-1-84882-957-2_9,

TABLE 9–1. Diagnostic criteria for temporal arteritis (American College of Rheumatology[3]).

Age greater than or equal to 50 years
New headache
Temporal artery abnormality on physical examination
Elevated ESR[a] ≥ 50 mm/h
Abnormal findings on temporal artery biopsy

[a]ESR, erythrocyte sedimentation rate.

Ultrasound Protocol

Duplex ultrasound permits localization of inflammation or stenosis of the temporal arteries and their branches. The presence of significant tenderness along the course of the superficial temporal artery may alter the examination, but generally ultrasound interrogation can be achieved along the full length of the temporal artery and its branches.

Patients are placed in a supine position with the head slightly elevated. The head is turned away from the side to be scanned. Color duplex ultrasound is performed bilaterally on the temporal arteries with a high-resolution linear transducer (L 10–5 MHz). The common superficial temporal arteries are established as a landmark medial to the ear and then followed inferiorly and superiorly to the frontal and parietal branches of the temporal artery. The vessels should be followed in longitudinal and transverse planes throughout the examination, with and without color flow, looking for the "halo" effect (Figures 9–1 and 9–2), arterial stenosis (Figure 9–3), and arterial occlusion. This can be challenging in many patients since the tortuosity of the artery may mean that keeping it in a single plane for visualization is difficult. Color flow imaging is used to facilitate following the anatomic course and branching of the artery and to define areas of flow disturbance or luminal narrowing. Color flow will allow for easier identification of the "halo" effect with the color settings adjusted appropriately. Care should be taken to prevent the color from "bleeding" over into the outer walls of the arteries and possibly obscuring the inflammation. This examination can be tedious due to the small size of the vessels, frequent tortuosity, and location of the arterial segments below the scalp above the hairline. Peak systolic velocities and end diastolic velocities should be obtained throughout the temporal arteries and branches, including the superficial temporal artery medial to the ear prior to the bifurcation, common temporal artery inferior to the ear, parietal branch coursing toward the scalp, and the frontal branch coursing toward the forehead. Care is taken to use appropriate angle correction between 45–60° with respect to the blood flow vector. A stenosis is defined as at least a two-fold increase of the peak systolic velocity accompanied by poststenotic turbulence.

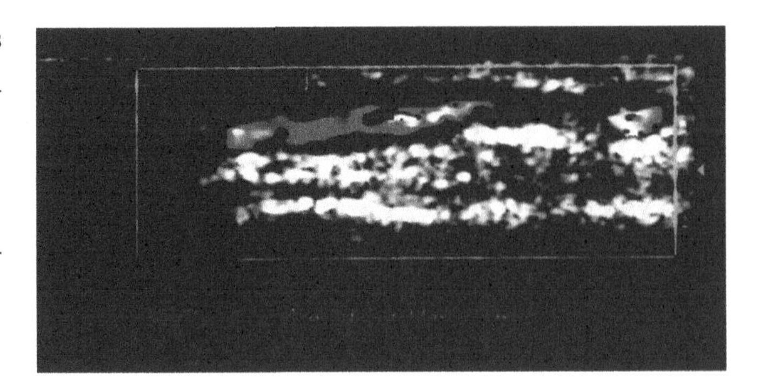

FIGURE 9–2. Halo seen in longitudinal cross-section.

B-mode imaging can define the areas of inflammation that represent edema within the arterial wall. The wall of the arterial segments affected with arteritis appears to be acoustically homogeneous and presents a "halo" around the lumen of the artery. These areas may be intermittent

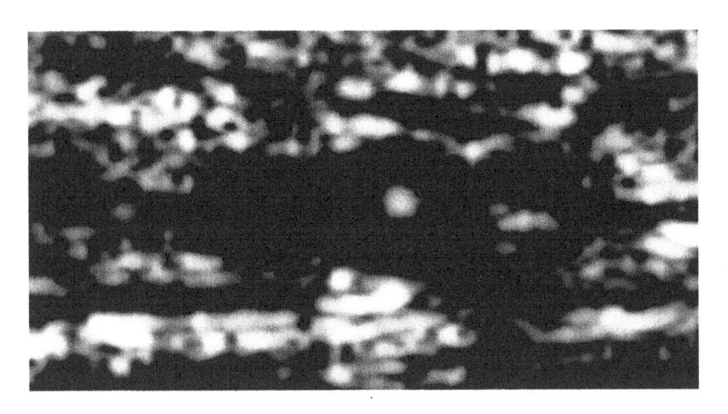

FIGURE 9–1. Halo seen in transverse.

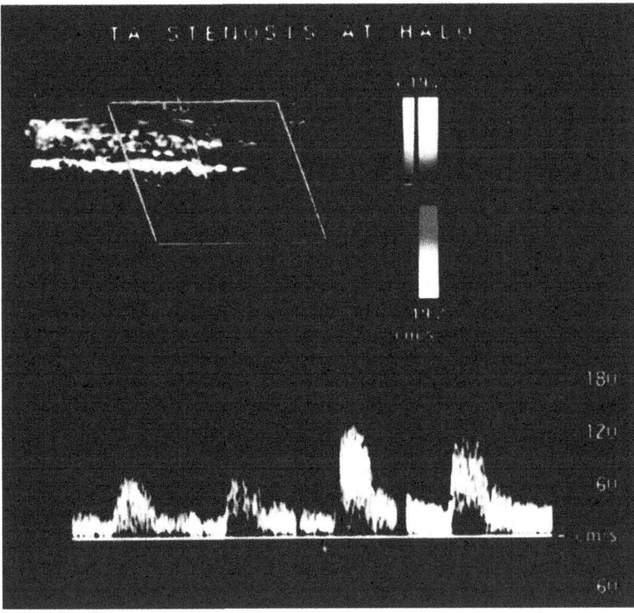

FIGURE 9–3. Spectral Doppler evaluation for stenosis.

or focal within the branches; therefore a thorough evaluation of all branches is necessary. More echogenic, diffuse plaque is probably atherosclerosis, not inflammation, but may also represent areas of "burned out" arteritis. Elevations in peak systolic velocities may be noted in these areas. Alternatively, occlusions of segments of the artery may represent similar issues and should also be noted for reporting.

Once the arteries are fully interrogated, a map should be generated for each side imaged. This map of pathologic findings on ultrasound should be used as a guide by the surgeon to allow accurate biopsy of the areas of concern. If no abnormalities are noted, then conventional blind biopsy is warranted.

Results of Duplex Ultrasound for Temporal Arteritis

While the diagnosis of temporal arteritis is clinical based on the ACR criteria outlined in Table 9–1, the presence of a biopsy consistent with giant cell arteritis is an important adjunct to reassure the patient and clinician of the diagnosis, justifying the initiation of steroid therapy to prevent progression or blindness. Unfortunately, biopsy is inexact, as temporal arteritis has a propensity for skip lesions with normal artery in the intervening segments as discussed earlier. Therefore, the challenge in diagnosis is in defining the inflammatory lesions in the artery responsible for the clinical consequences. Duplex ultrasound holds great promise in this regard since high-resolution ultrasound of the superficial temporal artery can often provide information about the likelihood of disease involvement as well as the extent of disease seen. Duplex ultrasound for directed biopsy was first proposed as early as 1982.[11] Unfortunately, no series using this strategy of ultrasound-directed biopsy has yet demonstrated efficacy, although some benefit has been suggested.[6] While this information has not yet been fully incorporated into the diagnostic algorithm for temporal arteritis, it seems likely that with further study and technical refinements, this noninvasive modality may ultimately be able to replace open biopsy in the diagnosis of temporal arteritis.

The halo effect seen around the artery correlates with areas of edema and giant cell formation surrounding the lumen. In these areas the artery appears enlarged clinically, with the bulk of the enlargement due to inflammation and edema. The main underlying pathology behind the clinical syndrome of temporal arteritis is small vessel ischemia. Therefore, the clinical consequences of temporal arteritis are associated with stenosis or occlusion rather than the halo formation associated with acute periarterial inflammation. Only as the inflammation progresses to fibrosis does the ischemic component begin, resulting in the symptoms associated with temporal arteritis. For this reason, the halo may not be as important as the presence of arterial stenosis or occlusion in the risk of visual changes associated with temporal arteritis.

One of the earliest reports suggesting utility of high-resolution color flow duplex ultrasound in temporal arteritis was by Williamson in 1992.[12] In this patient serial evaluation of ophthalmic artery blood flow was correlated with the changes in visual symptoms, showing return of blood flow and resolution of visual symptoms associated with increased immunosuppressive therapy. The fact that these changes in small artery blood flow could be qualitatively assessed noninvasively promised a new diagnostic modality for temporal arteritis.

Aburahma and Thaxton[13] reviewed their experience with duplex ultrasound in temporal arteritis in 21 patients, 19 of whom underwent temporal artery biopsy. In this series duplex was performed prebiopsy in only 8 of the patients, but the authors concluded that the use of duplex ultrasound might be beneficial in guiding the location and side of temporal artery biopsy in these patients.

The next step in evaluation of duplex ultrasound was a paper published by Schmidt in the *New England Journal of Medicine* in 1997.[14] This prospective evaluation of 30 patients, only 21 of whom had positive biopsies, evaluated three criteria: halo formation (a marker of inflammatory edema of the artery), arterial stenosis, and arterial occlusion. Using these three criteria, 28 of the 30 patients had a positive ultrasound evaluation. These results were compared to 30 age- and sex-matched controls, with any of the three ultrasound criteria demonstrated in only two patients.

While further research in duplex ultrasound for the diagnosis of temporal arteritis was clearly warranted, our group undertook a slightly different study published in 2002.[15,16] In this paper, we evaluated all patients referred to our practice for temporal artery biopsy by duplex ultrasound prior to biopsy. In these 32 patients only 7 met the criteria for the diagnosis of temporal arteritis. In this first attempt at applying duplex ultrasound diagnostic criteria to patients being evaluated for temporal arteritis, no positive biopsy was seen in any patient without one of the three criteria mentioned above. Therefore, we felt that temporal artery biopsy should be undertaken only on patients with ultrasound abnormalities, either halo or stenosis/occlusion.

Since these initial studies, multiple other studies have been published.[17–27] While the conclusions reached have often been contradictory (Table 9–2), ultrasound can clearly demonstrate abnormalities in the superficial temporal artery associated with temporal arteritis. The most recent meta-analysis published in 2005 attempted to review the world literature on ultrasound and temporal arteritis and reach conclusions based on the studies available. Karassa and his colleagues reviewed 23 studies

TABLE 9–2. Summary of studies using duplex ultrasound to diagnose temporal arteritis.

Study	Number of patients	Ultrasound findings evaluated: Halo formation	Stenosis	Occlusion	Conclusions
Schmidt[14]	30	+	+	+	May replace biopsy
Venz[28]	20	+			Halo alone not specific enough
LeSar[15]	32	+	+	+	May limit need for biopsy if negative
Nesher[27]	32	+			May limit need for biopsy if negative
Salvarani[26]	86	+			Did not improve upon physical examination
Murgatroyd[23]	26	+	+	+	May be helpful
Pfadenhauer[29]	67	+	+	+	Cannot replace biopsy
Reinhard[30]	48	+		+	May limit the need for biopsy if positive

totaling 2036 patients written in 5 different languages.[18] Their conclusions were that ultrasound may be helpful, but guidelines to its use and application were absent based on this heterogeneous collection of studies. Thus, we are left at this moment with more questions than answers, with great variability in the application of ultrasound techniques from site to site and no current potential for resolving these issues.

Future Directions

For us to define how better to use ultrasound for the diagnosis of giant cell arteritis, specifically temporal arteritis, we have to define what types of trials will be needed to demonstrate benefit. These trials are designed to embellish and define prospectively what can be done to diagnose temporal arteritis. While all of the strategies carry some risk, the overall benefit to patients with temporal arteritis may subsume the individual risk.

There are three basic approaches to trials to better define the use of ultrasound in the diagnosis of temporal arteritis. First is the use of duplex ultrasound to guide biopsy. For this strategy to be effective, a prospective predictive duplex ultrasound must be performed and then correlated with biopsy findings. The key to this study would be the interrogation of only those segments of the temporal artery appropriate for biopsy and the surgeon's focus on complete biopsy of those segments for correlation. Generally, this would include the common superficial temporal artery as well as the proximal portion of the parietal and frontal branches. A predictive score derived from the prebiopsy temporal artery duplex ultrasound would need to be correlated with carefully controlled biopsies with special attention to the anatomic location of disease. The anatomic correlations of biopsy and ultrasound would hopefully demonstrate the specific abnormalities seen on both. Areas of abnormality outside of the biopsy specimen would be excluded from this analysis. In this way accurate correlation of biopsy pathology in temporal arteries could be analyzed versus ultrasound findings in the same segment. Currently no series has accurately defined the abnormalities within the biopsy zone, and correlated this directly with ultrasound of the corresponding areas. In this study the only risk is the possibility of a positive ultrasound finding outside of the zone of biopsy, equivalent to the current risk when duplex ultrasound is used prior to biopsy. In this scenario, a decision to treat independent of biopsy would need to be reached.

The second approach is defining the criteria to help avoid unnecessary biopsies. In this study, all patients would undergo preprocedure duplex ultrasound scanning. If abnormalities were defined on the ultrasound scan in the zone of routine biopsy, then biopsy would be performed. If no abnormalities were seen in areas accessible for biopsy, then treatment would be based on clinical criteria and no biopsy would be performed. Using this strategy prospectively, patients would be followed for treatment outcomes, biopsy results, and the subsequent development of temporal arteritis. This study assumes that arterial pathology is present both in temporal arteritis and in degenerative atherosclerosis. Biopsy results would be used to refine the group of patients treated for temporal arteritis, excluding those patients with degenerative atherosclerosis alone. A negative ultrasound evaluation would be assumed to rule out either temporal arteritis or degenerative atherosclerosis, eliminating the need for biopsy. The risk of this study is the possibility of missing temporal arteritis in a patient with a false-negative duplex ultrasound evaluation. While in most series the risk of a false-negative ultrasound evaluation is quite small, it is not zero. In these patients the routine use of the five clinical criteria would be necessary to avoid undertreatment of patients with negative biopsies or ultrasounds.

A third approach to defining the value of duplex ultrasound in temporal arteritis would be its value as an indicator of positive biopsy results. Again, an ultrasound evaluation of the temporal arteries in the area of biopsy would be performed. If significant arterial pathology were found, then this would be viewed as a positive biopsy and the patient would be treated based on the diagnostic criteria outlined in Table 9–1. Instead of using surgical biopsy as one of the five criteria, either an abnormal duplex ultrasound or a positive surgical biopsy would be assumed to be equivalent. Since two additional criteria would be necessary for the diagnosis of temporal arteritis, this decreases the severity of a false-positive ultrasound study and requires additional criteria for the clinical diagnosis of temporal arteritis. By prospective assessment, the benefits of this diagnostic strategy could be objectively defined. Unfortunately since in most series the rate of positive biopsy is only about 25%, 75% of the patients would still require a biopsy to rule out the disease. Only in that less than 25% of patients with a positive ultrasound would biopsy be avoided and in those patients the risk of steroid therapy would be assumed. This strategy would result in every patient being exposed to either a biopsy or steroid therapy, both of which carry additional risk.

From our perspective and experience, either of the first two strategies seem to be the best next step in the use of ultrasound for temporal arteritis. In our opinion the third strategy exposes the patients to too much risk without adequate benefit. Ideally, the study should be undertaken as multicenter trials using a common protocol. Only in this manner can these data be generalized to the wider population of patients presenting with possible temporal arteritis to the clinician. In spite of these concerns ultrasound remains a viable diagnostic tool in the management of temporal arteritis.

References

1. Weyand CM, Goronzy JJ. Giant-cell arteritis and polymyalgia rheumatica. Ann Intern Med 2003;139(6):505–15.
2. Gonzalez-Gay MA, *et al.* Visual manifestations of giant cell arteritis. Trends and clinical spectrum in 161 patients. Medicine (Baltimore) 2000;79(5):283–92.
3. Hunder GG, *et al.* The American College of Rheumatology 1990 criteria for the classification of giant cell arteritis. Arthritis Rheum 1990;33(8):1122–8.
4. Lie JT. Illustrated histopathologic classification criteria for selected vasculitis syndromes. American College of Rheumatology Subcommittee on Classification of Vasculitis. Arthritis Rheum 1990;33(8):1074–87.
5. Pless M, *et al.* Concordance of bilateral temporal artery biopsy in giant cell arteritis. J Neuroophthalmol 2000;20(3): 216–8.
6. Ponge T, *et al.* The efficacy of selective unilateral temporal artery biopsy versus bilateral biopsies for diagnosis of giant cell arteritis. J Rheumatol 1988;15(6):997–1000.
7. van der Straaten D, *et al.* A case of biopsy-negative temporal arteritis—diagnostic challenges. Surv Ophthalmol 2004; 49(6):603–7.
8. Hoffman GS. Giant cell arteritis: Biopsy may not be diagnostic. Cleve Clin J Med 1998;65(4):218.
9. Lie JT. Temporal artery biopsy diagnosis of giant cell arteritis: Lessons from 1109 biopsies. Anat Pathol 1996;1: 69–97.
10. Hall S, *et al.* The therapeutic impact of temporal artery biopsy. Lancet 1983;2(8361):1217–20.
11. Barrier J, *et al.* The use of Doppler flow studies in the diagnosis of giant cell arteritis. Selection of temporal artery biopsy site is facilitated. JAMA 1982;248(17):2158–9.
12. Williamson TH, *et al.* Colour Doppler ultrasound in the management of a case of cranial arteritis. Br J Ophthalmol 1992;76(11):690–1.
13. AbuRahma AF, Thaxton L. Temporal arteritis: Diagnostic and therapeutic considerations. Am Surg 1996;62(6):449–51.
14. Schmidt WA, *et al.* Color duplex ultrasonography in the diagnosis of temporal arteritis. N Engl J Med 1997;337(19): 1336–42.
15. LeSar CJ, *et al.* The utility of color duplex ultrasonography in the diagnosis of temporal arteritis. J Vasc Surg 2002;36(6): 1154–60.
16. Nelms CR, Carter KA, Meier GH, *et al.* Diagnosis of temporal artery pathology using duplex ultrasonography. J Vasc Ultrasound 2002;26(4):273–7.
17. Schmidt WA, Blockmans D. Use of ultrasonography and positron emission tomography in the diagnosis and assessment of large-vessel vasculitis. Curr Opin Rheumatol 2005; 17(1):9–15.
18. Karassa FB, *et al.* Meta-analysis: Test performance of ultrasonography for giant-cell arteritis. Ann Intern Med 2005; 142(5):359–69.
19. Butteriss DJ, *et al.* Use of colour duplex ultrasound to diagnose giant cell arteritis in a case of visual loss of uncertain aetiology. Br J Radiol 2004;77(919):607–9.
20. Schmidt WA, Gromnica-Ihle E. Duplex ultrasonography in temporal arteritis. Ann Intern Med 2003;138(7):609; author reply 609–10.
21. Schmidt D, *et al.* Comparison between color duplex ultrasonography and histology of the temporal artery in cranial arteritis (giant cell arteritis). Eur J Med Res 2003;8(1):1–7.
22. Nicoletti G, *et al.* Colour duplex ultrasonography in the management of giant cell arteritis. Clin Rheumatol 2003; 22(6):508–9.
23. Murgatroyd H, *et al.* The use of ultrasound as an aid in the diagnosis of giant cell arteritis: A pilot study comparing histological features with ultrasound findings. Eye 2003;17(3): 415–9.
24. Hetzel SD, Reinhard M, Haedrich-Auw C. Comparison between color duplex ultrasonography and histology of the temporal artery in cranial arteritis. Eur J Med Res 2003; 8(2):91.
25. Schmidt WA, Gromnica-Ihle E. Incidence of temporal arteritis in patients with polymyalgia rheumatica: A

prospective study using colour Doppler ultrasonography of the temporal arteries. Rheumatology (Oxford) 2002;41(1): 46–52.
26. Salvarani C, *et al.* Is duplex ultrasonography useful for the diagnosis of giant-cell arteritis? Ann Intern Med 2002; 137(4):232–8.
27. Nesher G, *et al.* The predictive value of the halo sign in color Doppler ultrasonography of the temporal arteries for diagnosing giant cell arteritis. J Rheumatol 2002;29(6): 1224–6.
28. Venz S, *et al.* [Use of high resolution color Doppler sonography in diagnosis of temporal arteritis.] Rofo 1998;169(6): 605–8.
29. Pfadenhauer K, Weber H. Duplex sonography of the temporal and occipital artery in the diagnosis of temporal arteritis. A prospective study. J Rheumatol 2003;30(10): 2177–81.
30. Reinhard M, Schmidt D, Hetzel A. Color-coded sonography in suspected temporal arteritis—experiences after 83 cases. Rheumatol Int 2004;24(6):340–6.

10 Duplex Ultrasound Velocity Criteria for Carotid Stenting Patients

Brajesh K. Lal and Robert W. Hobson II

Introduction

Stroke is the third leading cause of death in the United States with over 783,000 strokes reported annually.[1] Over one-third of patients die and another one-third are severely disabled. The annual economic cost exceeds $30 billion.[2] Randomized trials have established the efficacy of carotid endarterectomy (CEA) in the prevention of stroke for patients with high-grade carotid stenosis (CS).[3–7] The advent of newer technologies and a desire for less invasive treatment have encouraged investigators to propose carotid artery stenting (CAS) as an alternative to CEA.[1,8–10] Our institution[1, 8,11–17] (Figure 10–1), along with others,[18–22] has demonstrated that CAS is technically feasible and safe in patients with restenosis after CEA, surgically inaccessible lesions, previous radiation, or significant medical comorbidities. The 30-day stroke and death rate in 190 CAS procedures at our institution was 4.15%, indicating a competitive alternative to CEA.[14] However, due to the proven efficacy of CEA, current indications for CAS have been limited to situations where CEA yields suboptimal results.[13,23]

Two randomized trials have compared CAS and CEA. The SAPPHIRE (Stenting and Angioplasty with Protection in Patients at High Risk for Endarterectomy) investigators randomized 334 high-risk patients to CAS or CEA.[24] The 30-day composite stroke, death, and myocardial infarction rate was not different between the two groups (CAS 12.2% vs. CEA 20.1%). The European CAVATAS (Carotid and Vertebral Artery Transluminal Angioplasty Study) investigators also reported comparable 30-day combined stroke and death rates (CEA 5.9% vs. CAS 6.4%).[25] The authors concluded that CAS was not inferior to CEA.

These trials were not powered to identify a difference between CAS and CEA. The NIH/NINDS-supported CREST (Carotid Revascularization Endarterectomy versus Stent Trial) is currently underway to make that determination.[26] In the lead-in phase of the trial, the combined stroke and death rate was 5.6% for symptomatic and 2.4% for asymptomatic patients undergoing CAS.[27] These preliminary results indicate low complication rates with CAS. The results of CREST may determine the role of CAS in future years. However, current data suggest clinical equipoise between CEA and CAS based on the three clinical end points of stroke, myocardial infarction (MI) and death. As a result of this information, the Food and Drug Administration (FDA) has approved the use of CAS in selected high-risk patients (significant medical comorbidities, post-CEA restenosis, anatomically inaccessible lesions above C_2, and radiation-induced stenoses).

In-Stent Restenosis: The Rationale for Post-Carotid Artery Stenting Surveillance

The incidences of in-stent restenosis (ISR) after bare metal stenting of the coronary and renal arteries have been reported as 20–35% and 15–25%, respectively.[13] It was therefore thought that ISR rates would be high with CAS too. Indeed, early reports noted post-CAS ISR in the ranges of 1–50%.[13] However, the reported rate of ISR depends on the definition of restenosis utilized, the duration of follow-up, and the methods of diagnosis and calculation used. Most studies have relatively short follow-up periods (≤12 months), and report absolute recurrence rates weighting each procedure equally regardless of the length of follow-up. This results in an underreporting of ISR rates. With longer follow-up (1–74 months) and the use of lifetable analysis, we reported more meaningful data on ISR after CAS. The majority of restenoses ≥40% occurred within 18 months (13/22, 60%) and the majority of clinically significant restenoses ≥80% occurred within 15

A.F. Aburahma, J.J. Bergan (eds.), *Noninvasive Cerebrovascular Diagnosis*, DOI 10.1007/978-1-84882-957-2_10,

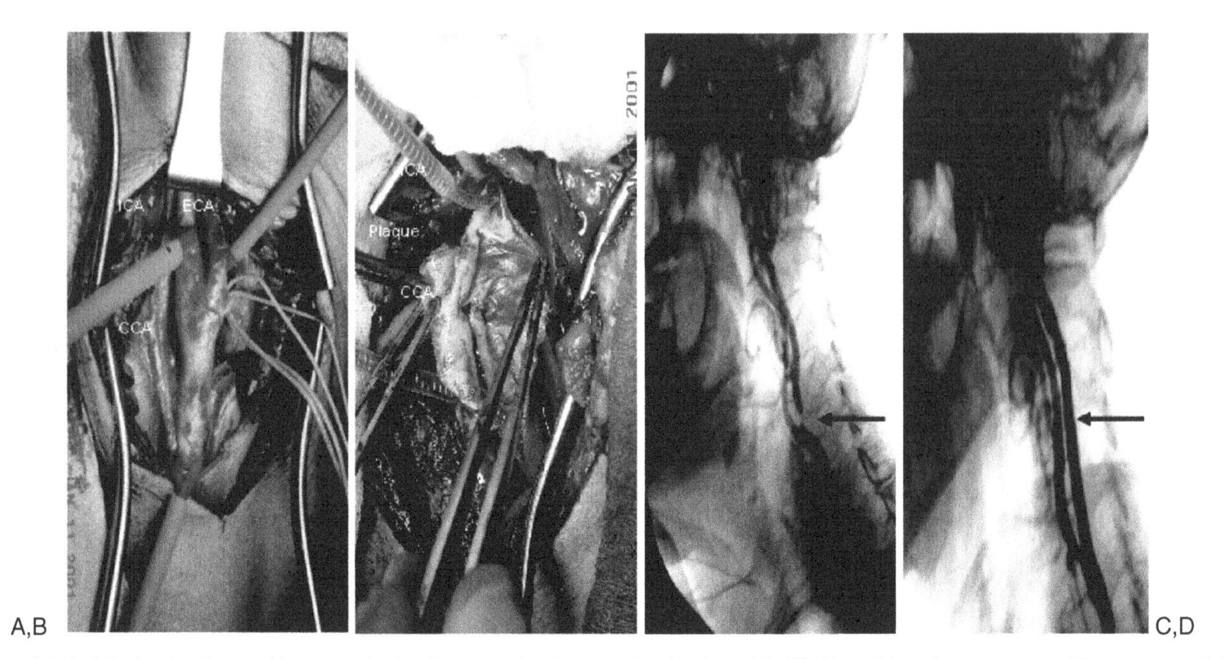

FIGURE 10–1. Methods of carotid revascularization practiced at our institution. (A, B) Carotid endarterectomy. Exposure and dissection of the plaque. CCA, common carotid artery; ICA, internal carotid artery; ECA, external carotid artery. (C, D) Carotid artery stenting. (B) Prestenting angiogram, arrow at stenosis in ICA; (C) poststenting angiogram, arrows at distal and proximal ends of stent.

months (3/5, 60%) of their intervention (Figure 10–2). The incidence of ISR ≥ 40 and ≥60% was 42.7% and 16.4%, respectively, at 48 months of follow-up. Our data also noted that hemodynamically significant (≥80%) ISR after CAS was 6.4% at 5 years (Figure 10–3). It is clear that a significant number of patients will develop moderate ISR after CAS, of which some will progress to high-grade stenosis. There is additional evidence that the placement of a stent induces continuing arterial remodeling. Nitinol self-expanding stents can continue to expand over a 2-year period poststenting.[28] Conversely, neointimal thickening has been reported to occur up to 1 year poststenting; further thickening may overwhelm positive remodeling of the arterial diameter from the stent and result in hemodynamically significant in-stent restenosis. This provides conclusive evidence that continued surveillance of patients is essential once CAS has been performed.

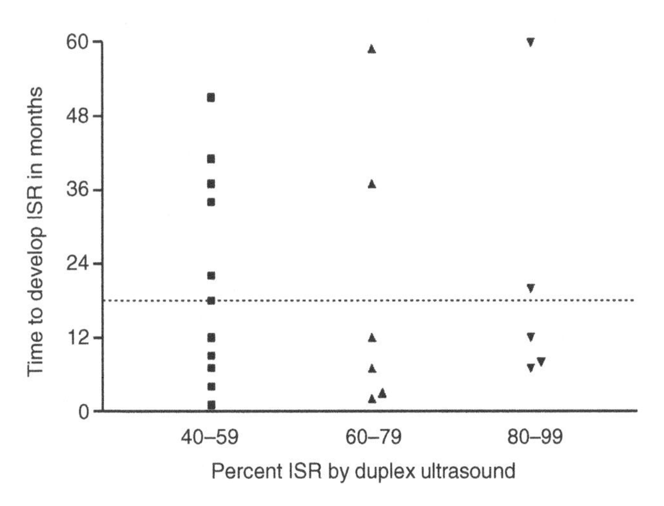

FIGURE 10–2. Distribution of in-stent restenosis cases based on time of diagnosis from initial carotid artery stenting procedure. Note that the majority of restenoses occurred within 18 months of the initial carotid artery stenting procedure. The dotted line identifies the 18 month postprocedure mark. ISR, in-stent restenosis. [Adapted from Lal B K, Hobson RW 2nd, Goldstein J, *et al.* In-stent recurrent stenosis after carotid artery stenting: Life table analysis and clinical relevance. J Vasc Surg 2003;38(6): 1162–8.]

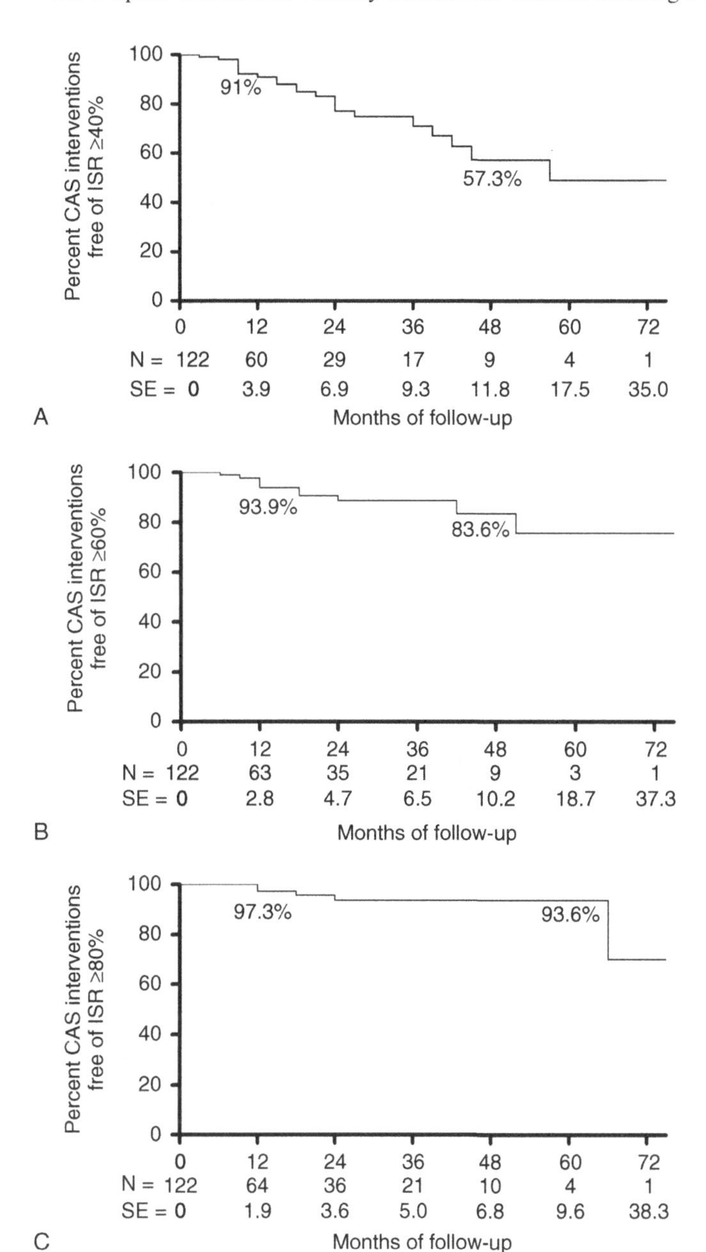

FIGURE 10–3. Kaplan–Meier cumulative event-free rates for clinically significant in-stent restenosis after CAS. (A) Event-free rate for ISR ≥ 80%. (B) Event-free rate for ISR ≥ 60%. (C) Event-free rate for ISR ≥ 40%. CAS, carotid artery stenting; ISR, in-stent restenosis; *N*, number at risk; SE, standard error. [Adapted from Lal BK, Hobson RW 2nd, Goldstein J, *et al.* In-stent recurrent stenosis after carotid artery stenting: Life table analysis and clinical relevance. J Vasc Surg 2003;38(6):1162–8.]

Duplex Ultrasonography: The Ideal Method for Post-Carotid Artery Stenting Surveillance

The characteristics of the ideal follow-up technique for CAS patients remain generally similar to that for CEA patients. The technique must be able to reliably identify changes in arterial diameter and stent morphology in an objective manner and be readily available, inexpensive, and associated with low observer variability. Computed tomography and magnetic resonance imaging may be considered: they are both expensive modalities and are associated with significantly reduced accuracy in determining diameter estimates of the carotid arteries. Therefore duplex ultrasonography (DU) remains the optimal imaging modality for post-CAS surveillance. It is noninvasive, safe, free of complications, readily available in vascular laboratories around the country, and is associated with a large experience with primary and recurrent carotid stenosis of the native carotid artery.

The utility of DU scanning in the detection of native carotid artery disease is well documented. Ultrasound velocities correlate with angiographic percent stenosis in the native unstented carotid artery.[29] The appropriate threshold velocities signifying different degrees of stenoses have been intensively analyzed and identified leading to the use of peak systolic velocity (PSV), end diastolic velocity (EDV), PSV/EDV ratio, or internal/common carotid artery (ICA/CCA) ratio, alone or in combination, to define normal and increasingly stenosed ICAs.[30] While thousands of carotid stents have been placed worldwide and in the United States, DU velocity criteria have not been well established for patients undergoing CAS. Robbin *et al.*[31] studied the use of DU in the follow-up of stented carotid arteries and noted that velocity measurements were unreliable after stenting. Similarly, Ringer *et al.*[32] reviewed their experience immediately after carotid stent placement and concluded that strict velocity criteria for restenosis were unreliable. Both groups applied limited, randomly selected velocity criteria to their data, and did not perform a systematic analysis to confirm their findings.

At our institution, we initially applied Intersocietal Commission for the Accreditation of Vascular Laboratories (ICAVL) accredited cutoff PSV and EDV criteria developed for native (unstented) carotid arteries to the follow-up of our first 90 CAS procedures.[17] Of these, 38 demonstrated a mean PSV ≥ 130 cm/s on postprocedure DU performed within 3 days. Using the velocity criteria established in our laboratory for unstented arteries, these patients would be characterized as technical failures of the procedure, having in-stent residual stenoses in the range of 20–49%. However, only six procedures demonstrated true angiographically proven residual stenosis ≥20%. We therefore concluded that stenting resulted in an elevation in measured DU velocities despite normal luminal diameters. Based on receiver operating characteristic (ROC) analysis of our data we found that a PSV ≥150 cm/s in combination with an ICA/CCA ratio ≥2.16 provides optimal sensitivity (100%), specificity (97.6%), positive predictive value (PPV) (75%), negative predictive value (NPV) (100%), and accuracy (97.7%) for differentiating 0–19% and ≥20% ICA in-stent residual stenosis after CAS[17] (Figure 10–4).

Compliance, a measure of arterial stiffness, is the relationship between strain (fractional deformation of wall) and stress (force per unit area of wall).[33] In an artery, it is described by the change in volume of a segment of artery in relation to pulsatile change in blood pressure. We reported, for the first time, a significant decrease in the compliance of the ICA after placement of a carotid stent (Figure 10–5). The enhanced stiffness of the stent-arterial wall complex renders the flow–pressure relationship of the carotid artery closer to that observed in a rigid tube[34] so that the energy normally applied to dilate the artery results in an increased velocity.

The new DU velocity criteria above define procedural success (<20% residual stenosis) and will most reliably discriminate normal from in-stent residual stenosis (≥20%) immediately after CAS. These proposed criteria can form the basis for additional prospective validation

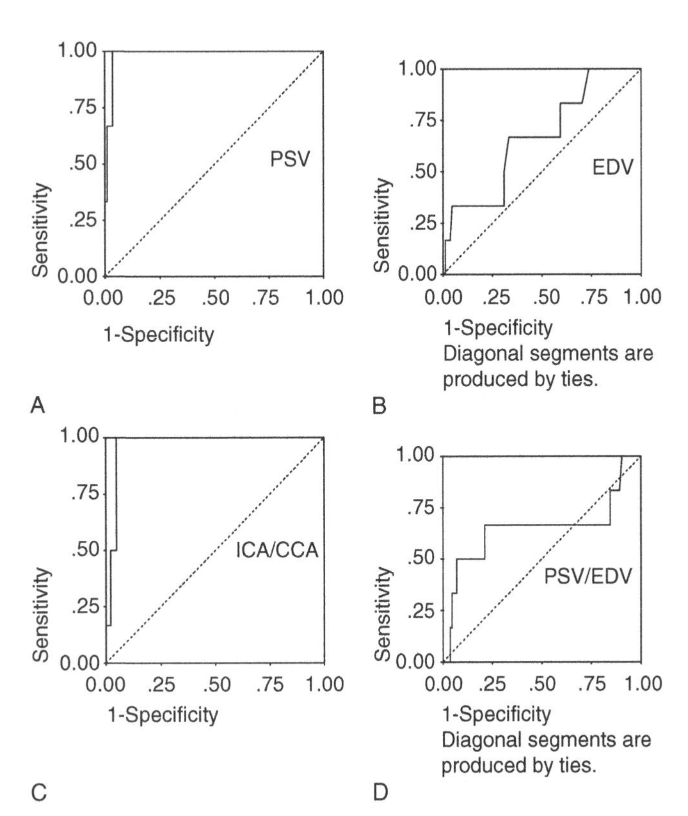

FIGURE 10–4. Receiver operating characteristics curves of various ultrasound velocity measurements (in cm/s) for differentiating between ≥20% or <20% angiographic in-stent residual stenosis immediately after carotid stenting. (A) In-stent PSV. (B) In-stent EDV. (C) In-stent PSV/EDV ratio. (D) In-stent PSV of ICA/CCA ratio. [Adapted from Lal BK, Hobson RW 2nd, Goldstein J, Chakhtoura EY, Duran WN. Carotid artery stenting: Is there a need to revise ultrasound velocity criteria? J Vasc Surg 2004;39(1):58–66.]

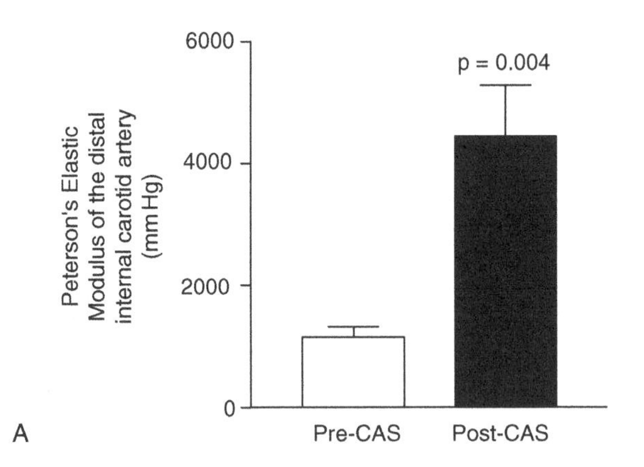

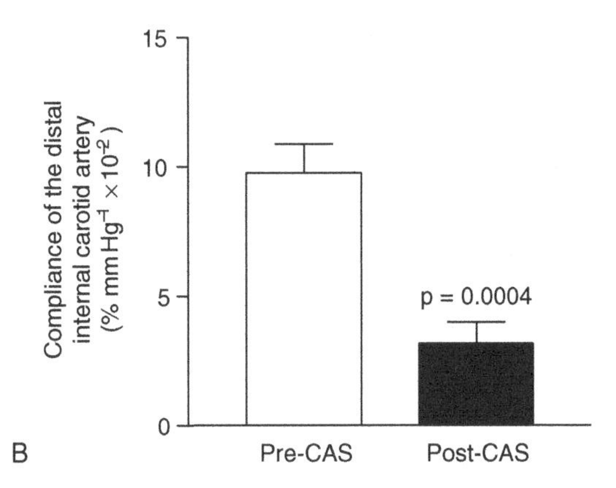

FIGURE 10–5. Measurement of elastic modulus (A) and compliance (B) demonstrates increased stiffness of the stented distal internal carotid artery post-CAS versus the native distal internal carotid artery (pre-CAS) (n = 20 for each measurement). Pre-CAS, prior to carotid artery stenting; post-CAS, after carotid artery stenting. [Adapted from Lal BK, Hobson RW 2nd, Goldstein J, Chakhtoura EY, Duran WN. Carotid artery stenting: Is there a need to revise ultrasound velocity criteria? J Vasc Surg 2004;39(1):58–66.]

studies to further develop criteria identifying post-CAS ISR of higher grades. Until these revised criteria are available, we recommend early registration of baseline velocity measurements after CAS against which future results should be compared.

While velocity criteria are being developed, increasing resolution of B-mode imaging is improving our ability to visualize the stent and luminal morphology. Further studies are required to establish the accuracy of luminal diameter measurements obtained by B-mode alone. However, it is possible that additional information derived from current B-mode imaging and spectral broadening may be used to supplement velocity measurements. For instance, in the presence of a PSV ≥ 150 cm/s and an ICA/CCA ratio ≥2.16, B-mode imaging may show no evidence of luminal encroachment in the stent, or there may be no spectral broadening. These data may therefore supplement the velocity criteria for determination of severity of in-stent stenosis.

Recommendations

1. All patients undergoing CAS must be placed in a regular follow-up protocol involving DU and clinical evaluation. The current risk of hemodynamically significant ISR is 6.4% over 4 years. Most ISR appears to occur early after CAS (18 months). Therefore follow-up must occur at baseline, 6 months, and annually thereafter.
2. The first follow-up DU after CAS must occur as soon after the procedure as possible, preferably during the same admission. Velocity criteria used to define residual stenosis ≥20% had to be revised to include a PSV ≥150 cm/s and an ICA/CCA ratio ≥2.16 in our laboratory. These values must be used as a guide to revise velocity criteria in individual vascular laboratories.
3. B-mode imaging of the arterial lumen and spectral waveform analysis must be used to supplement and enhance the accuracy of velocity criteria.
4. Revised velocity criteria defining higher grades of ISR are still under development; early registration of baseline velocities to compare subsequent follow-up velocities is the optimal surveillance protocol currently available. Elevations in PSV and/or ICA/CCA ratios may be indicative of developing ISR, which must then undergo angiographic evaluation and appropriate management.

References

1. Lal BK, Hobson IR. Carotid artery occlusive disease. Curr Treat Options Cardiovasc Med 2000;2(3):243–54.
2. Matcher DB, Duncan PW. Cost of Stroke. Stroke Clin Updates 1994;5:9–12.
3. Hobson RW 2nd, Weiss DG, Fields WS, *et al.* Efficacy of carotid endarterectomy for asymptomatic carotid stenosis. The Veterans Affairs Cooperative Study Group. N Engl J Med 1993;328(4):221–7.
4. North American Symptomatic Carotid Endarterectomy Trial Collaborators. Beneficial effect of carotid endarterectomy in symptomatic patients with high-grade carotid stenosis. N Engl J Med 1991;325(7):445–53.
5. Executive Committee for the Asymptomatic Carotid Atherosclerosis Study. Endarterectomy for asymptomatic carotid artery stenosis. JAMA 1995;273(18):1421–8.
6. Barnett HJ, Taylor DW, Eliasziw M, *et al.* Benefit of carotid endarterectomy in patients with symptomatic moderate or severe stenosis. North American Symptomatic Carotid Endarterectomy Trial Collaborators. N Engl J Med 1998; 339(20):1415–25.
7. Halliday A, Mansfield A, Marro J, *et al.* Prevention of disabling and fatal strokes by successful carotid endarterectomy in patients without recent neurological symptoms: Randomised controlled trial. Lancet 2004;363(9420):1491–502.
8. Hobson RW 2nd, Goldstein JE, Jamil Z, *et al.* Carotid restenosis: Operative and endovascular management. J Vasc Surg 1999;29(2):228–35; discussion 35–8.
9. Dorros G. Complications associated with extracranial carotid artery interventions. J Endovasc Surg 1996;3(2): 166–70.
10. Ferguson RD, Ferguson JG. Carotid angioplasty. In search of a worthy alternative to endarterectomy. Arch Neurol 1996;53(7):696–8.
11. Hobson RW 2nd, Lal BK, Chakhtoura E, *et al.* Carotid artery stenting: Analysis of data for 105 patients at high risk. J Vasc Surg 2003;37(6):1234–9.
12. Hobson RW 2nd, Lal BK, Chakhtoura EY, *et al.* Carotid artery closure for endarterectomy does not influence results of angioplasty-stenting for restenosis. J Vasc Surg 2002; 35(3):435–8.
13. Lal BK, Hobson RW 2nd, Goldstein J, *et al.* In-stent recurrent stenosis after carotid artery stenting: Life table analysis and clinical relevance. J Vasc Surg 2003;38(6):1162–8; discussion 9.
14. Cuadra S, Hobson R, Lal B, *et al.* Carotid artery stenting: Does the outcome depend on the indication? Abstract presented at the Vascular 2005, Annual conference of the Society for Vascular Surgery, Society for Vascular Technology, and Society for Vascular Medicine and Biology, Chicago, IL, 2005.
15. Choi HM, Hobson RW, Goldstein J, *et al.* Technical challenges in a program of carotid artery stenting. J Vasc Surg 2004;40(4):746–51; discussion 51.
16. Hobson RW 2nd. Carotid artery stenting. Surg Clin North Am 2004;84(5):1281–94, vi.
17. Lal BK, Hobson RW 2nd, Goldstein J, Chakhtoura EY, Duran WN. Carotid artery stenting: Is there a need to revise ultrasound velocity criteria? J Vasc Surg 2004;39(1):58–66.
18. Al-Mubarak N, Roubin GS, Vitek JJ, New G, Iyer SS. Procedural safety and short-term outcome of ambulatory carotid stenting. Stroke 2001;32(10):2305–9.
19. Roubin GS, New G, Iyer SS, *et al.* Immediate and late clinical outcomes of carotid artery stenting in patients with symptomatic and asymptomatic carotid artery stenosis: A 5-year prospective analysis. Circulation 2001;103(4):532–7.
20. Vitek JJ, Roubin GS, New G, Al-Mubarek N, Iyer SS. Carotid angioplasty with stenting in post-carotid endarterectomy restenosis. J Invasive Cardiol 2001;13(2):123–5; discussion 58–70.
21. Wholey MH, Wholey M, Mathias K, *et al.* Global experience in cervical carotid artery stent placement. Catheter Cardiovasc Interv 2000;50(2):160–7.
22. Ohki T, Veith FJ. Carotid artery stenting: Utility of cerebral protection devices. J Invasive Cardiol 2001;13(1): 47–55.
23. Veith FJ, Amor M, Ohki T, *et al.* Current status of carotid bifurcation angioplasty and stenting based on a consensus of opinion leaders. J Vasc Surg 2001;33(2 Suppl): S111–6.
24. Yadav JS, Wholey MH, Kuntz RE, *et al.* Protected carotid-artery stenting versus endarterectomy in high-risk patients. N Engl J Med 2004;351(15):1493–501.

25. Endovascular versus surgical treatment in patients with carotid stenosis in the Carotid and Vertebral Artery Transluminal Angioplasty Study (CAVATAS): A randomised trial. Lancet 2001;357(9270):1729–37.
26. Hobson RW 2nd. Update on the Carotid Revascularization Endarterectomy versus Stent Trial (CREST) protocol. J Am Coll Surg 2002;194(1 Suppl):S9–14.
27. Hobson RW 2nd, Howard VJ, Roubin GS, *et al.* Carotid artery stenting is associated with increased complications in octogenarians: 30-day stroke and death rates in the CREST lead-in phase. J Vasc Surg 2004;40(6):1106–11.
28. Willfort-Ehringer A, Ahmadi R, Gruber D, *et al.* Arterial remodeling and hemodynamics in carotid stents: A prospective duplex ultrasound study over 2 years. J Vasc Surg 2004;39(4):728–34.
29. Alexandrov AV, Brodie DS, McLean A, Hamilton P, Murphy J, Burns PN. Correlation of peak systolic velocity and angiographic measurement of carotid stenosis revisited. Stroke 1997;28(2):339–42.
30. Faught WE, Mattos MA, van Bemmelen PS, *et al.* Color-flow duplex scanning of carotid arteries: New velocity criteria based on receiver operator characteristic analysis for threshold stenoses used in the symptomatic and asymptomatic carotid trials. J Vasc Surg 1994;19(5):818–27; discussion 27–8.
31. Robbin ML, Lockhart ME, Weber TM, *et al.* Carotid artery stents: Early and intermediate follow-up with Doppler US. Radiology 1997;205(3):749–56.
32. Ringer AJ, German JW, Guterman LR, Hopkins LN. Follow-up of stented carotid arteries by Doppler ultrasound. Neurosurgery 2002;51(3):639–43; discussion 43.
33. Wilson KA, Hoskins PR, Lee AJ, Fowkes FG, Ruckley CV, Bradbury AW. Ultrasonic measurement of abdominal aortic aneurysm wall compliance: A reproducibility study. J Vasc Surg 2000;31(3):507–13.
34. Green JF. *Mechanical Concepts in Cardiovascular and Pulmonary Physiology,* 2nd ed. Philadelphia, PA: Lea & Febiger, 1977.

11 Use of Transcranial Doppler in Monitoring Patients during Carotid Artery Stenting

Mark C. Bates

Introduction

It has been over 20 years since Aaslid first described the technique of middle cerebral artery range gated Doppler interrogation via a low-frequency ultrasound transducer stationed just above the zygomatic arch.[1] Since that time insonation techniques with probe fixation headgear have made continuous real-time imaging much easier and advances in Doppler technology including "power Doppler" have improved signal clarity.[2] A detailed review of the physics and utility of transcranial Doppler (TCD) is eloquently presented in Chapter 6. The objective of this chapter is to expose the reader to some of the lessons learned from adjuvant transcranial Doppler during carotid stent-supported angioplasty.

Carotid endarterectomy has been proven in large randomized trials to reduce the risk of stroke or future neurologic events in patients with symptomatic and asymptomatic extracranial cerebrovascular disease.[3,4] The carotid endarterectomy techniques have matured and through the years we have learned that in the hands of experienced surgeons, the risk of a periprocedural neurologic event is very low.[5,6] The inherent risk of transcatheter interaction with the typical friable internal carotid artery lesion and resultant embolization of material to the brain was recognized early on as a limitation to carotid artery stenting.[7–10] The development of cerebral protection devices including distal occlusive balloons, distal filter systems, and proximal occlusive systems has rekindled enthusiasm about carotid artery stenting as an alternative to endarterectomy.[11–20]

Carotid artery stenting remains very controversial in many countries and currently there are no well-controlled randomized clinical trials that have shown clinical equipoise between carotid artery stenting and carotid endarterectomy.[21] There does appear to be a subgroup of patients that may benefit from this technology. These patients have been categorized as "high risk" for surgery based on anatomic and clinical criteria. At present there is one well-designed randomized trial evaluating carotid endarterectomy versus stenting in high-risk patients for endarterectomy.[22] While the SAPPHIRE trial did not show a statistically significant reduction in risk of periprocedural stroke in patients undergoing stenting versus surgery, there did seem to be an overall lower risk of serious adverse events when also considering myocardial infarction as an endpoint.[22] There have also been multiple registries of high-risk patients who have undergone carotid stenting with outcomes compared to historical controls. These studies also suggest carotid stenting may be a safe alternative to surgery in high-risk patients.[23–26] The recent approval by the United States Food and Drug Administration (FDA) for carotid artery stenting in patients that are considered high risk for surgery underscores the importance of better understanding the embolic risk of carotid artery stenting and TCD has given considerable insight to investigators on that front. In fact, TCD has provided early carotid stent pioneers with important feedback on embolic risks during different stages of the procedure and also significant insight into the physiology of the reperfusion syndrome.

Transcranial Doppler, Periprocedural Setup

The patient is placed in the normal supine position on the angiographic table. The TCD headgear (Figure 11–1A) is placed in a position such that the lateral Doppler transducer fixation gaits can be aligned just above the zygomatic arch along the temporal window. This allows for the continuous sampling of pulse wave Doppler signals from the middle cerebral distribution, as detailed in Figure 11–1B. Fortunately, the headgear is radiolucent, except for the lateral brackets and tightening apparatus as shown in Figure 11–2. Thus, digital subtraction intracerebral angiography can be performed without removal of the headgear. The patient is then prepped and

A.F. Aburahma, J.J. Bergan (eds.), *Noninvasive Cerebrovascular Diagnosis*, DOI 10.1007/978-1-84882-957-2_11,

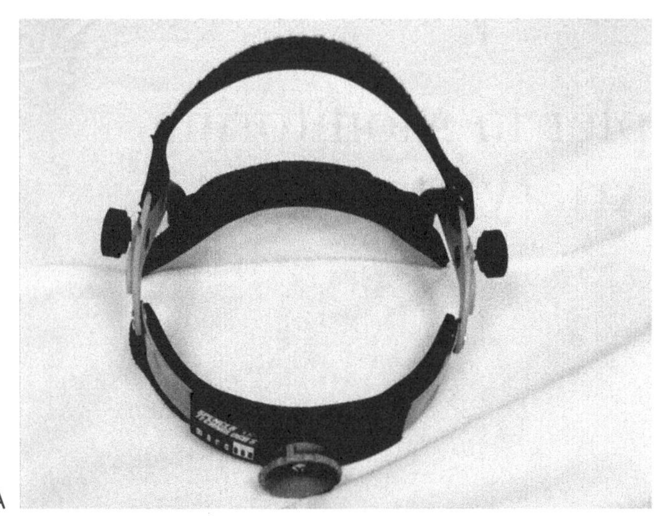

A

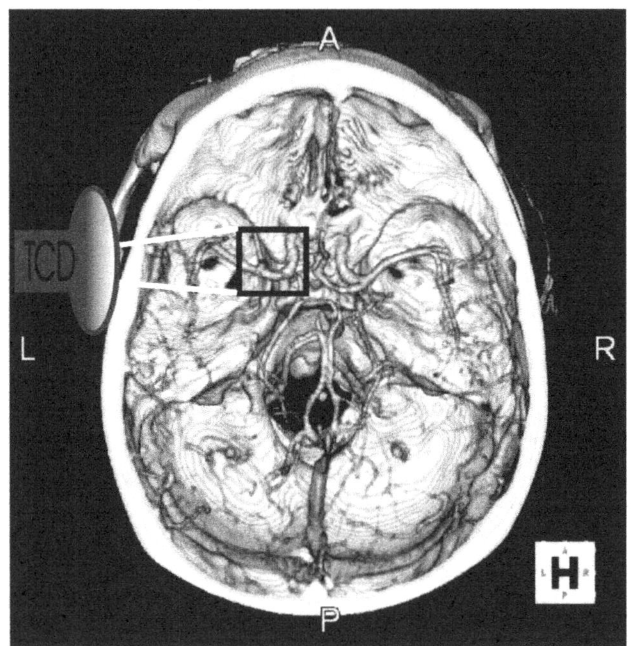

B

FIGURE 11–1. (A) The Spencer technologies headgear utilized for securing the transcranial Doppler probe for periprocedural imaging. The torque device in the front tightens the harness depending on the patient's cranial circumference. The lateral devices allow for positioning of the transcranial Doppler in a position appropriate for ideal insonation of the middle cerebral system. (B) A CT angiogram of a patient who subsequently underwent carotid artery stenting. The "TCD" represents the positioning of the probe and the square is the insonation window or area being monitored during carotid stenting.

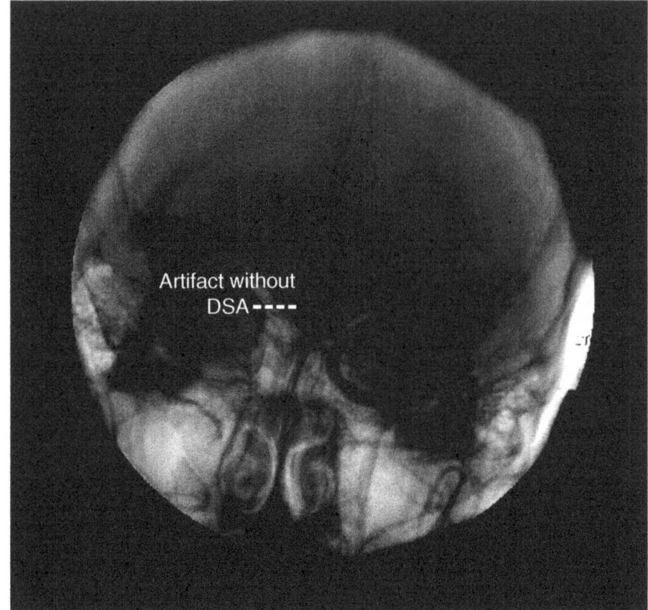

A

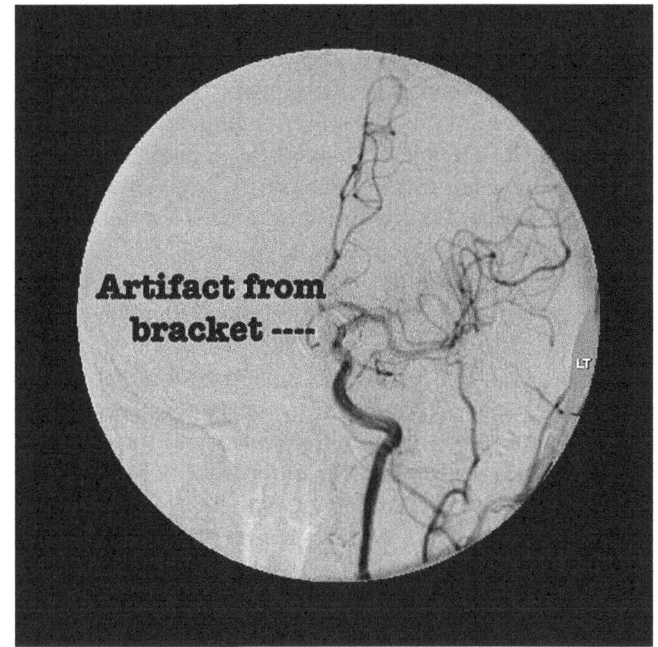

B

FIGURE 11–2. (A) A nonsubtracted image illustrating an artifact in the midline related to the ratchet device used to harness the transcranial Doppler. (B) During digital subtraction angiography the artifact silhouette persists but it is still possible to define the intracranial cerebral anatomy in the AP view without removing the transcranial Doppler harness.

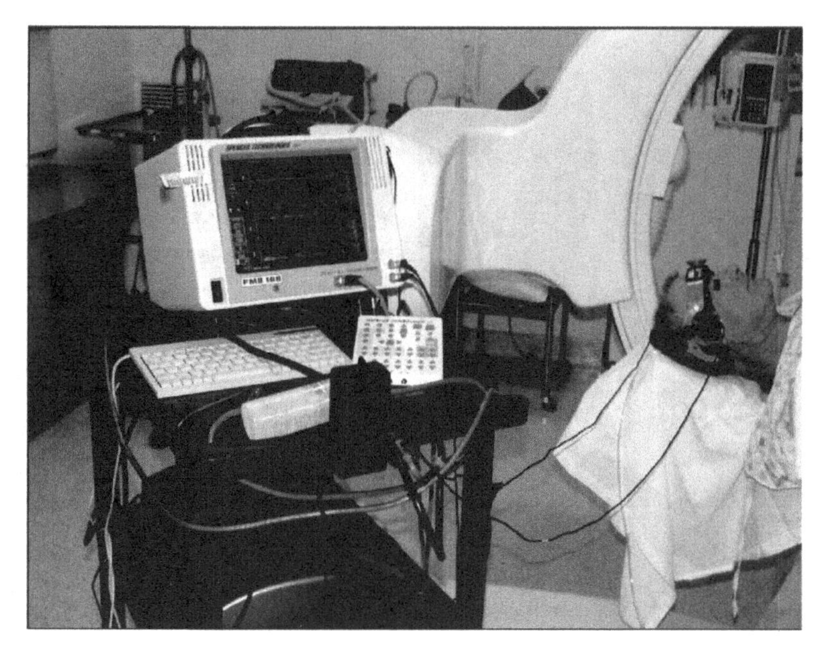

FIGURE 11–3. The typical setup during transcranial Doppler monitoring in the angiographic suite. The patient is placed in a supine position and the transcranial Doppler bracket is fixed to the head prior to baseline angiography.

draped in standard sterile fashion and baseline TCD interrogation is performed (Figure 11–3). Ideally, bilateral continuous pulse flow Doppler insonation of the middle cerebral arteries is monitored and digitally recorded throughout the procedure. It should be noted that anywhere from 9 to 16% of patients might not have an ideal window for accurate insonation of the middle cerebral artery.[27,28] In the case of an inadequate image of a window hand positioning of the probe and continuous monitoring are utilized versus continued attempts at repositioning the probe at different stages in the procedure.[27]

Preprocedural "Baseline" Transcranial Doppler Observations

The baseline TCD pattern may show blunting of the peak systolic wave in patients with severe extracranial disease.[28] More importantly, the TCD may give some insight into the collateral support via the Circle of Willis.[29,30] This information will help the operator better understand the patient's ability to tolerate cerebral protection systems that may arrest or even reverse ipsilateral internal carotid artery flow. Niesen *et al.* reported the utilization of baseline ratio between the peak systolic velocity in the ipsilateral middle cerebral vessel compared to the contralateral middle cerebral system as a reference for collateral support.[31] Also, the baseline intracranial flow characteristics could be important in predicting patients who are at risk for postprocedural reperfusion syndrome and intracranial hemorrhage. Mori *et al.* suggested the possibility of utilizing further hemodynamic testing in patients who are at increased risk for intracranial hemorrhage prior to placing them on the table.[32] This may include utilization of carbon dioxide reactivity or VMR testing with Diamox prior to interaction with the lesion.

Periprocedural Transcranial Doppler Observations

Transcranial Doppler provides two important parameters for continuous monitoring during carotid artery stenting. The first is related to ensuring preserved middle cerebral flow velocity and pulse volume. The utilization of a proximal or distal occlusive device for cerebral protection does result in interruption or reversal of flow in the ipsilateral internal carotid artery.[33] During internal carotid artery flow arrest or reversal a dramatic drop in middle cerebral flow velocity on TCD may precede the clinical hemispheric symptoms in patients with severe contralateral disease or inadequate collateral support due to an incomplete Circle of Willis. This provides the operator with additional insight as to how balloon occlusion will be tolerated and whether the procedure will need to be staged. Currently, the most widely tested distal occlusion balloon protection system is the guard wire (previously known as Percusurge). This device is a low-pressure balloon on a 0.014-inch wire that can be navigated across the lesion and then inflated to occlude the internal carotid artery during transcatheter intervention.[20] Utilization of this type of distal balloon occlusion system has proven to be effective in reducing the risk of embolization. However, Al-Mubarak *et al.* have shown with TCD

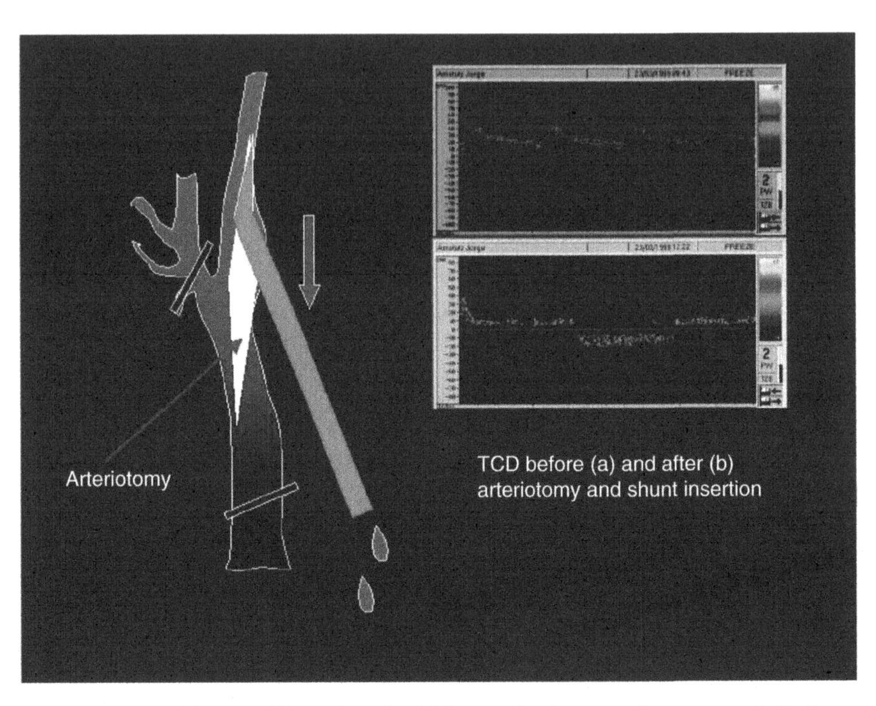

FIGURE 11–4. Transcranial Doppler evidence of intentional middle cerebral artery flow reversal during carotid endarterectomy. (Compliments of Dr. Juan Parodi.)

release of particles during balloon deflation that is likely related to inadequate particle retrieval from the cul-de-sac around the balloon.[34]

Parodi and Bates have shown with TCD the ability to completely reverse flow in the middle cerebral artery by transcatheter occlusion of the ipsilateral common and external carotid artery, while at the same time creating negative pressure at the tip of the guiding sheath as noted in Figure 11–4.[35] This may have significant implications for optimizing cerebral protection during carotid stenting and ultimately even facilitate clot retrieval during transcatheter treatment of acute stroke.

In patients with an intact Circle of Willis undergoing carotid stenting with a protection system that preserves flow (i.e., filter) the sudden interruption of flow to the ipsilateral middle cerebral artery could be an ominous finding suggesting a large embolic event or spasm in the internal carotid artery proper. Also, filter systems do have a threshold of particulate debris based on the filtered design and size.[36] If the volume of embolic debris exceeds the filter threshold then occlusion can occur and this may be heralded by changes on TCD. Similar changes can occur if there is spasm in the ipsilateral internal carotid artery system related to the distal protection filter.[27]

The second variable that is monitored by TCD during carotid artery stenting is the occurrence of microemboli signals (MESs). The reflective properties of microembolic material as it passes through the middle cerebral artery are translated into sudden signal shifts that are depicted as high velocity transient spikes on the continuous Doppler recording.[37–39] These high intensity signals may represent the egress of small particles or microembolic debris into the ipsilateral hemisphere.[40] It is difficult to differentiate artifact from small air bubbles from true embolic debris and that is one of the limitations of this technology.[41–43] *Ex vitro* studies by Coggia *et al.* and Ohki *et al.* have provided significant insight into when particles are released during different stages of the procedure.[44,45] The peak embolic risk during angioplasty in the *ex vitro* model appears to be during balloon deflation.[44] Similar findings are seen *in vivo* with continuous TCD during carotid stenting at the time of balloon deflation.[46,47] In our experience MESs are seen during all stages of carotid stenting with or without protection even with navigation of a 0.014-inch wire across the lesion (Figure 11–5).

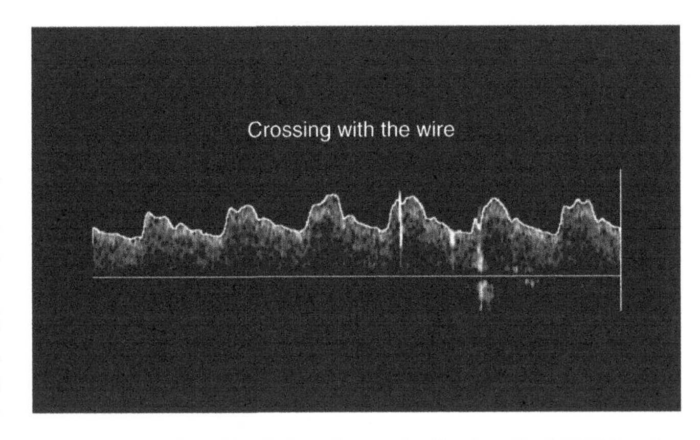

FIGURE 11–5. Small subtle microembolic signals (MESs) coincident with advancing the wire through the lesion. These MESs are shown as bright signals with the most prominent seen in the fourth complete Doppler pulse sequence.

Postprocedural Transcranial Doppler Observations

Some authors have followed TCD with serial interval studies during the first 12 h following carotid stenting.[48,49] Our center believes that this may be particularly important in patients who are at increased risk for intracranial hemorrhage. The preprocedural risk factors for reperfusion syndrome and/or intracranial hemorrhage include contralateral severe carotid disease or occlusion, baseline high-grade stenosis or "string sign" with slow flow, hypertension during the carotid stenting procedure, and baseline decrease of vasoreactivity.[50] Figure 11–6 details the TCD hemodynamic sequence of a patient who developed the typical reperfusion syndrome complicated by intra-

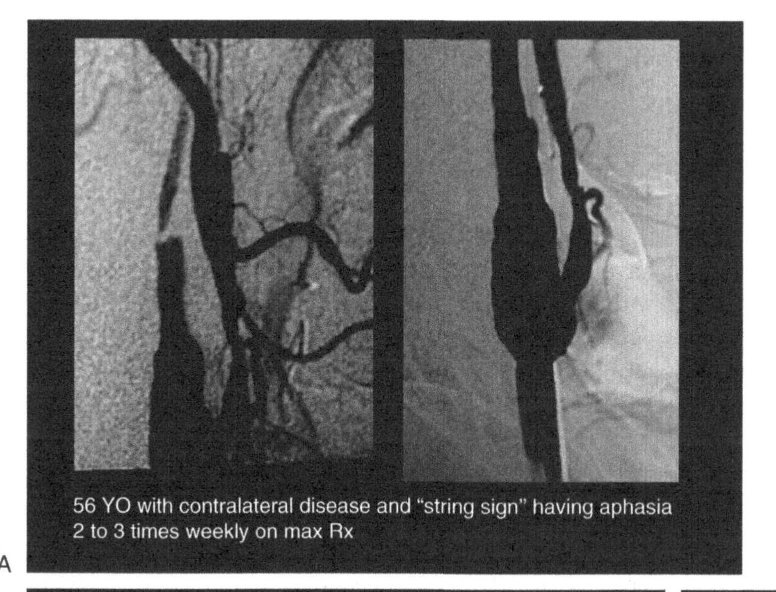

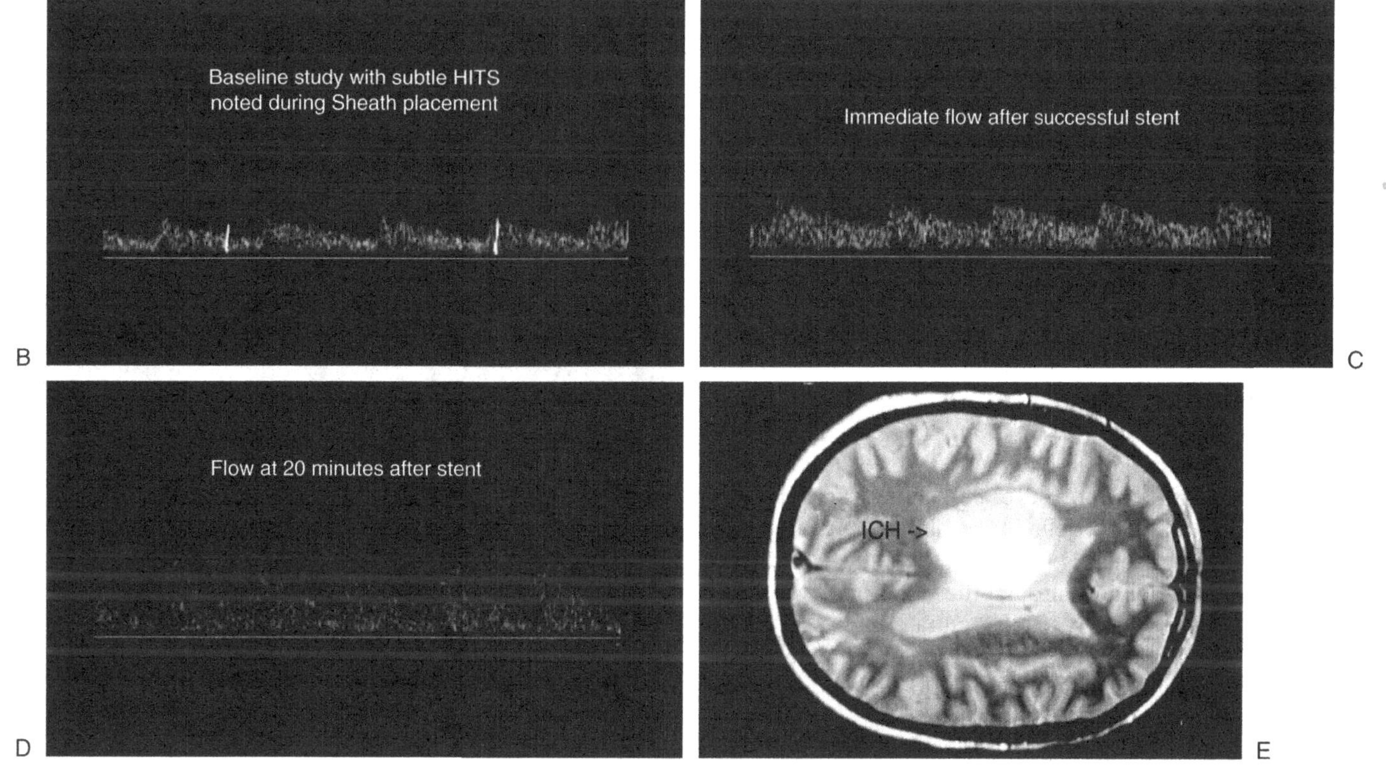

FIGURE 11–6. (A) Baseline angiography and follow-up angiography after carotid stenting in a patient with multiple risk factors for postprocedural intracranial hemorrhage. (B) Baseline low pulse volume middle cerebral artery Doppler in the patient illustrated in (A). (C) Immediate flow after carotid stent placement in the patient presented in (A). Note that the flow velocity has increased by approximately 30%. (D) The flow pattern in the same patient depicted in (A). This is 20 min following stent placement and note the flow velocity is now three times greater than the baseline velocity. (E) CT scan confirming a large intracranial hemorrhage depicted as an intracerebral hemorrhage (ICH) 12 h after stent placement.

cranial hemorrhage during our early experience with unprotected carotid stenting 10 years ago.

Few studies have actually reported continuous TCD in the early postoperative period after carotid stenting. However, it seems that MESs are uncommon during the recovery period after carotid stenting.[51]

Significance of Microemboli during Carotid Artery Stenting

Microembolic signals detected during carotid endarterectomy have been associated with a decrease in cognitive function.[52] Similarly, MESs with so-called "embolic storms" during different stages of carotid stent procedures are associated with ipsilateral defects on early follow-up diffusion weighted magnetic resonance imaging (MRI) scan.[53–57] Currently, there are very few data with regard to cognitive function in patients following protected carotid artery stenting, and this is a concern. Interestingly, in a small subgroup analysis of patients during the Carotid and Vertebral Artery Transluminal Angioplasty Study (CAVATAS) there were similar outcomes on neurologic testing in both the carotid endarterectomy and carotid stenting groups in spite of a higher number of MESs in the latter.[58]

The threshold or "safe" size for microemboli has not been clearly defined. Early work suggests that any particles more than 50 μm in size will not circulate to the venous cerebral system and thus by definition will cause some arteriolar occlusions.[59] Significant work on this front has been done to better understand the decrease in cognitive function that is seen after coronary artery bypass surgery. Based on a postmortem study by Moody *et al.* it appears that the particles causing decreased cognitive function after coronary artery bypass surgery are less than 70 μm in size.[60] This is particularly important to understand since most distal protection filters have a pore size of 100–120 μm.

Differentiating Microemboli from Air Bubbles

The differentiation of air bubbles from true atheroemboli has been very difficult. Several techniques have been described including a defined threshold of greater than 10 hits in a sequence.[27] Different mathematical sequences have also been defined through the years, however, there currently is no ideal way to differentiate these *in vivo*.[41–44]

There are certain stages of the procedure where contamination from an air artifact would be less likely. For example, crossing the lesion with the wire as noted in Figure 11–5 should not be associated with air embolization and is likely true microemboli. Also, many centers have reported that the highest numbers of emboli occur with predilatation or postdilatation as the balloon is deflated and it is also unlikely there is significant trapped air or artifact during this time as depicted in Figure 11–7. However, scattered MESs are typically seen during contrast injections, which is related to microbubbles in the contrast (Figure 11–8).

Most of the carotid stents used today are self-expanding stents made of nickel titanium with an outer constraining sheath. There is always a high volume of MES with retracting of the sheath housing the self-expanding stent and some authors have suggested that this is related to the shear force of a stent against the plaque.[27] However, we feel this is related to trapped air within the fabric of the stent and, thus, is less likely to be of pathologic concern (Figure 11–9).

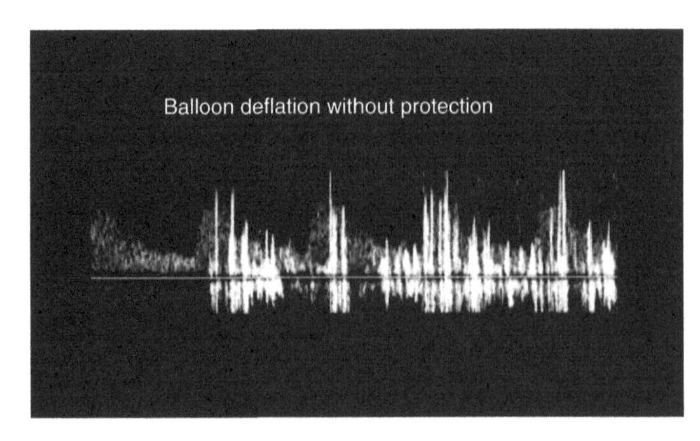

FIGURE 11–7. Multiple MESs in a patient after balloon deflation in our early experience before cerebral protection was available.

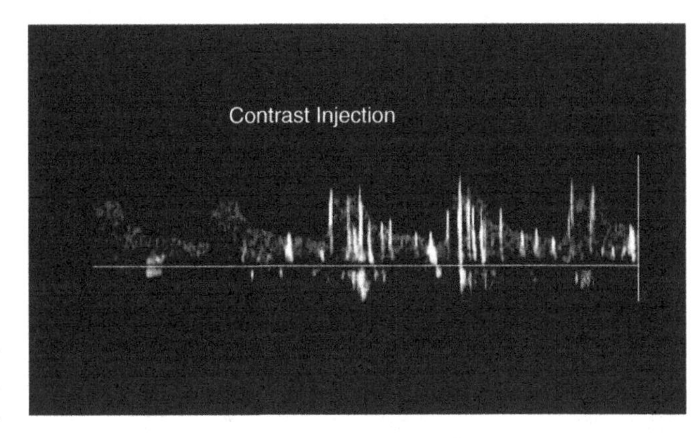

FIGURE 11–8. Multiple air bubble MESs during contrast injection.

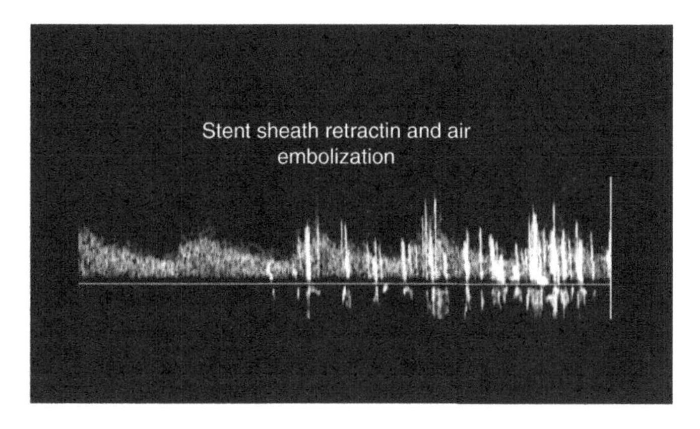

FIGURE 11–9. Fairly impressive air bubble microemboli during sheath retraction at the time of stent deployment.

Conclusions

Currently, TCD has not been declared mandatory for periprocedural adjuvant monitoring in patients undergoing carotid artery stenting based on consensus documents.[61] Many centers believe that transcranial Doppler is more of an academic tool to help understand the benefits and failure modes of current protection systems. Periprocedural transcranial Doppler is clearly indicated in patients who are at high risk for reperfusion syndrome and may also give additional insight into the long-term issues of decreased cerebral flow reserve and/or worsening cognitive function after carotid stenting. Obviously, there is much more to learn in terms of better understanding microemboli and the long-term consequences MESs have on the patients after carotid stenting. We believe TCD provides invaluable information during the procedure and should be applied to all patients undergoing carotid stenting. Clearly, the argument could be made that patients at high risk for reperfusion syndrome or those undergoing carotid stenting with internal carotid artery flow arrest or flow reversal should have TCD guidance. Only future studies will help us understand the importance of MESs in predicting issues related to cognitive function.

References

1. Aaslid R, Markwalder TM, Nornes H. Noninvasive transcranial Doppler ultrasound recording of flow velocity in basal cerebral arteries. J Neurosurg 1982;57(6):769–74.
2. Bogdahn U, Becker G, Winkler J, *et al.* Transcranial color-coded real-time sonography in adults. Stroke 1990;21:1680–88.
3. North American Symptomatic Carotid Endarterectomy Trial Collaborators. Beneficial effect of carotid endarterectomy in symptomatic patients with high-grade carotid stenosis. N Engl J Med 1991;325:445–53.
4. European Carotid Surgery Trialists' Group. MRC European carotid surgery trial: Interim results for symptomatic patients with severe or with mild carotid stenosis. Lancet 1991;337:1235–43.
5. AbuRahma AF, Hannay RS. A study of 510 carotid endarterectomies and a review of the recent carotid endarterectomy trials. WV Med J 2001;97(4):197–200.
6. Bond R, Rerkasem K, AbuRahma AF, Naylor AR, Rothwell PM. Patch angioplasty versus primary closure for carotid endarterectomy. Cochrane Database Syst Rev 2004;(2):CD000160.
7. Diethrich EB. Indications for carotid artery stenting: A preview of the potential derived from early clinical experience. J Endovasc Surg 1996;3:132–9.
8. Naylor AR, Bolia A, Abbott RJ, Pye IF, Smith J, Lennard N, Lloyd AJ, London NJ, Bell PR. Randomized study of çarotid angioplasty and stenting versus carotid endarterectomy: A stopped trial. J Vasc Surg 1998;28(2):326.
9. Leisch F, Kerschner K, Hofman R, Bibl D, Engleder C, Bergmann H. Carotid stenting: Acute results and complications. Z Kardiol 1999;88:661–68.
10. Bettman MA, Katzen BT, Whisnant J, Brant-Zawadski MB, Broderick JP, Furlan AJ, Hershey LA, Howard V, Kuntz R, Loftus CM, Pearce W, Roberts A, Roubin G. Cartoid Stenting and Angioplasty. A statement for healthcare professionals from the councils on cardiovascular radiology, stroke, cardio-thoracic and vascular surgery, epidemiology and prevention, and clinical cardiology, American Heart Association. Stroke 1998;29:336–48.
11. Theron JG, Peyelle GG, Coskun O, *et al.* Carotid artery stenosis: Treatment with protected balloon angioplasty and stent placement. Radiology 1996;201:627–36.
12. Wholey MH, Al-Mubarak N, Wholey MH. Updated review of the global carotid artery stent registry. Catheter Cardiovasc Interv 2003;60:259–66.
13. Ohki T, Feith FJ. Carotid artery stenting: Utility of cerebral protection devices. J Invasive Cardiol 2001;13:47–55.
14. Henry M, Amor M, Klonaris C, *et al.* Angioplasty and stenting of the extracranial carotid arteries. Tex Heart Inst J 2000;27:150–58.
15. Reimers B, Corvaja N, Moshiri S, *et al.* Cerebral protection with filter devices during carotid artery stenting. Circulation 2001;104:12–15.
16. Parodi JC, Mura RL, Ferreira LM, *et al.* Initial evaluation of carotid angioplasty and stenting with three different cerebral protection devices. J Vasc Surg 2000;32:1127–36.
17. Al-Mubarak N, Colombo A, Gaines PA, *et al.* Multicenter evaluation of carotid artery stenting with a filter protection system. J Am Coll Cardiol 2002;39:841–46.
18. Mathur A, Roubin GS, Iyer SS, *et al.* Predictors of stroke complicating carotid artery stenting. Circulation 1998;97:1239–45.
19. Yadav JS, Roubin GS, Iyer S, *et al.* Elective stenting of the extracranial carotid arteries. Circulation 1997;95:376–81.
20. Al-Moubarak N, Roubin GS, Vitek JJ, *et al.* Effect of the distal-balloon protection system on microembolization during carotid stenting. Circulation 2001;104:199–200.
21. Zarins CK. Carotid endarterectomy: The gold standard. J Endovasc Surg 1996;3:10–15.
22. Yadav JS, WholeyMH, Kuntz RE, Fayed, P, Katzen, BT, Mishkel GJ, Bajwa TK, Whitlow P, Strickman NE, Jaff MR,

Popma JJ, Snead DB, Cutlilp DE, Firth BG, Ouriel K. Stenting and Angioplasty with Protection in Patients at High Risk for Endarterectomy Investigators. N Engl J Med 2004;351(15):1493–501.
23. Ireland JK, Chaloupka JC, Weigele JB, *et al.* Potential utility of carotid stent assisted percutaneous transluminal angioplasty in the treatment of symptomatic carotid occlusive disease in patients with high neurological risk. Stroke 2003;34:308.
24. Qureshi AI, Boulos AS, Kim SH, *et al.* Carotid angioplasty and stent placement using the Filterwire for distal protection: An international multicenter study. Stroke 2003;34:307.
25. Roubin GS, New G, Iyer SS, *et al.* Immediate and late clinical outcomes of carotid artery stenting in patients with symptomatic and asymptomatic carotid artery stenosis: A 5-year prospective analysis. Circulation 2001;103:532–37.
26. MacDonald S, Venables GS, Cleveland TJ, *et al.* Protected carotid stenting: Safety and efficacy of the MedNova NeuroSheild filter. J Vasc Surg 2002;35:966–72.
27. Benichou H, Bergeron P. Carotid angioplasty and stenting: Will periprocedural transcranial Doppler monitoring be important? J Endovasc Surg 1996;3:217–23.
28. (a) Hartmann A, Mast H, Thompson JL, Sia RM, Mohr JP. Transcranial Doppler waveform blunting in severe extracranial carotid artery stenosis. Cerebrovasc Dis 2000;10(1):33–8. (b) Gomez CR, Brass LM, Tegeler CH, *et al.* The transcranial Doppler standardization project. J Neuroimaging 1993;3:190–92.
29. Visser GH, Wieneke GH, van Huffelen AC, Eikelboom BC. The use of preoperative transcranial Doppler variables to predict which patients do not need a shunt during carotid endarterectomy. Stroke 2003;34:813–9.
30. Reinhard M, Muller T, Roth M, Guschlbauer B, Timmer J, Hetzel A. Bilateral severe carotid artery stenosis or occlusion—-cerebral autoregulation dynamics and collateral flow patterns. Acta Neurochir (Wien) 2003;145(12):1053–9.
31. Niesen WD, Rosenkranz M, Eckert B, Meissner M, Weiller C, Sliwka U. Hemodynamic changes of the cerebral circulation after stent-protected carotid angioplasty. AJNR Am J Neuroradiol 2004;25(7):1162–7.
32. Mori T, Fukuoka M, Kazita K, Mima T, Mori K. Intraventricular hemorrhage after carotid stenting. J Endovasc Surg 1999;6(4):337–41.
33. Tan W, Bates MC, Wholey M. Cerebral protection systems for distal emboli during carotid artery interventions. J Intervent Cardiol 2001;14(4):1–9.
34. Al-Mubarak N, Roubin GS, Vitek JJ, Iyer SS. Microembolization during carotid artery stenting with the distal-balloon antiemboli system. Int Angiol 2002;21(4):344–8.
35. Parodi JC, Bates MC. Angioplasty and stent with reversal of internal carotid flow as a cerebral protection device. In: Greenhalgh RM (ed). *ATLAS: Vascular and Endovascular Surgical Techniques*, 4th ed., pp. 198–213. Philadelphia: Saunders, 2001.
36. Kindel M, Spiller P. Transient occlusion of an Angioguard protection system by massive embolization during angioplasty of a degenerated coronary saphenous vein graft. Catheter Cardiovasc Interv 2002;55:2501–4.
37. Moehring MA, Ritcey JA. Microembolus sizing in a blood mimicking fluid using a novel dual-frequency pulsed Doppler. Echocardiography 1996;13(5):567–71.
38. Moehring MA, Ritcey JA. Sizing emboli in blood using pulse Doppler ultrasound—II: Effects of beam refraction. IEEE Trans Biomed Eng 1996;43(6):581–88.
39. Moehring MA, Klepper JR. Pulse Doppler ultrasound detection, characterization and size estimation of emboli in flowing blood. IEEE Trans Biomed Eng 1994;41(1):35–44.
40. Crawley F, *et al.* Comparison of hemodynamic cerebral ischemia and microembolic signals detected during carotid endarterectomy and carotid angioplasty. Stroke 1997;28(12):2460–64.
41. Devuyst G, Darbellay GA, Vesin JM, Kemeny V, Ritter M, Droste DW, Molina C, Serena J, Sztajzel R, Ruchat P, Lucchesi C, Dietler G, Ringelstein EB, Despland PA, Bogousslavsky J. Automatic classification of HITS into artifacts or solid or gaseous emboli by a wavelet representation combined with dual-gate TCD. Stroke 2001;32(12):2803–9.
42. Georgiadis D, Uhlmann F, Lindner A, Zierz S. Differentiation between true microembolic signals and artifacts using an arbitrary sample volume. Ultrasound Med Biol 2000;26(3):493–6.
43. Rodriguez RA, Giachino A, Hosking M, Nathan HJ. Transcranial Doppler characteristics of different embolic materials during in vivo testing. J Neuroimaging 2002;12(3):259–66.
44. Ohki T, Roubin GS, Veith FJ, *et al.* The efficacy of a filter in preventing embolic events during carotid artery stenting. An ex-vivo analysis. J Vasc Surg 1999;30:1034–44.
45. Coggia M, Goeau-Brissonniere O, Duval JL, *et al.* Embolic risk of the different stages of carotid bifurcation balloon angioplasty: An experimental study. J Vasc Surg 2000;31:550–57.
46. Antonius Carotid Endarterectomy, Angioplasty, and Stenting Study Group. Transcranial Doppler monitoring in angioplasty and stenting of the carotid bifurcation. J Endovasc Ther 2003;10(4):702–10.
47. Orlandi G, Fanucchi S, Fioretti C, Acerbi G, Puglioli M, Padolecchia R, Sartucci F, Murri L. Characteristics of cerebral microembolism during carotid stenting and angioplasty alone. Arch Neurol 2001;58(9):1410–3.
48. Abou-Chebl A, Yadav JS, Reginelli JP, Bajzer C, Bhatt D, Krieger DW. Intracranial hemorrhage and hyperperfusion syndrome following carotid artery stenting: Risk factors, prevention, and treatment. J Am Coll Cardiol 2004;43(9):1596–601.
49. Dalman JE, Beenakkers IC, Moll FL, Leusink JA, Ackerstaff RG. Transcranial Doppler monitoring during carotid endarterectomy helps to identify patients at risk of postoperative hyperperfusion. Eur J Vasc Endovasc Surg 1999;18(3):222–7.
50. Morrish W, Grahovac S, Douen A. Intracranial hemorrhage after stenting and angioplasty of extracranial carotid stenosis. AJNR Am J Neuroradiol 2000;21:1911–16.
51. Censori B, Camerlingo M, Casto L, Partziguian T, Caverni L, Bonaldi G, Mamoli A. Carotid stents are not a source of microemboli late after deployment. Acta Neurol Scand 2000;102(1):27–30.

52. Gaunt ME, Martin PJ, Smith JL, Bell PR. Clinical relevance of intraoperative embolization detected by transcranial Doppler ultrasonography during carotid endarterectomy: A prospective study of 100 patients. AR Br J Surg 1994;81: 1435–9.
53. van Heesewijk HP, Vos JA, Louwerse ES, Van Den Berg JC, Overtoom TT, Ernst SM, Mauser HW, Moll FL, Ackerstaff RG. Carotid PTA and Stenting Collaborative Research Group. New brain lesions at MR imaging after carotid angioplasty and stent placement. Radiology 2002;224(2): 361–5.
54. Jaeger H, Mathias K, Drescher R, Hauth E, Bockisch G, Demirel E, Gissler HM. Clinical results of cerebral protection with a filter device during stent implantation of the carotid artery. Cardiovasc Intervent Radiol 2001;24(4): 249–56.
55. Wilkinson ID, Griffiths PD, Hoggard N, Cleveland TJ, Gaines PA, Macdonald S, McKevitt F, Venables GS. Short-term changes in cerebral microhemodynamics after carotid stenting. AJNR Am J Neuroradiol 2003;24(8): 1497–9.
56. Jaeger HJ, Mathias KD, Drescher R, Hauth E, Bockish G, Demirel E, Gissler HM. Diffusion-weighted MR imaging after angioplasty or angioplasty plus stenting of arteries supplying the brain. AJNR Am J Neuroradiol 2001;22(7): 1234–5.
57. Schluter M, Tubler T, Steffens JC, Mathey DG, Schofer J. Focal ischemia of the brain after neuroprotected carotid artery stenting. J Am Coll Cardiol 2003;42(6):1014–6.
58. Crawley F, Stygall J, Lunn S, *et al.* Comparison of microembolism detected by transcranial Doppler and neuropsychological sequelae of carotid surgery and percutaneous transluminal angioplasty. Stroke 2000;31:1329–34.
59. Sadoshima S, Heistad DD. Regional cerebral blood flow during hypotension in normotensive and stroke-prone spontaneously hypertensive rats: Effect of sympathetic denervation. Stroke. 1983;14(4):575–9.
60. Moody DM, Brown WR, Challa VR, Stump DA, Reboussin DM, Legault C. Brain microemboli associated with cardiopulmonary bypass: A histologic and magnetic resonance imaging study. Ann Thorac Surg 1995;59(5):1304–7.
61. Bettman MA, Katzen BT, Whisnant J, Brant-Zawadzki M, Broderick JP. Carotid stenting and angioplasty: A statement for healthcare professionals from the Councils on Cardiovascular Radiology, Stroke, Cardio-Thoracic and Vascular Surgery, Epidemiology, and Prevention, and Clinical Cardiology, American Heart Association. Circulation 1998;97(1): 121–3.

12 Use of an Angle-Independent Doppler System for Intraoperative Carotid Endarterectomy Surveillance

Manju Kalra, Todd E. Rasmussen, and Peter Gloviczki

Carotid Imaging

For the first few decades following the development and refinement of carotid endarterectomy in the 1950s through 1970s cerebral arteriography was the sole preoperative diagnostic modality and was considered the gold standard for carotid artery imaging. Cerebral arteriography, however, carries a risk of cerebrovascular events of 4% and permanent neurological deficit of approximately 1%.[1] Noninvasive techniques such as oculoplethysmography (OPG), Doppler waveform analysis, and supraorbital directional flow were extensively studied, showed poor or no correlation with arteriography, and were deemed unreliable for surgical decision making.[2,3] The Echoflow (Diagnostic Electronic Corp., Lexington, MA), a continuous wave directional Doppler velocity flowmeter that provided a velocity-sensitive color-coded computer-generated image of the extracranial carotid arteries developed in the 1970s was evaluated by several authors and showed merit as a screening tool for carotid stenosis.[3–7] It was not until the development of duplex ultrasonography (DUS) in the 1980s, however, that the supremacy of arteriography for surgical planning was seriously challenged.[8–12] DUS has become the most widely used screening tool for the detection of carotid stenosis, and in the majority of patients preoperative imaging with DUS alone is accurate, safe, and cost effective.[9,13–16]

Intraoperative Carotid Imaging

Assessment of technical perfection in the operating room is a necessary part of carotid endarterectomy. Historically, such assessment was limited to palpation of the reconstructed carotid artery. Continuous wave Doppler provides an audible assessment of arterial flow that is more sensitive than palpation and less invasive than arteriography, but it does not provide a quantitative measure and is therefore limited in its reliability and applicability.[17] The use of intraoperative contrast arteriography improves the ability to detect technical problems following endarterectomy and remains a common method for this evaluation. The routine use of intraoperative angiography has been shown to impact the results of carotid endarterectomy favorably by reducing operative mortality (2.9–1%), the permanent stroke rate (1.9–0.9%), and the temporary neurological deficit rate (6.3–1%) as well as the incidence of residual and recurrent stenotic lesions.[18] However, this technique is invasive and cumbersome and carries risk associated with vessel puncture and contrast injection.[18,19] It is routinely performed in a single projection and provides no functional assessment of flow within the reconstructed artery. Furthermore very few, if any, arterial reconstructions are followed with routine repeat arteriography in the months and years following the operation. These limitations of arteriography have accelerated the acceptance of duplex ultrasound for the intraoperative assessment of arterial reconstructions, especially in the carotid circulation.

The use of duplex ultrasonography in the operating room following carotid endarterectomy represents a significant advance that is less invasive than arteriography and provides more objective information than continuous wave Doppler and arteriography.[20,21] Duplex provides not only a grayscale or B-mode image of the vessel, but also a functional assessment of flow through the carotid artery using pulsed Doppler spectral analysis. Schwartz *et al.* in 1988 identified technical errors in 22% of patients undergoing intraoperative duplex scanning during carotid endarterectomy, with immediate corrective measures undertaken in 11%.[20] DUS has been shown to compare favorably with arteriography for the intaroperative assessment of carotid endarterectomy with false negative rates of 3.4% and 2.1%, respectively.[22] Panneton *et al.* reported abnormalities on intraoperative duplex examination in 41% of patients undergoing carotid endarterectomy; 30% of these defects were classified as minor and

A.F. Aburahma, J.J. Bergan (eds.), *Noninvasive Cerebrovascular Diagnosis*, DOI 10.1007/978-1-84882-957-2_12,

11% major hemodynamically significant based on the absence or presence of elevated peak systolic velocities, visible residual plaque-producing stenosis, thrombus, or intimal flap/dissection.[23] Ipsilateral perioperative neurological events occurred in two of three patients with unrevised significant defects identified on intraoperative duplex with none occurring following revision of the remaining 14 significant defects. In addition to improved immediate results, normal intraoperative duplex examination has been associated with improved late patency.[24] Even minor defects appeared to be associated with an increased incidence of late restenosis in this study.[24] Therefore, the sensitivity of intraoperative duplex has been shown to be similar to arteriography, it is safer and less cumbersome, and its routine use may decrease restenosis rates following carotid endarterectomy.[22–27]

Despite the usefulness of duplex ultrasound following carotid endarterectomy, this modality has limitations. Duplex requires B-mode imaging of the vessel in order to set or determine the angle of ultrasound insonation and perform pulsed Doppler sampling of arterial velocity. Such imaging requires training and experience in order to acquire accurate, reproducible readings, a skill that in some centers may necessitate a technologist or radiologist. Furthermore interpretation of the B-mode image in the operating room is often subjective and small defects are of unknown consequence and may be misleading. These facts combined with the cost of the duplex ultrasound equipment and the radiologist/technologist time may prohibit its use in the majority of centers performing carotid endarterectomy.

Angle-Independant Doppler System

Recent development and refinement of diffractive ultrasonic transducers have facilitated measurement of blood velocity independent of a B-mode image.[28–30] Thus a functional assessment of blood flow can be obtained with simpler, compact equipment that is easier to use and less expensive than conventional duplex. Traditionally only hemodynamically significant defects detected with duplex scanning have been routinely repaired.[20,23,24] The sensitivity of duplex scanning permits identification of even minor residual abnormalities, the significance of which remains unknown. Identification of elevated peak systolic velocities without a B-mode image with an angle-independent ultrasound would potentially enable detection of hemodynamically significant defects.

Concept of Angle-Independent Ultrasound

Based on the Doppler equation (Figure 12–1) an angle of insonation must be determined or known with a high degree of accuracy in order to determine the velocity of flowing blood. Standard duplex ultrasound combines a pulsed Doppler system with a B-mode scanner to allow the insonating beam to be aligned to the vessel at a desired or defined angle. The angle of insonation is set manually by the operator and requires training and experience to perform measurements in a reproducible manner.

$$\Delta f = \frac{2 f_0 V \cos \theta}{C}$$

FIGURE 12–1. Doppler equation calculating the magnitude of frequency shift (Δf) where f_0 = frequency of transmitted sound, V = velocity of blood, θ = the angle of insonation between the axis of the ultrasound beam and the direction of blood flow, and C = velocity of sound in tissue (~1.56×10^5 cm/s). (Reproduced from J Vasc Surg 2003;37:374–80. Copyright © 2003, with permission from Society of Vascular Surgery.)

The angle-independent ultrasound technology is based on a diffractive transducer that consists of a series of linear piezoelectric elements spaced a fraction of a wavelength apart. The diffracting conditions can be altered to generate multiple ultrasonic beams from a single insonating probe.[28–31] This diffractive transducer technology has led to the development of a new ultrasonic Doppler system that forms two ultrasound beams to insonate vessels and thereby functions to sample arterial velocities without an operator-determined angle (e.g., angle-independent) of insonation (Figure 12–2).

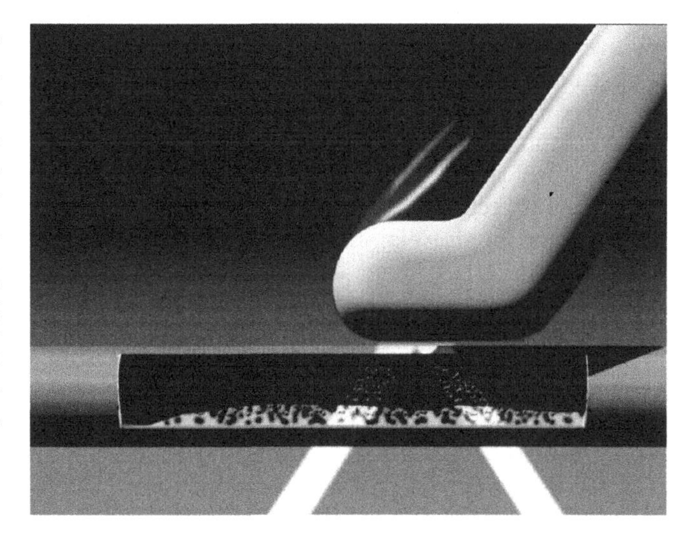

FIGURE 12–2. The diffractive transducer creates two continuous wave ultrasound beams that insonate the blood vessel and facilitates measurement of blood velocity without the need to set an angle of insonation.

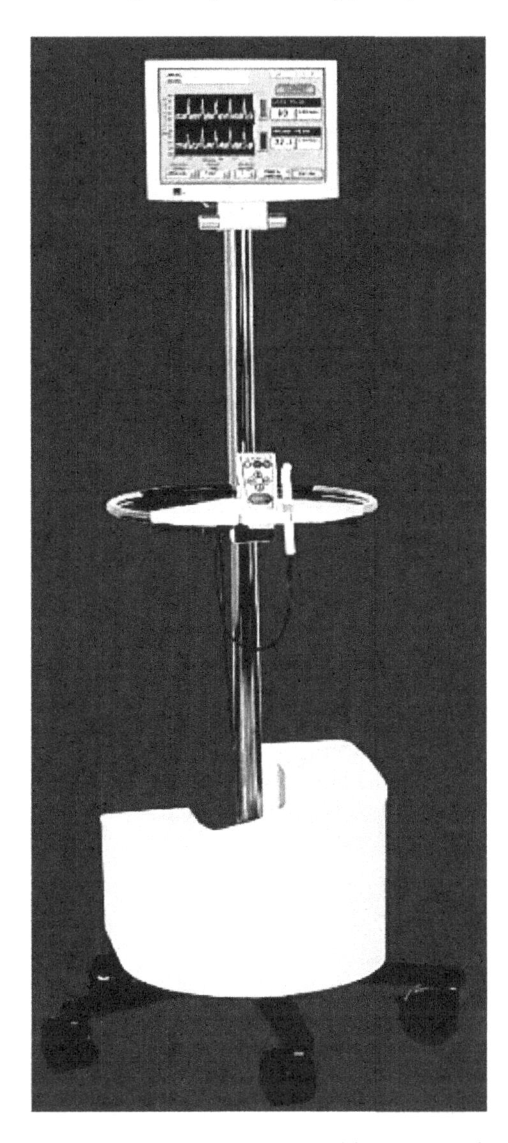

FIGURE 12–3. EchoFlow BVM-1 blood velocity meter (EchoCath, Inc, Princeton, NJ) with elevated display, remote control, printer capability, and mobile console. (Reproduced from J Vasc Surg 2003;37:374–80. Copyright © 2003, with permission from Society of Vascular Surgery.)

The commercially available EchoFlow BVM-1 blood velocity meter (EchoCath, Inc, Princeton, NJ) is a diffractive transducer-based technology that uses two ultrasonic beams and a 10-MHz probe to record blood velocity (Figure 12–3). The diffracting transducer in the EchoFlow device generates two beams to insonate the vessel at two distinct angles. The first ultrasound beam is at an unknown angle of insonation and the second beam differs from the first by a known degree. The two frequency measurements taken from the different ultrasound beams produce two Doppler shift equations with two unknowns (velocity and θ).[28–31] These equations can be solved to determine θ and ultimately blood velocity based on the mathematical equation or principle of two unknowns described by Daigle.[32] Thereby analysis of the two ultrasound beams and their respective Doppler equations allows the EchoFlow system to provide blood velocity measurements without the need to preset an angle of insonation as is necessary with standard duplex ultrasound.

In addition, based on velocity measured and the size of the vessel insonated this flowmeter also allows flow to be measured independently of the angle of insonation. Its use was initially reported in animal studies.[33] Skladany *et al.* made 65 flow determinations in the carotid arteries of five pigs. Flow measurements were obtained in arteries bled into a calibrated vessel and compared with the true volume of the blood captured. The flowmeter measured flow-volume rates in milliliters per minute were found to be within ± 15% of the cylinder captured volume.[33]

Clinical Evaluation of the Angle-Independent Doppler System

The small size and portability, low operator dependency, and low cost of this ultrasonic flowmeter suggested potential for widespread clinical applicability. There is no need for the operator to hold the probe at a predetermined angle to measure flow velocity in the carotid artery. The system is therefore easier to use, does not require a technologist or a radiologist, and is less expensive than conventional duplex scan. To measure velocity intraoperatively in the carotid artery, one probe can be used for all patients and all size vessels. The probe is placed over the surface of the vessel and a single switch is pushed to obtain a measurement (Figure 12–2). The waveform and velocity measurements are displayed on an LCD screen (Figure 12–4).

The EchoFlow angle-independent ultrasonic Doppler system was evaluated by us for intraoperative surveillance following carotid endarterectomy in 65 consecutive patients (36 female, 29 male; mean age, 71 years). Velocity measurements of the common, internal, and external carotid arteries were performed in 65 patients after carotid endarterectomy Three velocity measurements were obtained by the vascular surgeon from each of the arteries with the EchoFlow device and compared with the velocity measurements obtained with the duplex ultrasound scan performed by a radiologist.[34]

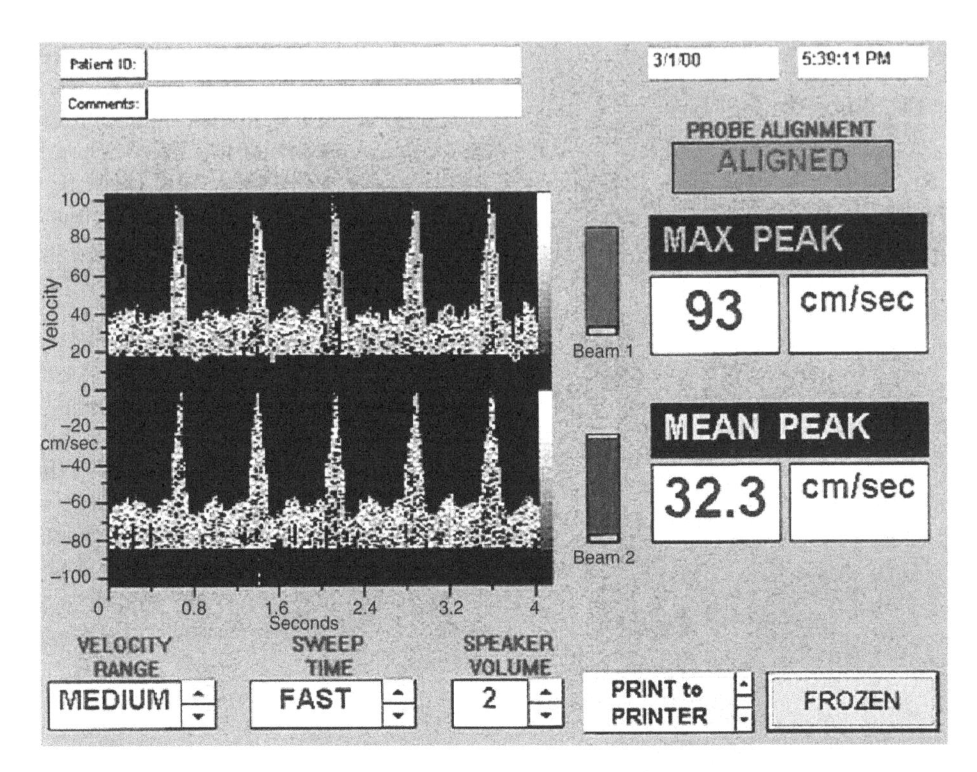

FIGURE 12–4. EchoFlow system projects the arterial Doppler waveform on the left of the display screen and the velocity readings on the right. It also provides an audible Doppler signal and has the capability to send readings to a printer.

Reliability of Angle-Independent Velocity Measurement

Velocity measurements obtained using the angle-independent system were reproducible in the common, internal, and external carotid arteries with intrapatient correlation coefficients of 0.95, 0.96, and 0.95, respectively (Table 12–1).

Comparison to Duplex Ultrasound

Mean velocity measurement difference (bias) between EchoFlow and duplex was −12 cm/s for the common carotid artery, −8 cm/s for the internal carotid artery, and −11 cm/s for the external carotid artery (Table 12–2). Intraclass correlation coefficients were 0.60, 0.69, and 0.73 for the common, internal, and external carotid arteries, respectively. Within-patient differences showed a significant correlation with increasing velocity measurements in each of the three arteries measured ($p < 0.05$).

The vast majority of velocity measurements from the common, internal, and external carotid arteries fell within two standard deviations of the mean differences between EchoFlow and duplex. The majority of velocity measurements from each of the three carotid arteries with EchoFlow were within an error of ±25 cm/s compared to velocity measurements obtained by duplex ultrasound (Figure 12–5). Seventy-five percent of common, 88% of internal, and 78% of external carotid velocity measurements obtained with the angle-independent ultrasound scan device were within 25 cm/s of the velocities measured with duplex ultrasound scan. Differences between the EchoFlow device and duplex scan velocity measurements correlated with increasing arterial velocities in each of the three arteries measured ($p < 0.05$).

When interpreting these results, it is important to recall the limitations of the study. Only peak systolic velocity was

TABLE 12–1. Intrapatient reliability of EchoFlow carotid velocity measurements.

Vessel[a]	Within patient standard deviation (cm/s)	Intraclass correlation coefficient
CC	4.65	0.95
IC	4.42	0.96
EC	6.81	0.95

[a]CC, common carotid; IC, internal carotid; EC, external carotid.

TABLE 12–2. Comparison of carotid velocity measurements between EchoFlow and duplex.

Vessel[a]	Mean difference (bias) (Echoflow-duplex)	Standard deviation of differences (Echoflow-duplex)	Limits of agreement (95%)	Diff ≤25 cm/s (%)	Intraclass correlation coefficient
CC	−11.91	22.0	−55 to 31	75.4	0.60
IC	−8.33	20.0	−47 to 31	87.5	0.69
EC	−11.35	30.6	−71 to 49	77.5	0.73

[a]CC, common carotid; IC, internal carotid; EC, external carotid.

measured; the study included only a limited number of patients and an assessment on outcome was not reported. Also, the specific point of insonation on the artery from which velocities were sampled may have varied between the EchoFlow and duplex scan probes, making agreement between these two methods difficult to confirm.[34]

Based on the results of this preliminary study application of the angle-independent ultrasound system should be viewed as a supplement to and not a replacement for standard duplex ultrasound at the present time. This new system represents an initial or screening modality available in the operating room to assess arterial reconstruction or bypass much like continuous wave Doppler is currently used. If a technical defect is suspected duplex ultrasound or intraoperative arteriography should continue to be performed.

The noninvasive and compact nature of the angle-independent ultrasound device combined with its simple operating system make its potential application broad. The manufacturing cost of this unit has been contained and is less than $10,000 for a fully equipped unit, significantly less expensive than the standard duplex ultrasound machine.[33] Furthermore, elimination of the need for a specially trained person to operate the device substantially reduces the operating cost of the unit.

By providing an objective velocity measurement with an audible Doppler signal this technology significantly extends continuous wave Doppler yet is nearly as

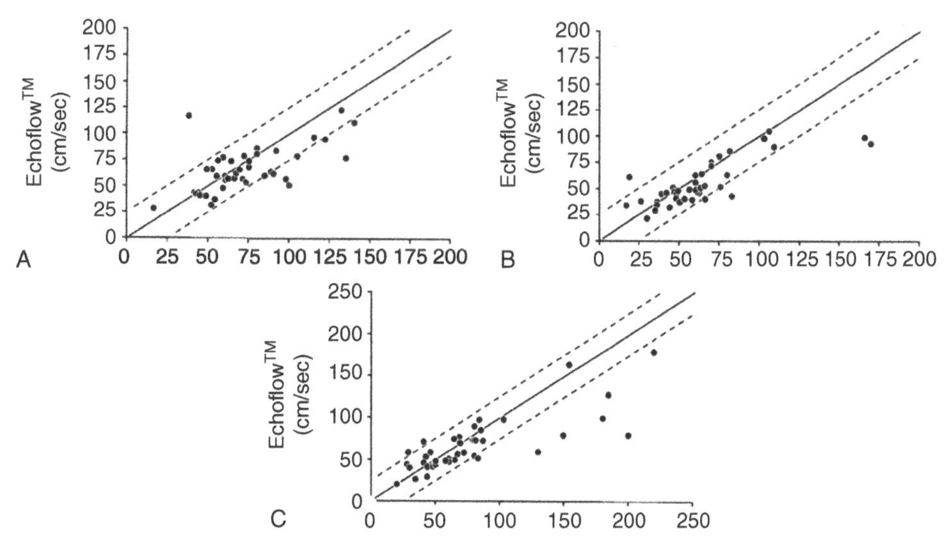

FIGURE 12–5. (A) Comparison of peak systolic velocity measurements between EchoFlow (y-axis) and duplex (x-axis) from the common carotid artery. Dashed reference lines represent error of ±25 cm/s. (Reproduced with permission from J Vasc Surg 2003;37:374–80). (B) Comparison of peak systolic velocity measurements between EchoFlow (y-axis) and duplex (x-axis) from the internal carotid artery. Dashed reference lines represent error of ±25 cm/s. (Reproduced with permission from J Vasc Surg 2003;37:374–80). (C) Comparison of peak systolic velocity measurements between EchoFlow (y-axis) and duplex (x-axis) from the external carotid artery. Dashed reference lines represent error of ± 25 cm/s. (Reproduced from J Vasc Surg 2003;37:374–80. Copyright © 2003, with permission from Society of Vascular Surgery.)

simple to use. This technology may provide surgeons who do not otherwise have access to duplex ultrasound machines and the expertise necessary to use them with a comparable means of assessing arterial velocity in the operating room. It has potential broad applicability in the intraoperative assessment of arterial velocities following reconstruction or bypass.

References

1. Hankey GJ, Warlow CP, Sellar RJ. Cerebral angiographic risk in mild cerebrovascular disease. Stroke 1990;21(2):209–22.
2. Lefemine AA, Broach J, Woolley TW. Comparison of arteriography and noninvasive techniques for the diagnosis of carotid artery disease. A statistical analysis of 140 patients. Am Surg 1986;52(10):526–31.
3. Persson AV, O'Leary DH, Kovacs A, Dyer VE. Clinical use of noninvasive evaluation of the carotid artery. Surg Clin North Am 1980;60(3):513–26.
4. Curry GR, White DN. Color coded ultrasonic differential velocity arterial scanner (Echoflow). Ultrasound Med Biol 1978;4(1):27–35.
5. Oliva L, Gemma GB, Bertoglio C, Rezzo R, Stabilini L. [Doppler ultrasonic arteriography with colorimetric morpho-function analysis of frequency (Echoflow). Preliminary trials]. Minerva Med 1981;72(37):2465–71.
6. Schain FB, Balzer K, Carstensen G. Non-invasive studies of the extra-cranial cerebral arteries: Indication for angiography and operation. Thorac Cardiovasc Surg 1982;30(1):2–6.
7. Torvaldsen S, McCauley J, Patel AS, Chakera TM. Assessment of cervical carotid artery disease. A comparison between the Doppler "Echoflow" and conventional angiography. Med J Aust 1985;142(10):542–5.
8. Hames TK, Humphries KN, Ratliff DA, Birch SJ, Gazzard VM, Chant AD. The validation of duplex scanning and continuous wave Doppler imaging: A comparison with conventional angiography. Ultrasound Med Biol 1985;11(6): 827–34.
9. Dawson DL, Zierler RE, Strandness DE Jr, Clowes AW, Kohler TR. The role of duplex scanning and arteriography before carotid endarterectomy: A prospective study. J Vasc Surg 1993;18(4):673–80; discussion 680–3.
10. Taylor DC, Strandness DE Jr. Carotid artery duplex scanning. J Clin Ultrasound 1987;15(9):635–44.
11. Londrey GL, Spadone DP, Hodgson KJ, Ramsey DE, Barkmeier LD, Sumner DS. Does color-flow imaging improve the accuracy of duplex carotid evaluation? J Vasc Surg 1991;13(5):659–63.
12. Bray JM, Galland F, Lhoste P, Nicolau S, Dubas F, Emile J, *et al.* Colour Doppler and duplex sonography and angiography of the carotid artery bifurcations. Prospective, double-blind study. Neuroradiology 1995;37(3):219–24.
13. Wagner WH, Treiman RL, Cossman DV, Foran RF, Levin PM, Cohen JL. The diminishing role of diagnostic arteriography in carotid artery disease: Duplex scanning as definitive preoperative study. Ann Vasc Surg 1991;5(2):105–10.
14. McKittrick JE, Cisek PL, Pojunas KW, Blum GM, Ortgiesen P, Lim RA. Are both color-flow duplex scanning and cerebral arteriography required prior to carotid endarterectomy? Ann Vasc Surg 1993;7(4):311–6.
15. Chervu A, Moore WS. Carotid endarterectomy without arteriography. Ann Vasc Surg 1994;8(3):296–302.
16. Shifrin EG, Bornstein NM, Kantarovsky A, Morag B, Zelmanovich L, Portnoi I, *et al.* Carotid endarterectomy without angiography. Br J Surg 1996;83(8):1107–9.
17. Seifert KB, Blackshear WM Jr. Continuous-wave Doppler in the intraoperative assessment of carotid endarterectomy. J Vasc Surg 1985;2(6):817–20.
18. Courbier R, Jausseran JM, Reggi M, Bergeron P, Formichi M, Ferdani M. Routine intraoperative carotid angiography: Its impact on operative morbidity and carotid restenosis. J Vasc Surg 1986;3(2):343–50.
19. Blaisdell FW, Lim R Jr, Hall AD. Technical result of carotid endarterectomy. Arteriographic assessment. Am J Surg 1967;114(2):239–46.
20. Schwartz RA, Peterson GJ, Noland KA, Hower JF Jr, Naunheim KS. Intraoperative duplex scanning after carotid artery reconstruction: A valuable tool. J Vasc Surg 1988; 7(5):620–4.
21. Bandyk DF, Mills JL, Gahtan V, Esses GE. Intraoperative duplex scanning of arterial reconstructions: Fate of repaired and unrepaired defects. J Vasc Surg 1994;20(3):426–32; discussion 432–3.
22. Dilley RB, Bernstein EF. A comparison of B-mode real-time imaging and arteriography in the intraoperative assessment of carotid endarterectomy. J Vasc Surg 1986; 4(5):457–63.
23. Panneton JM, Berger MW, Lewis BD, Hallett JW Jr, Bower TC, Gloviczki P, *et al.* Intraoperative duplex ultrasound during carotid endarterectomy. Vasc Surg 2001;35(1):1–9.
24. Baker WH, Koustas G, Burke K, Littooy FN, Greisler HP. Intraoperative duplex scanning and late carotid artery stenosis. J Vasc Surg 1994;19(5):829–32; discussion 832–3.
25. Coelho JC, Sigel B, Flanigan DP, Schuler JJ, Spigos DG, Tan WS, *et al.* An experimental evaluation of arteriography and imaging ultrasonography in detecting arterial defects at operation. J Surg Res 1982;32(2):130–7.
26. Seelig MH, Oldenburg WA, Chowla A, Atkinson EJ. Use of intraoperative duplex ultrasonography and routine patch angioplasty in patients undergoing carotid endarterectomy. Mayo Clin Proc 1999;74(9):870–6.
27. Papanicolaou G, Toms C, Yellin AE, Weaver FA. Relationship between intraoperative color-flow duplex findings and early restenosis after carotid endarterectomy: A preliminary report. J Vasc Surg 1996;24(4):588–95; discussion 595–6.
28. Vilkomerson DL, Lyons D, Chilipka T. Diffractive transducers for angle-independant velocity measurements. *Proceedings of the 1994 Ultrasonics Symposium,* pp. 1677–1682. Piscataway: IEEE Press, 1994.
29. Vilkomerson D, Chilipka T, Lyons D. Higher-order diffracting-grating transducers. Med Imaging (SPIE) 1997;3037: 206–12.
30. Palachon PV, Lyons D, Chilipka T, Shung K. Improved diffracting grating transducers. Med Imaging (SPIE) 1999; 3664:155–60.

31. Vilkomerson DL, Lyons D, Domagala P, Chilipka T. Considerations in design of angle-independent Doppler instruments using diffracting-grating transducers. *Proceedings of the 1999 Ultrasonics Symposium,* pp. 1459–1464. Piscataway: IEEE Press, 1999.
32. Daigle R. Aortic flow sensing using an ultrasonic esophageal probe. Doctoral thesis, Colorado State University, 1974.
33. Skladany M, Vilkomerson D, Lyons D, Chilipka T, Delamere M, Hollier LH. New, angle-independent, low cost Doppler system to measure blood flow. Am J Surg 1998; 176(2):179–82.
34. Rasmussen TE, Panneton JM, Kalra M, Hofer JM, Lewis BD, Rowland CM, *et al.* Intraoperative use of a new angle-independent Doppler system to measure arterial velocities after carotid endarterectomy. J Vasc Surg 2003;37(2):374–80.

13 Clinical Implications of the Vascular Laboratory in the Diagnosis of Cerebrovascular Insufficiency

Ali F. AbuRahma

Various noninvasive tests for the evaluation of cerebrovascular insufficiency have been described in previous chapters. Most forms of noninvasive testing pose less stress and less expense to the patient than angiography. While early forms of noninvasive testing depended on the presence of severe disease, the current techniques, especially carotid artery imaging, demonstrate the opposite characteristic. Carotid imaging is able to detect minimal disease that is not hemodynamically significant; in fact, overestimation of the degree of stenosis in these cases has been a consistent problem. Nevertheless, any test intended for screening must have a high degree of sensitivity to be used appropriately in the initial assessment of disease. Noninvasive assessment, therefore, combines low risk, low cost, and high sensitivity.

Although we agree that patients should be evaluated by careful history and physical examination, our policy tends to rely on noninvasive vascular testing as an initial step in the diagnosis of carotid artery disease. The results of noninvasive tests may also help in obtaining optimal angiograms. An example is the patient with noninvasive evidence of severe stenosis who has no significant stenosis demonstrated in standard views of the carotid artery bifurcation. The results of the noninvasive tests indicate the need for additional projections, and if the bifurcation region does not show the expected lesion, there is a strong indication for obtaining adequate siphon views.

Prior to the advent of digital techniques, standard angiograms were routinely used in the evaluation of patients with cerebral ischemic attacks in order to determine whether vascular reconstructive surgery was indicated. Standard angiography was of limited clinical value, particularly as a means of diagnostic screening in asymptomatic patients, because of prohibitive costs, poor patient acceptance, and the risk of arterial catheterization. As a result, noninvasive vascular tests became established as the preferred means of diagnostic screening in asymptomatic patients, because they provided an objective method of determining the hemodynamic significance of carotid disease in a safe and relatively cost-efficient manner.

Recent studies have questioned the role of arteriography as the "gold standard" in the evaluation of carotid artery occlusive disease.[1–5] Contrast arteriography has also been noted to have an 1–4% incidence of neurologic complications with about a 1% incidence of stroke reported in the Asymptomatic Carotid Atherosclerosis Study (ACAS).[6] Other complications of arteriography that were reported include complications at the arterial puncture site (5%), and contrast-induced renal dysfunctions in 1–5%. With this in mind, it would be beneficial and cost-effective if these patients could be safely evaluated without invasive arteriography. Color duplex ultrasonography of the carotid arteries and magnetic resonance angiography (MRA) are two noninvasive modalities that can detect and grade carotid artery stenosis.

Carotid Angiography, Magnetic Resonance Angiography, and/or Color Duplex Ultrasound in the Diagnosis of Carotid Artery Disease (Single or Combined)

Carotid duplex ultrasound (DUS) is readily available, noninvasive, inexpensive, fast, repeatable with good resolution of carotid plaque morphology, and has excellent accuracy in most experienced medical centers. One of its limitations is that there is no suitable acoustic access to certain vessels of interest in the body. For example, it cannot directly visualize the origin of the left carotid artery, the distal internal carotids, or the Circle of Willis (Figure 13–1). Therefore, a screening examination based on ultrasound alone may be incomplete for certain surgical patients. Ultrasound is also highly operator

A.F. Aburahma, J.J. Bergan (eds.), *Noninvasive Cerebrovascular Diagnosis*, DOI 10.1007/978-1-84882-957-2_13,

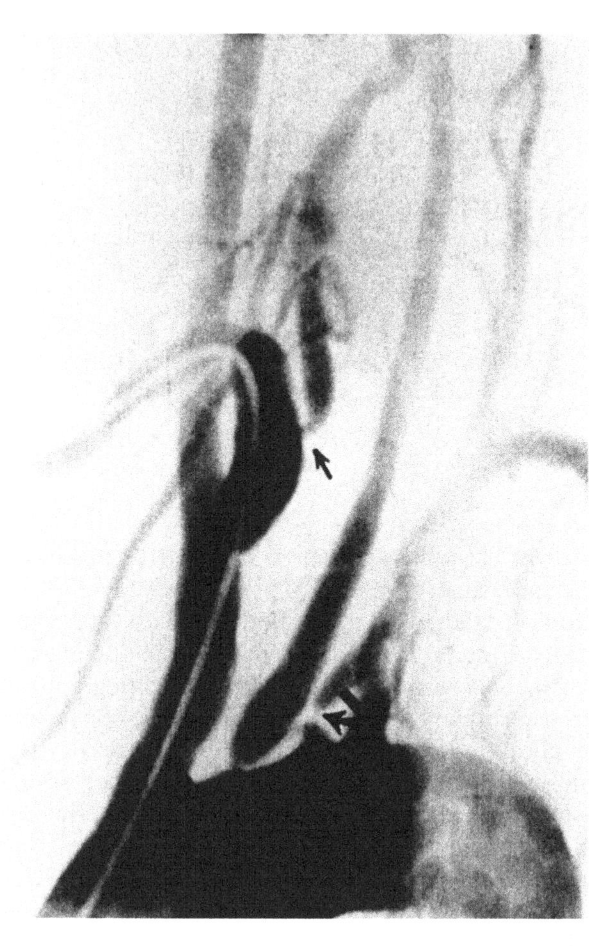

FIGURE 13–1. Four vessel arch aortogram showing tight stenosis at the origin of the left common carotid artery (open arrow), a tight stenosis of the right vertebral artery (straight arrow), and a tight stenosis of the left vertebral artery (curved arrow) which originates from the arch of the aorta.

dependent, with a skilled technologist providing more reliable information than the novice.

The weaknesses of color DUS as a noninvasive screening examination are complemented by MRA. MRA is also a noninvasive modality and can access almost any place in the body, e.g., the carotid artery from the arch to the Circle of Willis, and is not obscured by overlying bone or dense vascular calcification. It is repeatable and less costly than conventional angiography with excellent resolution for severe to total occlusion or minimal carotid artery disease. It can display vessel anatomy as a rotating three-dimensional angiogram that can be readily interpreted by those who did not perform the study (Figure 13–2). Severe or tight stenoses (≥70%) are usually seen as a flow gap (Figure 13–3). Like ultrasound, it can be used to measure blood flow volumes and blood velocity, although it lacks the temporal resolution of Doppler devices. MRA can also be combined with cerebral magnetic resonance imaging at the same time. Since it is noninvasive, it can be applied safely on patients with compromised renal functions or severe contrast allergies. There is no danger of thromboembolic phenomena as might occur with catheter manipulation during conventional contrast angiography. However, there are several instances in which MRA is likely to be unsuccessful: patients who require intensive monitoring or mechanical respiration are difficult to study by MRA, patients who are claustrophobic will require sedation before the study, and patients who cannot hold still for approximately 4–8 min at a time will have images that are considerably degraded. The images are also degraded by the presence of small pieces of metal in the body near the vessel of interest, e.g., surgical clips and small fragments from surgical instruments. Patients with intracranial aneurysms, clips, or cardiac pacemakers are excluded from having a magnetic resonance angiogram. Other disadvantages of MRA include poor plaque morphology and overestimation of stenoses in certain patients (Figure 13–4). MRA is extremely sensitive to the presence of vascular stenosis. When there is a difficulty, it is usually in specificity, i.e., the stenosis may be overestimated, but rarely missed or underestimated. This overestimation may result from turbulence. Whenever there is a mixing flow or chaotic flow (blood flow that is accelerating and decelerating rapidly), the vascular signal may be lost, and this loss of signal may be misinterpreted as a stenosis.

Cerebral arteriography, on the other hand, has the following advantages: it is relatively accurate and is capable of describing the extent of the lesion or the pathology (Figure 13–1). However, as indicated earlier, it is invasive with a definite small risk of neurologic complications, expensive, with only a fair description of the plaque morphology, and it may also underestimate the pathology or stenosis if proper filming is not undertaken (Figure 13–5).

Several studies have reported satisfactory results of carotid endarterectomy performed with color DUS alone or in combination with MRA.[7–15] Jackson *et al.* prospectively evaluated carotid MRA and compared its accuracy with color-flow duplex.[16] Fifty patients were prospectively evaluated with conventional angiography and MRA after clinical and color-flow duplex findings indicated the need for carotid angiography. Using receiver-operating characteristic (ROC) curves, the probability of correctly predicting a ≥60% stenosis using various color-flow duplex thresholds and MRA was assessed. Sensitivity, specificity, positive predictive value (PPV), and negative predictive value (NPV) in determining ≥60% stenoses were estimated. For MRA the sensitivity was 85% [95% confidence interval (CI) = 69–94%], specificity 70% (CI = 56–81%), PPV 68% (CI = 53–80%), and NPV 86% (CI = 72–94%). For color-flow duplex, the sensitivity was 89% (CI = 74–96%), specificity 93% (CI = 82–98%), PPV 89% (CI = 74–96%), and NPV 93% (CI = 82–98%). When MRA and color-flow duplex results were concordant (n = 64), the sensitivity was 100% (CI = 89–100%), specificity 95% (CI = 81–99%), PPV 94% (CI = 77–99%), and NPV 100% (CI = 92–100%).

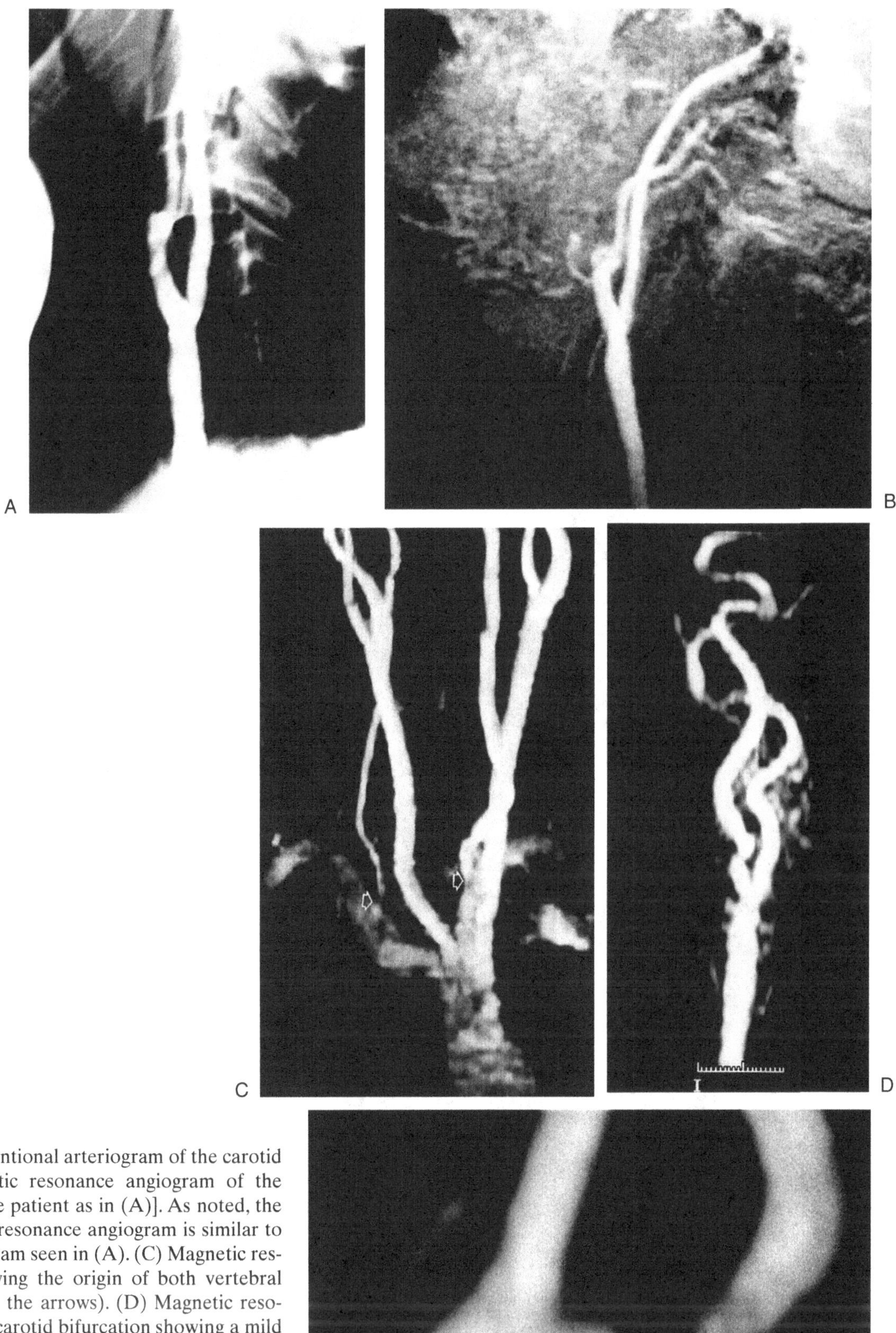

FIGURE 13–2. (A) Conventional arteriogram of the carotid bifurcation. (B) Magnetic resonance angiogram of the carotid bifurcation [same patient as in (A)]. As noted, the quality of this magnetic resonance angiogram is similar to the conventional angiogram seen in (A). (C) Magnetic resonance angiogram showing the origin of both vertebral arteries (as indicated by the arrows). (D) Magnetic resonance angiogram of the carotid bifurcation showing a mild to moderate degree of stenosis of the proximal internal carotid artery. (E) Magnetic resonance angiogram of the carotid artery bifurcation showing moderate to severe stenosis of the internal carotid artery (white arrow).

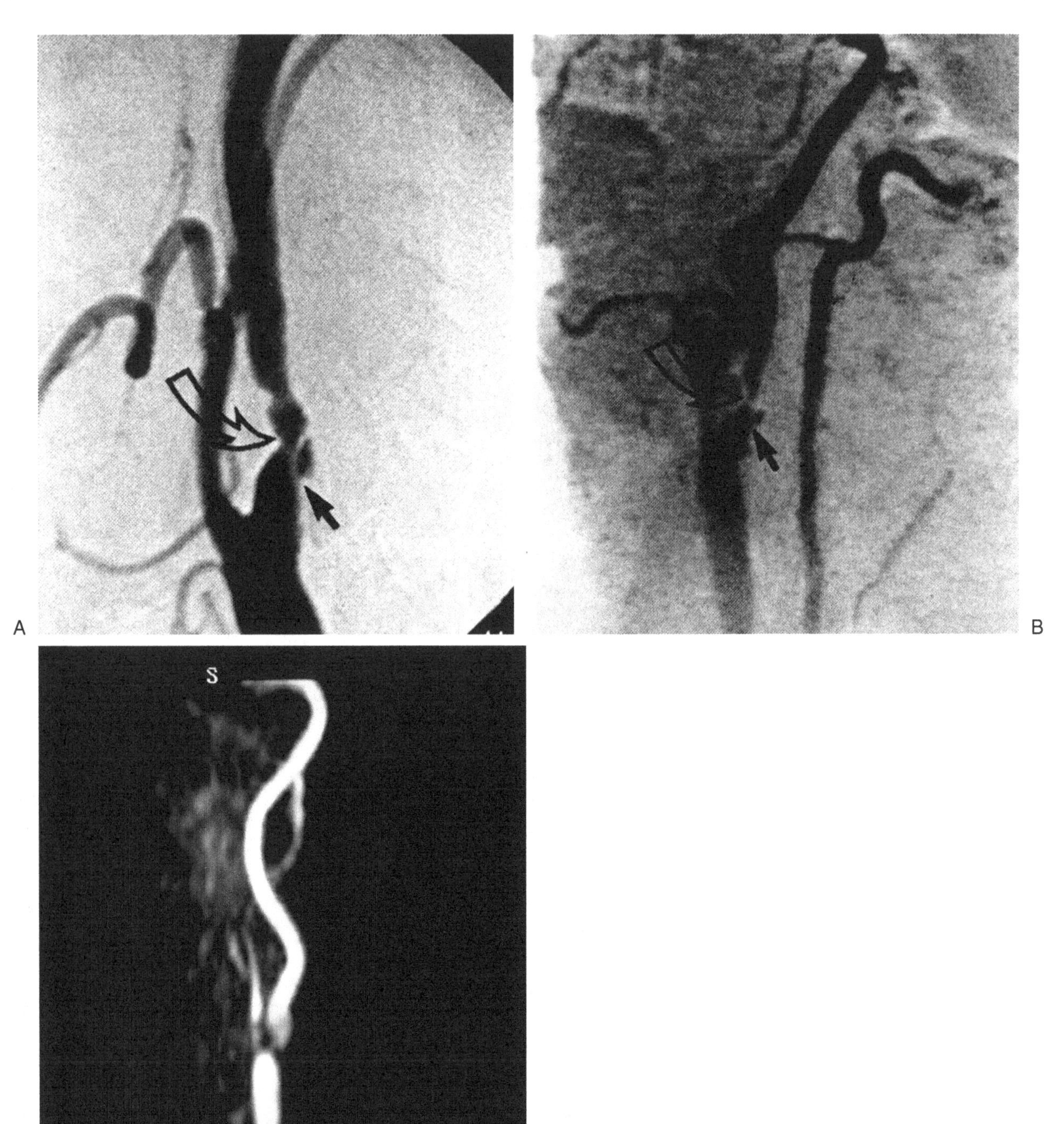

FIGURE 13–3. (A) Conventional arteriogram showing severe to tight stenosis of the proximal internal carotid artery (curved white arrow) with associated ulceration (black arrow). (B) Three-dimensional TOF magnetic resonance angiogram of the same patient showing the same tight stenosis with ulceration. (C) Carotid magnetic resonance angiogram showing severe to tight stenosis of the internal carotid artery without ulceration as indicated by flow gap (black arrow).

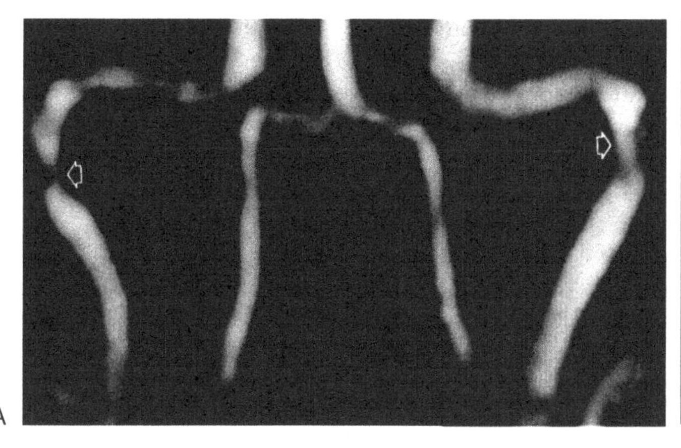

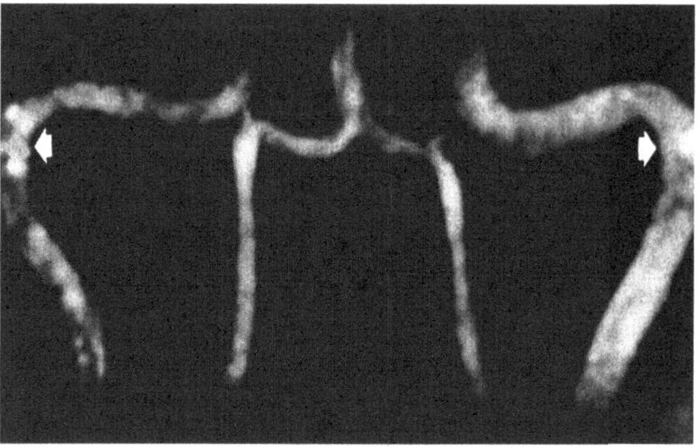

FIGURE 13–4. (A) Two-dimensional time of flight (TOF) magnetic resonance angiogram of the carotid arteries showing flow artifacts at the base of the skull (open arrows). (B) Three-dimensional TOF magnetic resonance angiogram of the same patient showing that the narrowing is no longer evident (white arrows).

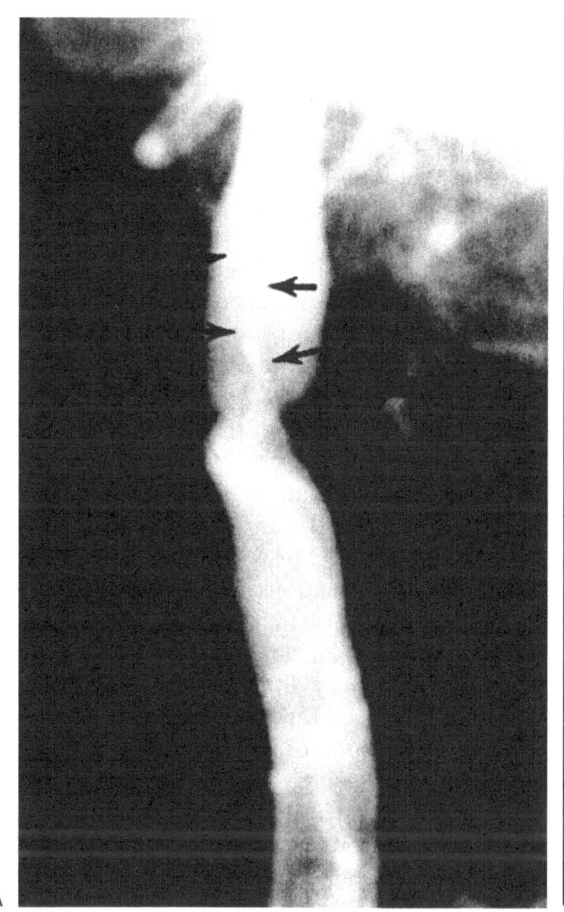

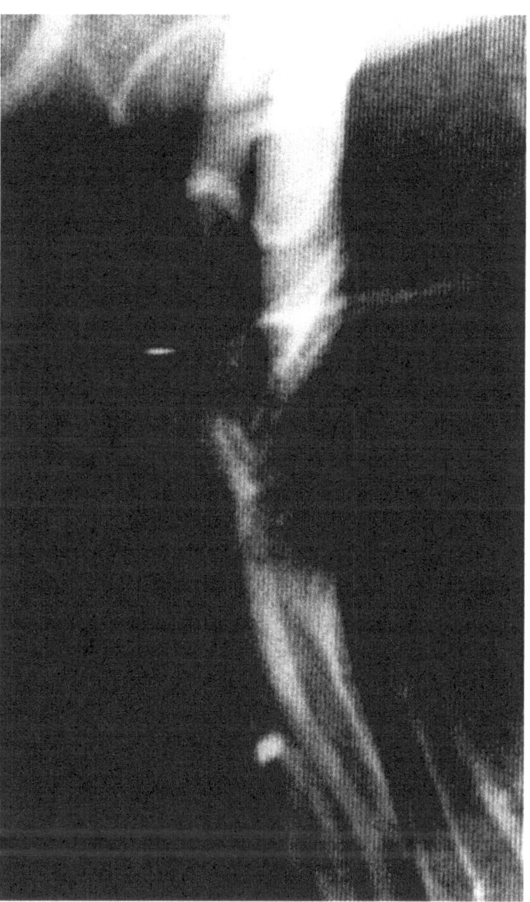

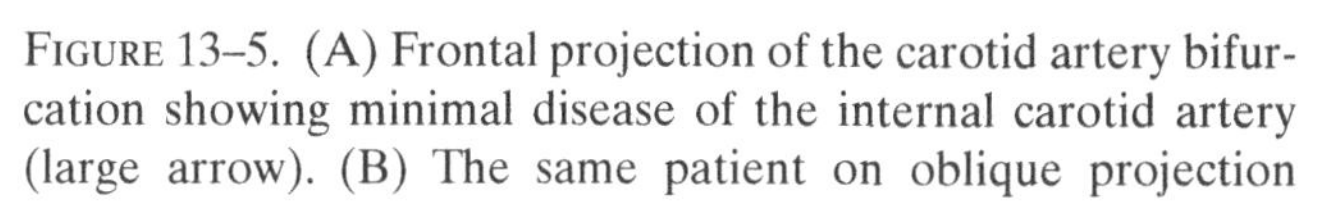

FIGURE 13–5. (A) Frontal projection of the carotid artery bifurcation showing minimal disease of the internal carotid artery (large arrow). (B) The same patient on oblique projection showing tight stenosis of the origin of the internal carotid artery (solid black arrow).

The area under the ROC curve for color-flow duplex was 95%, compared to 83% for MRA ($p = 0.0005$). They concluded that the low specificity of MRA precludes its use as the definitive imaging modality for carotid stenosis. The 93% specificity of color-flow duplex alone warrants its consideration as a definitive carotid imaging study. By ROC curve analysis, color-flow duplex offers superior accuracy to MRA. The data of Jackson *et al.* support noninvasive preoperative carotid imaging for detecting a threshold stenosis of ≥60% whether color-flow duplex is used alone, or in combination with the selective use of MRA.

In a prospective diagnostic study, Nederkoorn *et al.*[13] investigated the accuracy of noninvasive testing compared with digital subtraction angiography (DSA). They performed DUS, MRA, and DSA on 350 consecutive symptomatic patients. Separate and combined test results of DUS and MRA were compared with the reference standard DSA. DUS had a sensitivity of 87.5% (95% CI, 82.1–92.9%) and a specificity of 75.7% (95% CI, 69.3–82.2%) in identifying severe 70–99% internal carotid artery stenosis. MRA yielded a sensitivity of 92.2% (95% CI, 86.2–96.2%) and a specificity of 75.7% (95% CI, 68.6–82.5%). When MRA and DUS results were combined, agreement between these two modalities (84% of patients) gave a sensitivity of 96.3% (95% CI, 90.8–99.0%) and a specificity of 80.2% (95% CI, 73.1–87.3%) for identifying severe stenosis. It was concluded that MRA showed a slightly better accuracy than DUS in the diagnosis of carotid artery stenosis, however, to achieve the best accuracy, both tests should be performed subsequently.

Westwood *et al.*[15] conducted a study to determine if sufficient evidence exists to support the use of MRA as a means of selecting patients with recently symptomatic severe carotid stenosis for carotid endarterectomy (CEA). A systematic review of published research on the diagnostic performance of MRA was analyzed. One hundred and twenty-six potentially relevant articles were identified, but many articles failed to examine the performance of MRA as a diagnostic test at the surgical decision thresholds used in major clinical trials on CEA. Twenty-six articles were included in a meta-analysis that showed a maximal joint sensitivity and specificity of 99% (95% CI, 98–100%) for identifying 70–99% stenosis and 90% (81–99%) for identifying 50–99% stenosis. Only four articles evaluated contrast-enhanced MRA. They concluded that MRA was accurate for selecting patients for CEA at the surgical decision thresholds established in the major endarterectomy trials, but the evidence was not very robust because of the heterogeneity of the studies included.

Recently, Nederkoorn *et al.*[14] performed a systematic review of published studies retrieved through PUBMED, from bibliographies of review papers, and from experts. The English-language medical literature (between 1994 and 2001) was searched for studies that met the selection criteria: (1) DUS and/or MRA was performed to estimate the severity of carotid artery stenosis, (2) DSA was used as the standard of reference, and (3) the absolute numbers of true positives and negatives and false positives and negatives were available or derivable for at least one definition of disease (degree of stenosis).

Sixty-three publications on DUS, MRA, or both were included in the analysis, yielding the test results of 64 different patient series on DUS and 21 on MRA. For the diagnosis of 70–99% versus <70% stenosis, MRA had a pooled specificity of 90% (95% CI, 86–93) and a pooled sensitivity of 95% (95% CI, 92–97). These numbers were 87% (95% CI, 84–90) and 86% (95% CI, 84–89) for DUS, respectively. For recognizing occlusion, MRA yielded a sensitivity of 98% (95% CI, 94–100) and a specificity of 100% (95% CI, 99–100), and DUS had a sensitivity of 96% (95% CI, 94–98) and a specificity of 100% (95% CI, 99–100). A multivariable summary ROC curve analysis for diagnosing 70–99% stenosis demonstrated that the type of MR scanner predicted the performance of MRA, whereas the presence of verification bias predicted the performance of DUS. For diagnosing occlusion, no significant heterogeneity was found for MRA; for DUS, the presence of verification bias and type of DUS scanner were explanatory variables. MRA had a significantly better discriminatory power than DUS in diagnosing 70–99% stenosis (regression coefficient, 1.6; 95% CI, 0.37–2.77). No significant difference was found in detecting occlusion (regression coefficient, 0.73; 95% CI, −2.06–3.51). These results suggest that MRA has a better discriminatory power compared with DUS in diagnosing 70–99% stenosis and is a sensitive and specific test compared with DSA in the evaluation of carotid artery stenosis. For detecting occlusion, both DUS and MRA are very accurate.

Several other studies reported on the value of MRA[17–22] and CTA[23,24] in the diagnosis of carotid artery stenosis.

Doppler ultrasound is likely to remain the initial screening method of the carotid bifurcation in most centers. However, MRA may be used as a screening method in two situations: (1) when obtaining a magnetic resonance image of the brain to assess prior ischemic events, screening images of the bifurcation can easily be included with very little additional expense; and (2) MRA may be used for patients whose findings are equivocal by ultrasound, e.g., patients with unfavorable anatomy, such as high bifurcation, tortuous vessels that are difficult to identify, considerable overlying adipose tissue that may obscure the vessel, or dense vascular calcifications that cause acoustic shadowing. MRA can also provide a noninvasive assessment of those portions of the carotid that are not accessible to the ultrasound transducer, which can be manifested by an ultrasound showing a dampened waveform consistent with the presence of a tandem lesion or proximal stenosis or occlusion.

Specific application of any of these three modalities, i.e., color duplex ultrasonography, MRA, and conventional contrast angiography, are described in the following sections.

Asymptomatic Carotid Bruit

Although some asymptomatic carotid bruits radiate from the heart or the great vessels, a considerable proportion of them originate from the carotid artery bifurcations. Fell *et al.*[25] reported on 100 patients with 165 asymptomatic carotid bruits. Duplex scanning showed a normal internal carotid artery in 12 cases (7%), <50% stenosis in 83 (50%), ≥50% stenosis in 61 (37%), and occlusion in 9 (6%). Thus, although the majority of neck bruits were associated with some degree of carotid stenosis, only 43% had ≥50% stenosis, which may justify further work-up in selected patients. Noninvasive carotid testing permits separation of earlier, moderate atheromatous lesions from advanced, flow-reducing lesions. Most authorities agree that the early lesions require no treatment, but the patient should be followed at yearly intervals with repeat noninvasive testing to detect possible progression to more advanced stenosis. Identification of advanced stenosis of the internal carotid artery indicates a patient who is at an increased risk for subsequent stroke.

As indicated earlier, the ACAS study concluded that patients with ≥60% stenoses who were treated medically had a higher stroke rate over a 5-year period in comparison to patients who underwent a CEA. With this in mind, most authorities recommend screening for asymptomatic carotid stenoses, particularly in patients who are good candidates for a potential CEA. Figure 13–6 summarizes a practical approach in patients with asymptomatic carotid bruits or nonhemispheric symptoms. After the initial step of carotid DUS, if <60% stenosis was detected, it is recommended that the test be repeated in 6 months.

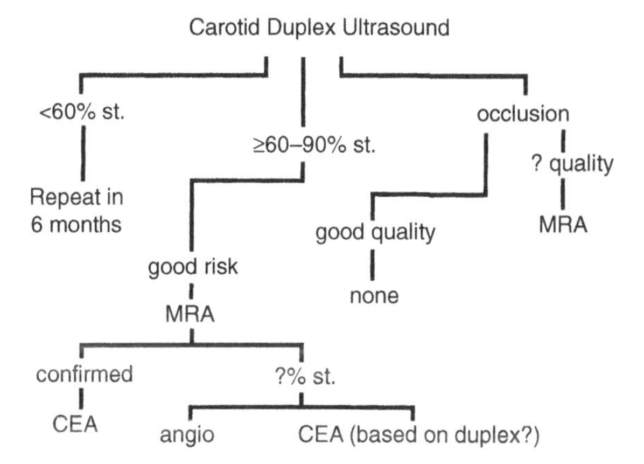

FIGURE 13–6. Management protocol for patients with asymptomatic carotid bruit or nonhemispheric symptoms. MRA, magnetic resonance angiography; CEA, carotid endarterectomy; st., stenosis.

If stenosis of ≥60–99% was detected and the patient is a good risk, a magnetic resonance angiogram can be done to complement the findings of the ultrasound, and if confirmed, a CEA is recommended. If the magnetic resonance angiogram was not conclusive or contradicted the ultrasound findings, then angiography may be considered in centers with a minimal stroke risk rate from angiography. However, in patients with a good quality carotid DUS, an endarterectomy may be considered based on ultrasound findings only. Several authorities would not recommend CEA in asymptomatic patients unless carotid stenosis exceeds 70–80%. In patients who had a good quality ultrasound showing total occlusion, no further follow-up is needed. However, if the quality of the ultrasound was limited, a magnetic resonance image is recommended to confirm occlusion.

Another indication for studying asymptomatic patients is to screen patients with advanced coronary artery disease or peripheral vascular diseases. Due to the diffuse nature of atherosclerosis, many of these patients have occult carotid bifurcation lesions with a resulting increased risk of stroke. This type of screening is carried out most often in patients who are being considered for cardiac or major peripheral arterial operations in order to detect carotid stenoses that may substantially increase the risk of intraoperative and postoperative stroke.

Patients with Atypical or Nonhemispheric Symptoms

Patients with atypical or nonhemispheric symptoms often do not have a clear indication for angiography. Some of these patients' symptoms include dizziness, blackouts, bilateral visual disturbances, or bilateral motor or sensory deficits. Since a variety of nonvascular causes, such as orthostatic hypotension, cardiac arrhythmias, and medications, may be responsible for these symptoms, noninvasive carotid testing is important in identifying these patients with hemodynamically significant carotid stenosis. Our management protocol for this group of patients is outlined in Figure 13–6.

Patients with Focal Neurologic Deficits (Transient Ischemic Attacks or Strokes)

A major proportion of transient ischemic attacks (TIAs) or permanent focal neurologic deficits in hemispheric distribution or with amaurosis fugax is caused by embolization from ulcerations and atheromatous plaques. Therefore, the purpose of carotid screening in patients with hemispheric neurologic symptoms is to identify lesions that could be the source of cerebral emboli or could reduce cerebral hemispheric blood flow. In the North American Symptomatic Carotid Endarterectomy Trial (NASCET) study,[26] carotid endarterectomy was highly beneficial for patients with

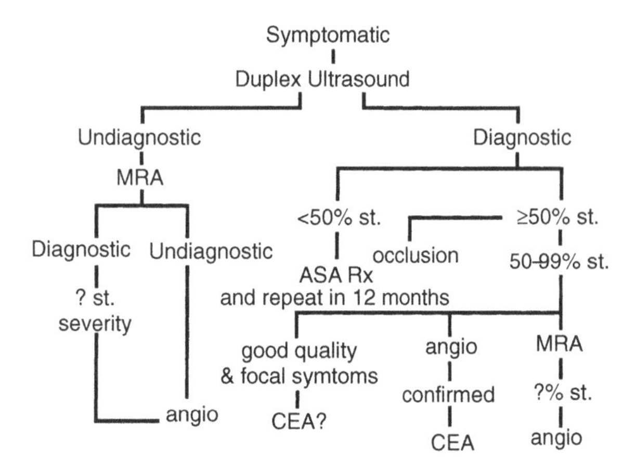

FIGURE 13–7. Management protocol for patients with suspected hemispheric symptoms (cerebrovascular disease). For <50% stenosis, repeat ultrasound in 12 months. MRA, magnetic resonance angiography; CEA, carotid endarterectomy; ASA Rx, acetylsalicylic acid treatment; st., stenosis.

recent hemispheric TIAs or mild strokes and >70–99% and 50–69% stenoses of the ipsilateral internal carotid artery. Based on these results, patients with symptoms of severe stenoses of the carotid artery should be treated by CEA unless their medical condition makes the risk of surgery prohibitive. Our management protocol for this group of patients is outlined in Figure 13–7. As noted in Figure 13–7, the initial step is to obtain a color DUS, and if the study is diagnostic and shows <50% stenosis, the patient is treated medically (e.g., aspirin therapy and repeat color DUS in 12 months). If the stenosis is ≥50%, the ultrasound is of good quality, and the patient has classical focal hemispheric symptoms, a CEA can be done based on the carotid DUS findings alone; or MRA can be done to complement the ultrasound findings, and if the diagnosis is confirmed, surgery may be considered without angiography. Angiography is reserved for patients with a marginal quality DUS or magnetic resonance angiogram, or in patients with contradictory magnetic resonance angiogram and DUS results. If the DUS shows total occlusion and the ultrasound was of good quality, no further work-up is usually necessary. For patients with a DUS that is not diagnostic, an arteriogram or magnetic resonance angiogram is done, and if it is diagnostic and the severity of stenosis is established, surgery can be done accordingly. If the MRA is not diagnostic, angiography is recommended.

Specific Duplex Criteria for Specific Clinical Situations

In choosing our criteria for peak systolic velocity and end diastolic velocity, we chose the values that gave the highest overall accuracy. However, which criteria to use should depend on the "outcome" desired by the clinician. Although some surgeons have advocated CEA based on duplex criteria alone,[5,12,16] the decision to proceed with an arteriogram is based on the duplex findings in the majority of patients. The mortality and morbidity of arteriography vary from institution to institution, but can be significant.[6,27] We propose that vascular laboratories at institutions with significant mortality and morbidity in relation to carotid arteriography use duplex criteria

TABLE 13–1. Selected optimal criteria with best PPV (≥95%) and overall accuracy in detecting ≥60–99% and 70–99% ICA stenosis.[a]

Best PPV	PPV	Overall accuracy	Sensitivity	Specificity	NPV
For ≥60% ICA stenosis					
ICA PSV ≥ 220 cm/s	96%	82%	64%	98%	76%
ICA EDV ≥ 80 cm/s	96%	87%	79%	97%	84%
ICA/CCA PSV ratio ≥4.25	96%	71%	41%	99%	65%
ICA PSV and EDV 150 and 65[b]	96%	90%	82%	97%	86%
For ≥70% ICA stenosis					
ICA PSV ≥ 300 cm/s	97%	80%	48%	99%	76%
ICA EDV ≥ 110 cm/s[b]	100%	91%	75%	100%	87%
ICA/CCA PSV ≥ none	—	—	—	—	—
ICA PSV and EDV 150, 110[b]	100%	91%	75%	100%	87%

[a]PPV, positive predictive value; NPV, negative predictive value; ICA, internal carotid artery; PSV, peak systolic velocity; EDV, end diastolic velocity; CCA, common carotid artery.
[b]These values have the best PPV and overall accuracy.

TABLE 13–2. Selected optimal criteria with best NPV (≥95%) and overall accuracy in detecting ≥60–99% and 70–99% ICA stenosis.[a]

Best NPV	NPV	Overall accuracy	Sensitivity	Specificity	PPV
For ≥60% ICA stenosis					
ICA PSV ≥ 135 cm/s[b]	99%	80%	99%	64%	71%
ICA EDV—none	—	—	—	—	—
ICA/CCA PSV ratio ≥ 1.62	95%	71%	97%	47%	62%
ICA PSV and EDV—none	—	—	—	—	—
For ≥70% ICA stenosis					
ICA PSV > 150 cm/s[b]	99%	80%	99%	69%	65%
ICA EDV ≥ 60 cm/s	96%	83%	94%	77%	71%
ICA/CCA PSV ≥ none	—	—	—	—	—
ICA PSV and EDV—none	—	—	—	—	—

[a]NPV, negative predictive value; PPV, positive predictive value; ICA, internal carotid artery; PSV, peak systolic velocity; EDV, end diastolic velocity; CCA, common carotid artery.
[b]These values have the best NPV and overall accuracy.

with 95% or greater PPV and the best overall accuracy in order to minimize the number of patients undergoing unnecessary arteriography (Table 13–1). These criteria can also be utilized when CEA is performed without preoperative arteriography. In those institutions where arteriography does not significantly add to the mortality and morbidity of the overall treatment of carotid disease, we suggest using the criteria described in Table 13–2. These criteria have the highest negative predictive value to ensure that only a minimum number of patients with equal to or greater than 60% or 70% stenoses are missed.

A new classification was proposed by us which would consist of lesions <30% stenosis, ≥30–49% stenosis, ≥50–59% stenosis, ≥60–69% stenosis, and ≥70% stenosis. This new duplex classification would fit into the existing trials [NASCET, ACAS, and Veteran's Administration Cooperative Study (VA)], and may be of benefit as new conclusions are released.[28] By reporting results using these criteria, the clinician will be better able to make decisions regarding the need for CEA or arteriogram based on the risks and benefits for individual patients. With the added risks of arteriography, decisions to operate would be better based on duplex findings alone. Having PPVs of 90–97% and accuracies of 87–93% can eliminate many unnecessary arteriograms.

It is important to note that the data obtained by individual vascular laboratories will vary as a result of differences in equipment, abilities, and consistencies of vascular technicians and reader interpretations.[28] Therefore, each laboratory must adapt a method that employs the equipment they use and has validated their method when using proposed new duplex criteria.

Intraoperative Assessment of Carotid Endarterectomy

Intraoperative use of the B-mode ultrasound imaging system for completion evaluation of the CEA has been advocated by Sigel *et al.*[29] The development of smaller scanning heads and probes together with techniques of sterilization has made this application feasible. The ultrasound examination can be performed quickly and, unlike angiography, requires no delay for film processing. Nor is it necessary to inject contrast material. Angiography is also associated with the risks of subintimal injections, thromboembolic complications, and allergic reactions.

Despite careful operative techniques, certain vascular defects can be missed, e.g., intimal flaps, luminal thrombus/platelet aggregation, stricture, etc. that occur in the course of carotid repair (Figure 13–8). These defects can escape visual inspection and palpation of the repair. If these defects are left undetected, they can result in stroke secondary to thrombus formation, platelet aggregation, or arterial thrombosis; or they may result in postoperative recurrent carotid stenoses. Blaisdell *et al.* reported the fallibility of clinical assessment by routine completion angiography, which revealed unsuspected defects in 25% of cases.[30] A number of investigators have subsequently confirmed the observations of Blaisdell *et al.* by using angiography, alone or in combination with various ultrasound techniques, such as continuous-wave Doppler examination, pulse Doppler spectral analysis, or duplex ultrasonography. Intraoperative monitoring has consistently documented severe defects in the internal carotid artery (ICA) or the common carotid artery (CCA) that warranted immediate correction in approximately

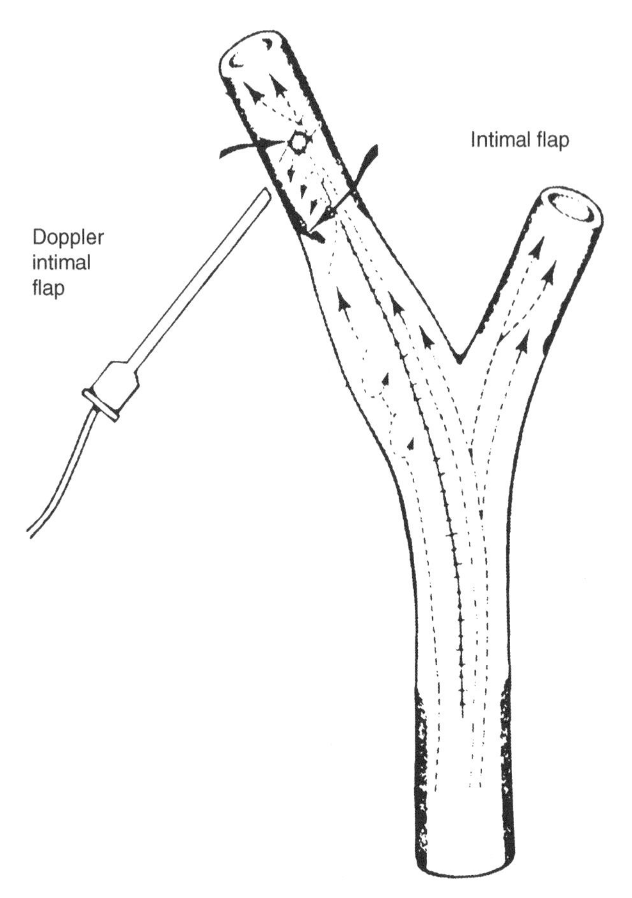

FIGURE 13–8. The application of Doppler probe to detect defects of a repaired internal carotid artery (intimal flap).

2–10% of all repairs.[31–37] Although the percentage of patients with residual repair defects in whom a postoperative stroke would develop if the defects were left untreated is not known, prudent surgical practice dictates that detection and revision of these defects should be done at the primary operation, since the sequelae of an ICA thrombosis are frequently catastrophic.

Baker *et al.*[33] reported that recurrent stenoses (>75%) developed in 17% of patients with abnormal unrepaired CEAs by intraoperataive imaging compared with 4.3% in normal CEAs ($p < 0.001$). This suggests that abnormalities detected by intraoperative DUS, if not corrected, may contribute to recurrent carotid stenosis after CEA.

Kinney *et al.*[34] showed the importance of intraoperative scanning in a prospective study of 461 CEAs. They correlated the results of intraoperative assessment by clinical inspection, ultrasound, or arteriography with an end point of stroke. The CEA site was assessed by ultrasound and arteriography in 268 cases, by ultrasound and Doppler spectral analysis alone in 142 cases, and with clinical inspection in only 51 cases. Based on intraoperative assessment, 26 endarterectomies (6%) were revised at the time of the surgery. Perioperative morbidity was similar in cases with normal, mildly abnormal, or no ultrasound. There were 12 temporary (3%) and six permanent (1%) neurologic deficits and six deaths (four strokes and two cardiac events). Based on life-table analysis, the incidence of >50% ICA stenosis or occlusions was increased ($p < 0.007$) in patients with residual flow abnormality or no study. However, patients with normal intraoperative studies had a significantly lower rate of late ipsilateral stroke compared with the other patients ($p = 0.04$). The incidence of stroke was increased ($p = 0.00016$) in patients with ICA restenosis or occlusion (3 of 35) compared with patients without recurrent stenosis (3 of 426) during a mean follow-up of 30 months. It was concluded that a normal intraoperative duplex scan may prevent recurrent stenosis as well as stroke after CEA in the long-term.

Most authorities rely on imaging or Doppler flow detection technique to exclude technical defects. The diagnostic signal analysis is highly sensitive and specific (>90%), particularly if pulse Doppler analysis is performed. This technique is simple, widely available, and relatively inexpensive. Although abnormalities of the Doppler flow signal are readily apparent by audible interpretation, quantitative spectral analysis is preferable. With flow and pressure reducing lesions, a spectral broadening is present throughout the pulse cycle, and a peak systolic velocity (PSV) exceeding 150 cm/s is noted. Visual inspection of velocity spectra and calculation of PSV can be obtained by a high-frequency pulse Doppler probe or duplex scanning, which permits classification of flow patterns into three categories: normal flow, mild to moderate flow disturbance, and severe flow disturbance.[31] When a significant residual flow abnormality is identified, angiography is usually recommended to delineate the abnormality before reexploration of the repair.

Recently, intraoperative duplex ultrasonography has been advocated because of its ability to provide both anatomic and hemodynamic information.[35–38] Improvements in linear ray scan head design and electronic signal processing, including color-coded velocity display, have made duplex scanning feasible in the operating room and an ideal modality for intraoperative assessment of CEA. Duplex scanning has an advantage over Doppler flow analysis alone, in that the structure of the anatomic defects associated with severe flow disturbance can usually be determined. B-mode imaging is sensitive in detecting small intimal defects in flaps, however, most authorities have not repaired these minor lesions, and the outcome of the procedure has not been adversely influenced.[37]

A comparison of intraoperative and early postoperative duplex findings after CEA indicated that a majority of these abnormalities identified by duplex scanning

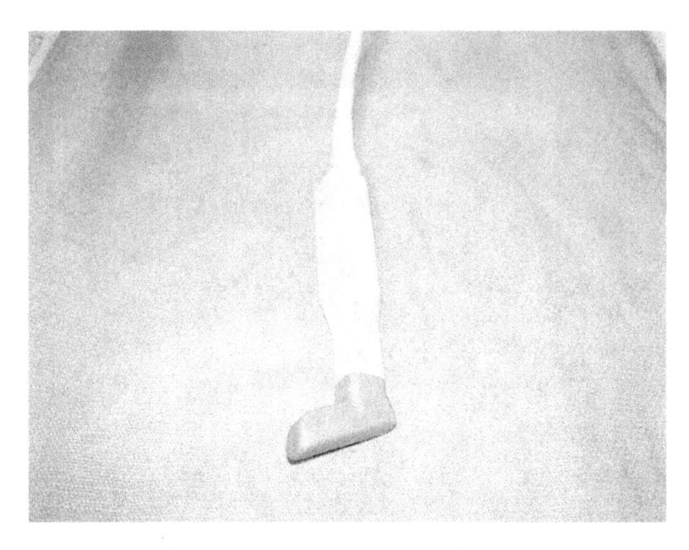

FIGURE 13–9. Transducer covered by sterile disposable plastic sleeve that contains acoustic gel.

within 3–6 months of CEA represent residual rather than recurrent stenoses.[36]

Recently, Ascher *et al.*[39] reported on the value of intraoperative carotid artery duplex scanning in a modern series of 650 consecutive primary endarterectomy procedures (April 2000 to April 2003). Major technical defects at intraoperative duplex scanning (>30% luminal ICA stenosis, free-floating clot, dissection, arterial disruption with pseudoaneurysm) were repaired. CCA residual disease was reported as wall thickness and percent stenosis (16–67%; mean 32% ± 8%) in all cases. Postoperative 30-day TIA, stroke, and death rates were analyzed. There were no clinically detectable postoperative thromboembolic events in this series. All 15 major defects (2.3%) identified with duplex scanning were successfully revised. These included seven intimal flaps, four free-floating clots, two ICA stenoses, one ICA pseudoaneurysm, and one retrograde CCA dissection. Diameter reduction ranged from 40% to 90% (mean, 67 ± 16%), and peak systolic velocity ranged from 69 to 497 cm/s (mean, 250 ± 121 cm/s). Thirty-one patients (5%) with the highest residual wall thickness (>3 mm) in the CCA and 19 (3%) with the highest CCA residual diameter reduction (>50%) did not have postoperative stroke or TIA. Overall postoperative stroke and mortality rates were 0.3% and 0.5%, respectively; combined stroke and mortality rate was 0.8%. One stroke was caused by hyperperfusion, and the other occurred as an extension of a previous cerebral infarct. It was concluded that intraoperative duplex scanning had a major role in these improved results, because it enabled detection of clinically unsuspected significant lesions. Residual disease in the CCA does not seem to be a harbinger of stroke or TIA.

Color duplex scanning with a 7.5- to 10-MHz linear ray transducer has been used for intraoperative studies. These studies are conducted with the transducer covered by a sterile disposable plastic sleeve that contains acoustic gel (Figure 13–9). The probe is generally positioned in the cervical incision directly over the exposed carotid repair. A sterile solution is instilled into the incision for acoustic coupling. As the surgeon scans the arterial repair, the technologist adjusts the instrument to optimize the Doppler angle, sample volume, color-coded image, and recorded velocity spectra. Vessel walls are imaged at 90°, but blood flow patterns should be evaluated at Doppler angles of <60°.

For CEAs with primary closure, the entire CEA segment should be examined with duplex ultrasound. The point in the CCA at which the lesion is transected should be examined. Normally, this should leave a distinct shelf, which can be appreciated on B-mode imaging. This can be easily visualized in both transverse and longitudinal views. The velocity data proximal to, in, and distal to the endarterectomy site should also be done in longitudinal view and sampling of the PSVs in the endarterectomy site should be obtained. Similarly, scanning of the proximal ICA in the bulb and beyond it should be done and attention should be called to the point of the transaction of the plaque or the end of the plaque distally. The external carotid artery should also be examined for the first few centimeters, looking for residual plaques or areas of thrombus. In patients who have CEAs closed with a patch, either polytetrafluoroethylene (PTFE) or Dacron, it is impossible to scan through the patch itself because of the air within the wall of the patch. However, it is possible to scan along the side of the artery, either posterior or anterior to the patch, which may yield the necessary information (Figures 13–10 and 13–11).

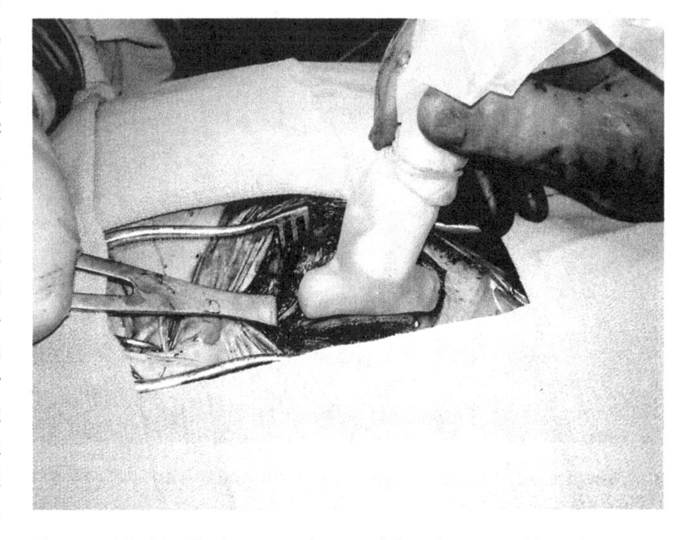

FIGURE 13–10. Probe scanning position for carotid endarterectomy closed with a patch. It is impossible to scan through the PTFE patch, but the operator can scan along the side of the artery, either posterior or anterior to the patch.

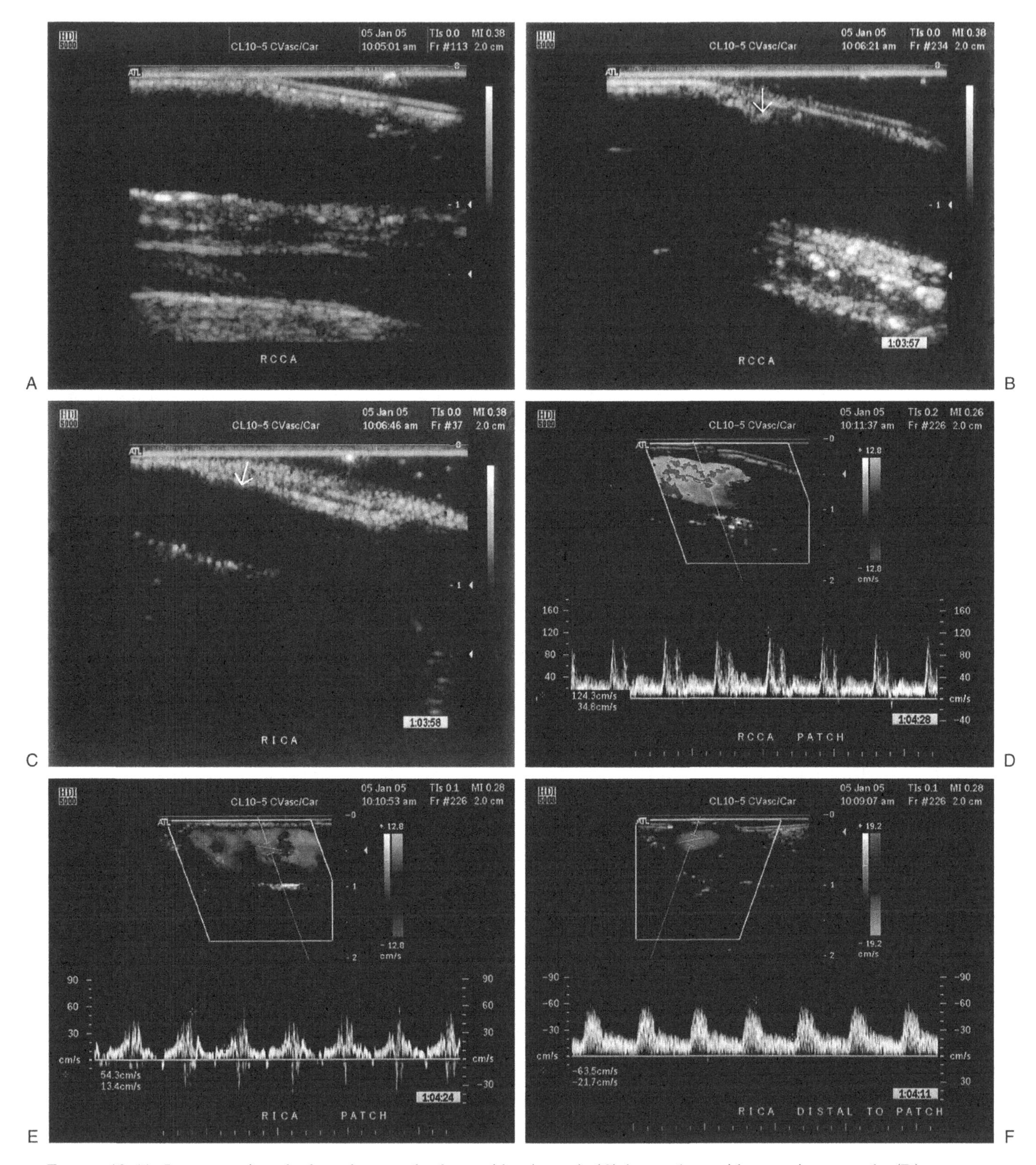

FIGURE 13–11. Intraoperative duplex ultrasound of carotid endarterectomy: (A) common carotid artery in grayscale. Note the shelf of the proximal end of carotid endarterectomy (arrow), (B) common carotid artery bifurcation in grayscale (arrow), (C) internal carotid artery in grayscale, (D) common carotid artery with color flow, (E) internal carotid artery with patch with color flow, and (F) distal internal carotid artery with color flow.

The limitations of this technique are largely related to lack of experience, correct measurement of duplex derived flow velocities, recognition of abnormal flow patterns, and transducer size. Intraoperative duplex imaging has the following advantages over angiography: comparable or higher accuracy, safety, ease of repeated use after reexploration, and low cost. Color duplex scanning is also sensitive to variations in anatomy and minor vascular defects that may alter blood flow streamlines. Certain flow patterns produced by carotid patch angioplasty should be noted and should not be regarded as abnormal. Some authorities have reported vascular defects in as many as one-third of their repairs, but only one-third of these appear to justify reexploration.

Intraoperative Monitoring of Carotid Endarterectomy with Transcranial Doppler Sonography

Transcranial Doppler (TCD) sonography has the advantage of allowing monitoring of both hemodynamic and embolic events, primarily in the middle cerebral artery distribution during CEA. The middle cerebral artery cannot be insonated in 5–15% of patients, most commonly because of the lack of a window for Doppler signal penetration of the skull. Severe cerebral ischemia is considered present in the first minute after carotid occlusion if the middle cerebral artery velocity decreases to 15% of the baseline or lower, and mild ischemia if it drops to 15–40% of the baseline. An adequate perfusion is present if the velocity is >40% of the baseline.[40] Following insertion of the shunt or upon declamping, a brisk recovery in middle cerebral artery velocity should be seen, usually >80%. Absolute mean velocities of 15 cm/s or even 30 cm/s have been alternatively suggested. A middle cerebral artery velocity of 30 cm/s has correlated roughly with a carotid artery stump blood pressure of 50 mm Hg. Some authorities reported that TCD detects critically low flow that results in neurologic deficits, even in the absence of electroencephalographic changes. The converse is also true: a pronounced drop in mean velocity has been observed in conjunction with a normal EEG and no resultant cerebral infarction, the cortex surviving from the other cerebral and laptomeningeal vessels.

In a recent study, Ackerstaff *et al.*[41] concluded that in CEA, TCD-detected microemboli during dissection and wound closure, ≥90% middle cerebral artery velocity decrease at cross-clamping, and ≥100% pulsatility index increase at clamp release are associated with operative stroke. In combination with the presence of preoperative cerebral symptoms and ≥70% ipsilateral ICA stenosis, these four TCD monitoring variables can reasonably discriminate between patients with and without operative stroke. This supports the use of TCD as a potential intraoperative monitoring modality to alter the surgical technique by enhancing a decrease of the risk of stroke during or immediately after the operation.

TCD can also be used in the postoperative period to detect early thrombosis of the carotid artery, continued embolization, or the hyperperfusion syndrome. It has been reported that markedly increased mean velocity (150% of the baseline) may herald an intracranial hemorrhage. The use of TCD monitoring during CEA has led some surgeons to modify their operative techniques based on hearing a distressing frequency of emboli while operating with the continuously audible TCD.

Patients Who Develop a Neurologic Deficit After Leaving the Operating Room

If patients wake up well after CEA and then develop a neurologic deficit, emergent reexploration is indicated. If the deficit proves to be a TIA as symptoms resolve prior to the return to the operating room, heparin anticoagulation followed by duplex scan is preferred. A thrombosed ICA may be treated operatively or medically (anticoagulation), particularly in patients with dense deficits. A patent carotid without apparent pathology is immediately followed by CT scanning to identify intracranial hemorrhage or other pathology. If negative, an angiogram should be done to confirm the duplex findings and assess the intracranial vasculature. If negative, oral anticoagulation is started. Thromboembolism of inaccessible intracranial vasculature has been treated with selective catheterization and lytic therapy, although this is still considered investigational. Blood clots found at the endarterectomy site are treated by emergency reexploration.

Post-Carotid Endarterectomy Surveillance

Restenosis is a known entity that occurs after CEA and may vary between 12 and 36%, but the frequency of restenosis varies depending on the diagnostic method used and the frequency of follow-up examinations.[42–52] Several studies have reported on the value of postoperative carotid duplex surveillance, but no consensus has been reached.[42–52] The advantages that have been cited are detection of significant restenosis prior to the onset of neurologic events, which aids in the prevention of potential strokes, and follow-up on the contralateral carotid artery to document the development of surgically correctable stenosis. Opponents of routine postoperative carotid duplex surveillance claim that restenosis is benign in nature, therefore, a large number of strokes may not be prevented by this surveillance.[45,46,48,49,52] Despite the high rate of restenosis, symptoms attributed to restenoses are rare, therefore several authorities have suggested that routine surveillance of patients after CEA is not efficacious.[44–46,49]

Mattos *et al.*[46] described their experience with postoperative carotid duplex surveillance and found an equal stroke-free survival at 5 years between patients with or without >50% restenosis. In addition, only one of 380 patients suffered a stroke in their study, suggesting a benign clinical significance of recurrent carotid artery stenosis. Mackey *et al.* claim a low rate of clinically significant restenosis.[45] Their retrospective series of 258 patients (348 arteries) show a potential 4% incidence of late strokes, but this included all patients who underwent repeat CEA for asymptomatic restenosis. They also noted that the majority of restenoses (53%) remained asymptomatic and did not progress to occlusion throughout follow-up. Of 10 documented late occlusions, eight did not result in stroke. Eight patients with operable restenosis had TIAs and underwent reoperation. They found that even patients with 75–99% restenosis most often remained asymptomatic (37%) or had TIAs (32%). Only two (11%) of 19 patients with 75–99% restenosis had an unheralded stroke. They felt that postoperative carotid duplex surveillance was not justified due to the low incidence of symptomatic restenosis.

In spite of these findings, investigators have been reluctant to advise that postoperative carotid duplex surveillance be abandoned because the cost-effectiveness of this surveillance has not been formally investigated. Others have reported that high-grade stenosis (>75%), whether caused by myointimal hyperplasia of the CEA site or progressive atherosclerosis of the contralateral carotid artery, is associated with an increased risk of late stroke.[34,52]

Ouriel *et al.* reported an 11% incidence of restenotic lesions greater than 80%. Although the incidence of symptoms with restenotic lesions was low (12%), the onset of symptoms at the time of occlusion was significant.[47] Forty-two percent of patients became symptomatic at the time of occlusion, with 33% resulting in a stroke. This led to the observation that critical restenoses are precursors to stroke, even if asymptomatic, and, therefore, the detection of >80% restenosis allows future stroke prevention, if operative intervention is undertaken.[47] Mattos *et al.* also described the outcome for >80% restenosis. In their group, one of three patients with >80% restenosis suffered a stroke, one had a TIA, and one remained asymptomatic. This suggests a more serious course once restenosis reaches >80%.[46]

So far, a consensus has not yet been reached in the surgical literature regarding the usefulness, cost-effectiveness, or timing of postoperative carotid duplex surveillance.

Timing of Postoperative Carotid Duplex Surveillance

Several authors have recommended an initial surveillance duplex on the operative carotid system within the first 6 months[43,46–48,52] to detect residual stenosis from the operative procedure or early restenosis.[47] For example, Roth *et al.*[52] recently recommended an initial DUS to ensure a technically successful CEA, with subsequent postoperative carotid duplex surveillance at 1–2 years, as long as restenosis and contralateral stenoses remain <50%. More frequent follow-up (every 6 months) is warranted if >50% stenosis is noted, or with the onset of symptomatic disease.[52]

Several studies have reported that the majority of restenoses occurs during the first 1–2 years after CEA. Mattos *et al.*[43] noted that 70% of restenoses were detected within 1 year after the CEA, and 96% developed within 15 months. Thomas *et al.*[42] reported that 70% of restenoses in their study occurred within 1 year of the CEA. Similar observations were noted by us previously.[50]

Ricco *et al.*[53] reported on the need for follow-up duplex scan 1 year after CEA was performed with prosthetic patching and intraoperative completion arteriography. A total of 605 CEA procedures with prosthetic patch closure and intraoperative completion arteriography were performed in 540 patients. All patients underwent duplex scan at 4 days and then yearly after the procedure. Intraoperative completion arteriography showed abnormalities in 114 cases, including 17 involving the ICA and 73 involving the external carotid artery. Successful revision was achieved in all cases and confirmed by repeat arteriography. Postoperative duplex scans at 4 days detected three abnormalities involving the ICA (0.5%), including asymptomatic occlusion in one case and residual stenosis >50% in two cases. Ninety-eight percent of patients were stenosis-free at 1 year. Actuarial stroke-free survival was 98.3% at 3 years. Diameter reduction of the contralateral carotid artery progressed over 70% within 1 year after CEA in 22.9% of patients with contralateral carotid stenosis over 50% at the time of the initial intervention. The findings of this study indicate that duplex scan follow-up 1 year after CEA with intraoperative completion arteriography is unnecessary unless postoperative duplex scan demonstrates residual stenosis of the ICA. However, duplex scan at 1 year is beneficial for patients presenting with contralateral carotid artery disease with diameter reduction >50% at the time of CEA.

Lovelace *et al.*[54] conducted a study on optimizing duplex follow-up in patients with an asymptomatic ICA stenosis of <60%. All patients who underwent initial carotid duplex examination for any indication since January 1, 1995, with at least one patent, asymptomatic, previously nonoperated ICA with <60% stenosis; with 6 months or greater follow-up; and with one or more repeat duplex examinations were entered into the study. On the basis of the initial duplex examination, ICAs were classified into two groups: those with a PSV <175 cm/s and those with a PSV of 175 cm/s or more. Follow-up duplex examinations were performed at varying intervals to detect progression from <60% to 60–99%. A total of 407 patients (640 asymptomatic ICAs with <60% stenosis) underwent serial duplex scans (mean follow-up, 22 months). Three ICAs (0.5%) became symptomatic and progressed to 60–99% ICA stenosis at a mean of 21 months, whereas four other ICAs occluded without stroke during follow-up. Progression to 60–99% stenosis without symptoms was detected in 46 ICAs (7%) (mean, 18 months). Of the 633 patent asymptomatic arteries, 548 ICAs (87%) had initial PSVs <175 cm/s, and 85 ICAs (13%) had initial PSVs of 175 cm/s or more. Asymptomatic progression to 60–99% ICA stenosis occurred in 22 (26%) of 85 ICAs with initial PSVs of 175 cm/s or more, whereas 24 (4%) of 548 ICAs with initial PSVs <175 cm/s progressed ($p < 0.0001$). The Kaplan–Meier method showed freedom from progression at 6 months, 12 months, and 24 months was 95%, 83%, and 70% for ICAs with initial PSVs of 175 cm/s or more versus 100%, 99%, and 95%, respectively, for ICAs with initial PSVs <175 cm/s ($p < 0.0001$).

They concluded that patients with <60% ICA stenosis and PSVs of 175 cm/s or more on initial duplex examination are significantly more likely to progress asymptomatically to 60–99% ICA stenosis, and progression is sufficiently frequent to warrant follow-up duplex studies at 6-month intervals. Patients with <60% ICA stenosis and initial PSVs <175 cm/s may have follow-up duplex examinations safely deferred for 2 years.

Cost-Effectiveness of Postoperative Carotid Duplex Surveillance

There have been reports that postoperative carotid duplex surveillance is not cost-effective since there is such a low incidence of symptomatic restenosis. Patel *et al.* evaluated the cost-effectiveness of postoperative carotid duplex surveillance.[51] They concluded that postoperative carotid duplex surveillance after CEA has an unfavorable cost-effectiveness ratio. In the process of their analysis, they identified a subset of patients in which postoperative carotid duplex surveillance may be cost-effective. These included patients in whom the rate of progression to >80% stenosis exceeded 6% per year. In their analysis, they felt that some groups of patients could potentially have a rate of disease progression that approaches or exceeds the level at which postoperative carotid duplex surveillance becomes cost-effective. Some of these include patients with multiple risk factors, e.g., smoking, hypertension, hyperlipidemia, diabetes mellitus, coronary artery disease, female gender, and a young age. In addition, they concluded that with postoperative carotid duplex surveillance, the rate of carotid artery occlusion could be reduced by 15% per year. Our evaluation of the cost of postoperative carotid duplex surveillance agrees with these conclusions (see Our Clinical Experience).

Our Clinical Experience

Three hundred and ninety-nine CEAs were randomized into 135 with primary closure, 134 with PTFE patch closures, and 130 with vein patch closures and followed for a mean of 47 months. Postoperative carotid duplex surveillance was done at 1, 6, and 12 months, and every year thereafter (a mean of 4.0 studies/artery). A Kaplan–Meier analysis was used to estimate the rate of ≥80% restenosis over time and the time frame of progression from <50% to 50–79% and ≥80% stenosis.

Greater than or equal to 80% restenosis developed in 24 (21%) with primary closure and nine (4%) with patching. A Kaplan–Meier estimate of freedom from 50–79% restenosis at 1, 2, 3, 4, and 5 years was 92%, 83%, 72%, 72%, and 63% for primary closure and 99%, 98%, 97%, 97%, and 95% for patching A Kaplan–Meier estimate of freedom from ≥80% restenosis at 1, 2, 3, 4, and 5 years was 92%, 83%, 80%, 76%, and 68% for primary closure and 100%, 99%, 98%, 98%, and 91% for patching ($p < 0.01$).

Out of 56 arteries with 20–50% restenosis, 2/28 patch closures and 10/28 primary closures progressed to 50–<80% restenosis ($p = 0.02$) and 0/28 patch closures and 6/28 primary closures progressed to ≥80% ($p = 0.03$). In primary closures, the median time to progression from <50% to 50–79%, <50% to ≥80%, and 50–79% to ≥80% was 42, 46, and 7 months, respectively. Of the 24 arteries with ≥80% restenosis in primary closures, 10 were symptomatic. Thus, assuming that symptomatic restenosis would have undergone duplex examinations anyway, there were 14 asymptomatic arteries (12%)

that could have been detected only by postoperative carotid duplex surveillance (estimated cost of $139,200) and would have been candidates for redo CEA. Of the nine arteries with patch closures (three PTFE and six vein patch closures) with ≥80% restenosis, six asymptomatic arteries (four vein patch closure and two PTFE, 3%) could have been detected by postoperative carotid duplex surveillance. In patients with a normal duplex at the first 6 months, only 4/222 (2%) patched arteries (two asymptomatic) developed ≥80% restenosis versus 5/13 (38%) in patients with abnormal duplex examinations ($p < 0.001$).

Assuming a 5% stroke rate for the 14 repeat CEAs for asymptomatic ≥80% restenosis in the primary closure group in our series,[55] 0.7 strokes would be associated with the 14 repeat CEAs and approximately 4.7 strokes would have been prevented through surgical intervention prior to occlusion (assuming a similar outcome of ≥80% restenosis as described by Mattos *et al.*[46]). There was a net reduction of four strokes in patients with primary closure and an approximate cost of $56,150 per stroke prevented.

Also, assuming a similar outcome of >80% restenosis as described by Ouriel *et al.*,[47] and if one-half of these >80% restenosis would progress to total occlusion (7 patients), and assuming one-third of patients with total occlusion would suffer a stroke, then approximately 2.3 strokes would be prevented by doing the 14 redo CEAs. Since 0.7 strokes would result from repeating 14 CEAs,[55] the net effect would be prevention of 1.6 strokes at a cost of $224,600, i.e., $140,250 per stroke prevented. This analysis does not take into consideration the value of duplex screening of the contralateral nonoperated side.

The justification for this cost is unclear without a definite estimate of the economic burden for caring for these stroke victims. Considering the low incidence of >80% restenosis in patients with patch angioplasty closure, the cost-effectiveness of postoperative carotid duplex surveillance appears to be unfavorable and, therefore, should be limited to a single DUS to detect residual stenosis. Subsequent follow-up should be dictated by the results found on the initial scan and the onset of neurologic symptoms.

Our randomized prospective studies confirm that carotid restenosis is a known entity that follows a percentage of patients who undergo carotid surgery. In the past, the clinical significance of carotid restenosis has led some investigators to conclude that postoperative carotid duplex surveillance is not warranted. We showed that based on the incidence of >80% restenosis, postoperative carotid duplex surveillance may be beneficial in patients with primary closure with examinations at 6 months and at 1–2 year intervals for several years. For patients with patching, a 6-month postoperative duplex examination, if normal, is adequate.

Duplex Ultrasound Surveillance of Carotid Stents

Kupinski *et al.*[56] conducted a study to evaluate the DUS characteristics of carotid stents including comparing hemodynamic to B-mode and color-flow imaging data in 40 carotid stents placed in the common or internal carotid arteries of 37 patients. DUS examinations included PSV and end diastolic velocity (EDV) taken proximal to the stent (prestent), at the proximal, mid, and distal regions of the stent, and distal to the stent (poststent). The stents were evaluated at 1 day, and 3, 6, and 12 months post-procedure and yearly thereafter. The average follow-up interval was 6 ± 1 month. In 31 patient ICA stents, the PSV proximally within the stent was 92 ± 6cm/s with an EDV of 24 ± 2cm/s. The mid stent PSV was 86 ± 5cm/s with an EDV of 24 ± 2cm/s. The distal stent PSV was 90 ± 4 with an EDV of 26 ± 2cm/s. Proximal to the stent, the PSV was 70 ± 3cm/s with an EDV of 17 ± 1cm/s. Distal to the stent, the PSV was 77 ± 4cm/s with an EDV of 25 ± 2cm/s. There were no defects observed on B-mode image and no areas of color turbulence. Three stents developed stenotic areas with PSVs of 251, 383, and 512cm/s. The EDV was 50, 131, and 365cm/s, respectively. Poststenotic turbulence was present in each of these stents. An elevated PSV of >125cm/s was found in 32% of the stents (9 of 28) without evidence of stenosis on B-mode image of post-stenotic turbulence. These data demonstrate that velocities within stented carotid arteries can be elevated above established ranges for normal. They concluded that velocity criteria may need to be adjusted when applied to stented carotid arteries. It has been suggested that focal velocity increase at the point of maximal narrowing >150cm/s and a prestenotic (or present) to stenotic segment PSV ratio of 1:≥2 are suggestive of significant in-stent restenosis.[57]

Determination of Progression

It has now become clear that it is possible to determine major progression of disease in two different categories with duplex scanning technology. Progression of disease from a mild form (20–50% diameter reduction) to a severe form (50–99% diameter reduction) can be accurately detected based on significant changes in peak frequency.[58] In addition, in severe stenosis, it is possible to identify the development of extreme degrees of stenosis (>80% diameter reduction) by the changes in the ratio between peak systolic and end diastolic frequencies. The ability to identify such disease progression without invasive arteriographic studies will contribute to our understanding of the natural history of the disease process.

Natural History of Carotid Artery Stenosis, Contralateral to Carotid Endarterectomy

A few nonrandomized studies have reported on the natural history of carotid artery stenosis contralateral to CEA. Recently, we analyzed the natural history of carotid artery stenosis contralateral to CEA from two randomized prospective trials.[50,59]

The contralateral carotid arteries of 534 patients who participated in two randomized trials comparing CEA with primary closure versus patching were followed clinically and had DUSs at 1 month and every 6 months. Carotid artery stenoses were classified into <50%, ≥50–<80%, ≥80–99%, and occlusion. Late contralateral CEAs were done for significant carotid artery stenoses. Progression of carotid artery stenosis was defined as progress to a higher category of stenosis. A Kaplan–Meier life table analysis was used to estimate freedom from progression of carotid artery stenosis. The correlation of risk factors and carotid artery stenosis progression was also analyzed.

Out of 534 patients, 61 had initial contralateral CEAs, within 30 days of the ipsilateral CEA, and 53 had contralateral occlusions. Overall, 109/420 (26%) progressed at a mean follow-up of 41 months (range: 1–116 months). Progression of contralateral carotid artery stenosis was noted in 5/162 (3%) patients who had baseline normal carotids; 56/157 (36%) patients with <50% carotid artery stenosis progressed versus 45/95 (47%) patients with 50–<80% carotid artery stenosis ($p = 0.003$). The median time for progression was 24 months for <50% carotid artery stenosis and 12 months for ≥50–<80% carotid artery stenosis ($p = 0.035$). Freedom from progression for patients with baseline <50% and ≥50–<80% carotid artery stenosis at 1, 2, 3, 4, and 5 years was 95%, 78%, 69%, 61%, 48%; and 75%, 61%, 51%, 43%, and 33%, respectively ($p = 0.003$). Freedom from progression in patients with baseline normal carotid arteries at 1, 2, 3, 4, and 5 years was 99%, 98%, 96%, 96%, and 94%. Late neurologic events referable to the contralateral carotid artery were infrequent in the whole series (28/420, 6.7%) and included 10 strokes (2.4%) and 18 TIAs (4.3%) (28/258, 10.9% in patients with contralateral carotid artery stenosis); however, late contralateral CEAs were done in 62 patients (62/420, 15%, in the whole series, 62/258, 24%, in patients with contralateral carotid artery stenosis). The survival rates were 96%, 92%, 90%, 87%, and 82% at 1, 2, 3, 4, and 5 years.

We concluded that progression of contralateral carotid artery stenosis was noted in a significant number of patients with baseline contralateral carotid artery stenosis. Serial carotid DUSs every 6–12 months for patients with ≥50–<80% carotid artery stenosis and every 12–24 months for ≤50% carotid artery stenosis are adequate.

Carotid Endarterectomy Based on Carotid Duplex Ultrasonography Without Angiography

In many centers, carotid evaluation by angiography is no longer done routinely, even when planning for surgery, to eliminate the risk of neurologic events during angiography. The risk of stroke from angiography is around 1%.[6]

Although standard conventional angiography is still generally considered to be the definitive diagnostic test for carotid artery stenosis, there has been an increasing interest in performing CEA based on clinical evaluation and duplex scanning only.[3–5,7–12,60–63] This has been stimulated by improvement in the accuracy and reliability of color carotid duplex scanning, along with the increasing demands to minimize both the risk of carotid angiography and the cost of medical care. CEAs are generally indicated for high-grade stenoses of asymptomatic patients and in moderate to severe stenoses in patients with hemispheric neurologic events. These stenoses can usually be accurately detected by duplex scanning.

Dawson *et al.*[60] reviewed arteriograms and duplex scans in 83 patients and found that in 87% the clinical presentation and duplex findings were adequate for patient management. They concluded that arteriography was necessary in 13% that (1) showed an unusual or atypical pattern of disease, (2) had technically inadequate duplex scans, or (3) had an internal carotid artery stenosis of <50%. This group[7] completed a subsequent prospective evaluation of 94 cases that showed that arteriography affected clinical management in only one case (1%). Dawson *et al.*[7] indicated that while specific indications for CEA without angiography remain controversial, the results of angiography rarely alter the clinical treatment plan when a technically adequate duplex scan shows an 80–99% stenosis in asymptomatic patients or an ipsilateral 50–99% stenosis in patients with hemispheric neurologic symptoms.[7]

The duplex and arteriogram results of 85 patients were prospectively evaluated by Moore *et al.* with a panel of neurologists, neurosurgeons, and vascular surgeons.[3] The duplex scan results were prospectively compared with arteriography. One hundred and fifty-nine of 170 carotid arteries were correctly characterized (94%); hemodynamically significant stenoses were correctly characterized in 100%. Thirty-two CEAs were performed by these authors in 29 patients without angiography. All duplex-predicted lesions were confirmed at surgery, and there were no perioperative strokes.

If arteriography is not done, there is a potential to miss significant lesions in the carotid siphon or an intracranial aneurysm or tumor as the cause of TIAs. However, it is unlikely that carotid siphon disease will produce significant symptoms,[64,65] and, therefore, does not impact the decision to perform CEA. Intracranial aneurysms occur in approximately 1–2% of patients undergoing arteriography,[66] but most are small and unlikely to be affected by CEA.[66] With the advances in imaging techniques, the concern for occult brain tumors has become less relevant.

In addition, associated costs are significant with some institutions reporting charges for cerebrovascular arteriography as high as $5000 to $6000. Strandness[67] has suggested that wider use of duplex scanning as the sole preoperative test could result in substantial savings. For instance, if 150,000 CEAs are done annually, with an average cost of angiography of $3000, the total cost of angiography alone would be $750 million dollars (not counting the costs of an estimated 7500 TIAs, 1500 strokes, and 100 deaths). If these same patients had duplex scanning alone, the total costs would be approximately $37 million; this represents a savings annually in the United States alone of $712 million.[67] We have already begun to see a shift in the testing that is done for a preoperative diagnosis. A report from the University of Vermont stated that 87% of their last 130 CEAs were performed without arteriography, with acceptable rates of stroke and death,[68]

CEA should not be attempted without arteriography unless the following criteria are met:[7]

1. The distal ICA is free of significant disease (disease is localized to the carotid bifurcation).
2. The CCA is free of significant disease.
3. Vascular anomalies, kinks, or loops are not present.
4. The duplex scan is technically adequate.
5. Vascular laboratory duplex accuracy is known.

Some potential pitfalls include patients with nonhemispheric symptoms, recurrent stenosis, or ICA stenosis of <50%.[7,60,68] However, as experience grows, indications may be expanded.

Therefore, angiography is most likely to be useful when the duplex scan is not diagnostic, in patients with atypical lesions that appear to extend beyond the carotid bifurcation, and for stenoses of <50% in patients with classical hemispheric neurologic symptoms.

Carotid Endarterectomy Based on Duplex Ultrasonography with Minimal Angiographic Findings

We published a report on CEA for symptomatic carotid artery disease and failed medical treatment with plaque associated with <60% stenosis by DUS.[69] All patients in this study underwent arteriography, which showed normal to <20% stenosis. CEA was uneventful in these 14 patients, and their symptoms resolved.

We found that carotid DUS is superior to carotid arteriography in detecting irregular or ulcerative heterogeneous plaques associated with mild degrees of stenosis. These patients should also be worked up to exclude other noncarotid causes of the TIAs or strokes.

Ultrasonic Carotid Plaque Morphology and Carotid Plaque Hemorrhage: Clinical Implications

The lack of neurologic symptoms in many patients with significant carotid stenosis has perplexed many scientists. It has been proposed that the character of the plaque may be as, or more important, than significant stenosis in producing neurologic events.

We[70] examined the importance of ultrasonic plaque morphology and its correlation to the presence of intraplaque hemorrhage and its clinical implications. We studied 152 carotid plaques associated with ≥50% ICA stenoses in 135 patients who had CEAs and characterized them ultrasonographically into irregular/ulcerative, smooth, heterogeneous, homogeneous, or not defined. Heterogeneous plaques were defined as a mixture of hyperechoic, isoechoic, and hypoechoic plaques. In contrast, homogeneous plaques were defined as consisting of only one of the three types of echogenic plaques. An isoechoic plaque was defined as having the ecogenicity of a normal intima-media complex. A hyperechoic plaque was brighter than an isoechoic plaque, and a hypoechoic plaque was not as bright as an isoechoic plaque. An irregular plaque was defined as a plaque that lacks a smooth surface with or without an intimal layer. A smooth plaque was defined as a plaque without surface irregularities or ulcerations. All plaques were examined pathologically for the presence of intraplaque hemorrhage. The ultrasonic morphology of the plaques included 63 with surface irregularity (41%), 48 smooth (32%), 59 heterogeneous (39%), 52 homogeneous (34%), and 41 (27%) not defined. Intraplaque hemorrhage was present in 57 out of 63 (90%) irregular plaques and 53 out of 59 (90%) heterogeneous plaques, in contrast to 13 out of 48 (27%) smooth plaques and 17 out of 52 (33%) homogeneous plaques ($p < 0.001$). Fifty-three out of 63 (84%) irregular plaques and 47 out of 59 (80%) heterogeneous plaques had TIAs/stroke symptoms, in contrast to 9 out of 48 (19%) for smooth plaques and 15 out of 52 (29%) for homogeneous plaques ($p < 0.001$). Fifty-four percent of the irregular plaques and 57% of the heterogeneous plaques had ipsilateral cerebral infarcts, in contrast to 12% of the smooth plaques ($p < 0.001$) and 14% of the homogeneous plaques ($p < 0.001$). We concluded that irregular and/or heterogeneous carotid plaques are more often associated with intraplaque hemorrhage, neurologic events, and cerebral infarcts. Therefore, ultrasonic plaque morphology may be helpful in selecting patients for CEA.

In another recent study, we[71] analyzed the natural history of 60–<70% asymptomatic carotid stenosis according to ultrasonic plaque morphology and its implication on treatment.

Patients with 60–<70% asymptomatic carotid stenosis during a 2-year period entered into a protocol of carotid duplex surveillance/clinical examination every 6 months. Their ultrasonic plaque morphology was classified as heterogeneous (Group A, 162) or homogeneous (Group B, 229). CEA was done if the lesion progressed to ≥70% stenosis or became symptomatic.

Three hundred and eighty-two patients (391 arteries) were followed at a mean follow-up of 37 months. The clinical/demographic characteristics were similar for both groups. The incidence of future ipsilateral strokes was significantly higher in Group A than in Group B: 13.6% versus 3.1% ($p = 0.0001$, odds ratio 5). Similarly, the incidence of all neurologic events (stroke/TIAs) was higher in Group A than in Group B: 27.8% versus 6.6% ($p = 0.0001$, odds ratio of 5.5). Progression to ≥70% stenosis was also higher in Group A than in Group B: 25.3% versus 6.1% ($p = 0.0001$, odds ratio 5.2). Forty-four (27.2%) late CEAs were done in Group A (16 for stroke, 21 for TIAs, and seven for ≥70% asymptomatic carotid stenosis) versus 13 (5.7%) for Group B (five for stroke, seven for TIAs, and one for ≥70% asymptomatic carotid stenosis ($p = 0.0001$, odds ratio 6.2).

We concluded that patients with 60–<70% asymptomatic carotid stenosis with heterogeneous plaquing were associated with a higher incidence of late stroke, TIAs, and progression to ≥70% stenosis than patients with homogeneous plaquing. Prophylactic CEA for 60–<70% asymptomatic carotid stenosis may be justified if associated with heterogeneous plaquing.

In another study[72] of the correlation of ultrasonic carotid plaque morphology and the degree of carotid stenosis, 2460 carotid arteries were examined using color DUS during a 1-year period. Carotid stenoses were classified into <50%, 50–<60%, 60–<70%, and >70–99%.

Heterogeneous plaques were noted in 138 of 794 arteries with <50% stenosis, 191/564 with 50–<60% stenosis, 301/487 with 60–<70% stenosis, and 496/615 with 70–99% stenosis. The higher the degree of stenosis, the more likely it is to be associated with heterogeneous plaques. Heterogeneous plaques were present in 59% of ≥50% stenoses versus 17% for <50% stenoses, 72% of ≥60% stenoses versus 24% for <60% stenosis, and 80% of ≥70% stenoses versus 34% for <70% stenoses ($p < 0.0001$ and odds ratios of 6.9, 8.1, and 8.0, respectively). Heterogeneous plaques were associated with a higher incidence of symptoms than homogeneous plaques in all grades of stenoses: 68% versus 16% for <50% stenosis; 76% versus 21% for 50–<60%; 79% versus 23% for 60–<70%, and 86% versus 31% for ≥70–99% ($p < 0.0001$ and odds ratios of 8.9, 11.9, 12.6, and 13.7, respectively). Heterogenosity of plaques was more positively correlated to symptoms than any degree of stenosis (regardless of plaque structure). Eighty percent of all heterogeneous plaques were symptomatic versus 58% for all ≥50% stenoses, 68% for all ≥60% stenoses, and 75% for all ≥70% stenoses ($p < 0.0001$, $p < 0.0001$, and $p = 0.02$, respectively).

We concluded that the higher the degree of carotid stenosis, the more likely it is to be associated with ultrasonic heterogeneous plaquing and cerebrovascular symptoms. Heterogenosity of the plaque was more positively correlated to symptoms than to any degree of stenosis. These findings suggest that plaque heterogenosity should be considered in selecting patients for CEA.[72]

Differentiating unstable from stable plaques by ultrasound has been hampered by the subjectiveness of interpreting such images.[73–76]

Biasi *et al.*[75] conducted a study to confirm that plaque echogenicity evaluated by computer analysis, as suggested by preliminary studies, can identify plaques associated with a high incidence of strokes. A series of 96 patients with carotid stenosis in the range of 50–99% were studied retrospectively (41 with TIAs and 55 asymptomatic). Carotid plaque echogenicity was evaluated using a computerized measurement of the median grayscale value (GSM). All patients had a CT brain scan to determine the presence of infarction in the carotid territory.

The incidence of ipsilateral brain CT infarctions was 32% for symptomatic plaques and 16% for asymptomatic plaques ($p = 0.076$). It was 25% for >70% stenosis and 20% for <70% stenosis ($p = 0.52$). It was 40% in those with a GSM of <50 and 9% for plaques with a GSM of >50 ($p < 0.001$) with a relative risk of 4.6 (95% CI 1.8–11.6).

It was concluded that a computer analysis of plaque echogenicity was better than the degree of stenosis in identifying plaques associated with an increased incidence of CT brain scan infarction and consequently useful for identifying individuals at high risk of stroke.

Kern *et al.*[74] investigated the value of real-time compound ultrasound imaging for the characterization of atherosclerotic plaques in the ICA. Thirty-two patients (22 men, 10 women; mean age, 75 years) with plaques of the ICA as identified by high-resolution B-mode scanning were investigated with real-time compound ultrasound imaging with the use of a 5- to 12-MHz dynamic range linear transducer on a duplex scanner. Two independent observers rated plaque morphology according to a standardized protocol. The majority of plaques were classified as predominantly echogenic and as plaques of irregular surface, whereas ulcerated plaques were rarely observed. The interobserver agreement for plaque surface characterization was good for both compound ultrasound (kappa = 0.72) and conventional B-mode ultrasound (kappa = 0.65). For the determination of plaque echogenicity, the reproducibility of compound ultrasound [kappa(w) = 0.83] was even higher than that of conventional B-mode ultrasound [kappa(w) = 0.74]. According to a semiquantitative analysis, real-time compound ultrasound was rated superior in the categories plaque texture resolution, plaque surface definition, and vessel wall demarcation. Furthermore, there was a significant reduction of acoustic shadowing and reverberations.

They concluded that real-time compound ultrasound was a suitable technique for the characterization of atherosclerotic plaques, showing good general agreement with high-resolution B-mode imaging. This advanced technique allows reduction of ultrasound artifacts and improves the assessment of plaque texture and surface for enhanced evaluation of carotid plaque morphology. This subject will be covered in depth elsewhere in this volume.

Intima-Media Thickness by Duplex Ultrasound

Poli *et al.*[76] reported on a study of ultrasonographic measurement of the CCA wall thickness in hypercholesterolemic patients, and they concluded that there was a correlation between the thickness of the carotid artery and the presence of cardiovascular risk factors. The measurement consists of determining the distance between the leading edge of the lumen-to-wall interface of the artery and the interface between the media and the adventitia on the artery wall. The combined width of this region is defined as intima-media thickness (IMT). It is believed that patients with larger IMTs had a greater number of cardiovascular risk factors than patients with thinner IMTs. O'Leary *et al.*[77] reported for the Cardiovascular Health Study Collaborative Research Group that thickening of the carotid wall was a marker for atherosclerosis in the elderly. This study clearly shows the strong cross-sectional relationships between risk factors and the thickness of the wall of both the ICA and the CCA. CCA wall thickening is a diffuse process whereas ICA wall thickness is a sonographic measurement of carotid plaque thickness and cholesterol deposition. Therefore, an increased internal carotid IMT corresponds to an increased degree of carotid artery stenosis, and the measurement of the ICA wall thickness correlates with the extent of subjectively graded percentage of stenosis.[78]

O'Leary *et al.*[79] showed a clear-cut scaling effect as well as excess risk with increasing thickening of the ICA and the CCA, as well as for a combined score adding measurement from the common and ICAs. IMT is felt to be a marker for future myocardial infarction as well as for stroke.

The Role of Carotid Duplex Scanning After Trauma

DUS can be used in evaluating vascular injuries of the neck. Although carotid trauma is not strictly a disease of the carotid bifurcation, developments in this area parallel the changes seen in surgery for atherosclerotic disease. Carotid duplex following cervical trauma was prospectively evaluated by Fry *et al.*[80] Fifteen patients had duplex scan and arteriography, and 11 of these had a region of interest in zone II and four in zone III. One injury was diagnosed by duplex scan in this group and this was confirmed by arteriography; both studies were normal in the remaining 14 patients. On the next 85 patients Fry *et al.* then performed duplex scan only, with arteriography reserved only for an abnormal duplex result. In this group, 62 patients had potential injuries in zone II and the remainder in zone III. Seven arterial injuries were identified by duplex scan and confirmed by arteriography. The remaining 76 patients had normal duplex scans and no sequelae up to 3 weeks postdischarge. It was concluded that DUS is a valuable tool in evaluating carotid injury.

Dissection of the Internal Carotid Artery

ICA dissection has been reported more often recently than was previously suspected. This disease can appear spontaneously, or may follow traumatic events accompanied by the fully developed picture of focal ischemia with facial and neck pain and Horner's syndrome (ptosis, miosis, and anhydrosis). It can also appear with very few symptoms, or may even be completely asymptomatic. Using a color flow DUS, the diagnosis can be made when the flow signal is carefully followed over the entire neck region. In the longitudinal section, forward and backward signal components in blue/red color coding are generally seen next to one another in the proximal ICA. Distally, an area free of flow signals marks the proximal end of the dissection. Corresponding Doppler signals characterize partial recanalization with systolic forward and backward signal components, but with diastolic forward flow preservation.[81–83] On angiography, proximally there is a thread-like occlusion/subtotal stenosis of the ICA without a connection to the intracranial vasculature (Figure 13–12). Monthly follow-up assessments are important, since the majority of the cases spontaneously recanalize.

Vertebrobasilar Insufficiency

During the 1970s and 1980s, there was limited clinical experience in regard to vertebrobasilar insufficiency, due in part to the difficulty in noninvasive study of vertebral artery flow. Furthermore, documented alterations in the

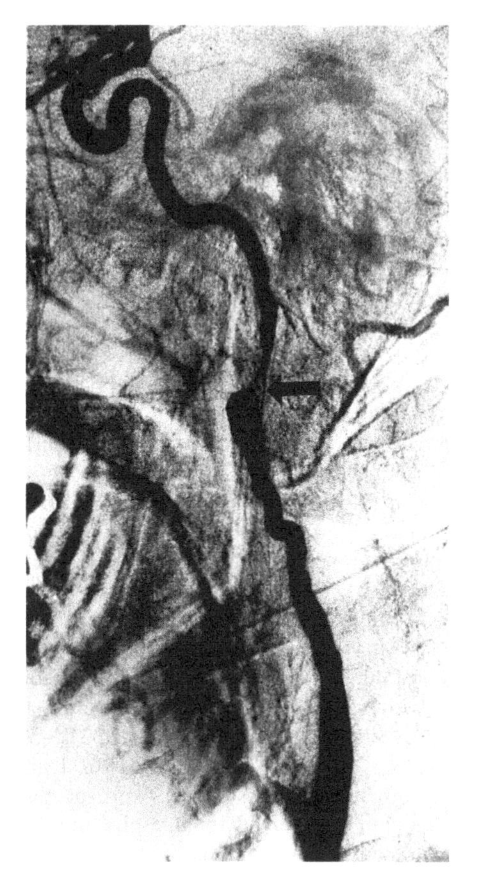

FIGURE 13–12. Carotid arteriogram showing internal carotid artery dissection of the higher cervical portion, as indicated by the black arrow.

vertebral flow may have little bearing on the clinical situation. Keller *et al.* studied vertebral artery flow using directional Doppler ultrasound in 90 patients, 40 of whom underwent subsequent arteriography.[84] The probe was positioned in the dorsal oropharynx after appropriate topical anesthesia, and the following four determinations were made: (1) the flow direction in each vertebral artery, (2) the related amplitude of both signals, (3) cessation of the flow in either vertebral artery during any part of the cardiac cycle, and (4) response of the vertebral flow to ipsilateral CCA compression. Under normal circumstances, the vertebral flow was always craniad and of equal amplitude in both vessels. It never reached zero during any phase diastole, and it did not change with CCA compression. Alteration of any of these normal observations was diagnostic of vertebral artery occlusive disease with a specificity of 82%. Kaneda *et al.*[85] simplified the previous technique by positioning the probe just below the mastoid process directed toward the contralateral eye. He reported a diagnostic accuracy of 92%. Others have found the mastoid approach unreliable, since spatial relationships between the probe and the vessel axis were poorly defined and more intervening structures were present.

Recent studies have shown that with adequate skill and patience on the operator's part, the innominate, subclavian, cervical, and prevertebral segment of the vertebral artery can be displayed with real-time, pulsed echo methods. Duplex scanning appears to be the most successful and accurate technique to diagnose atherosclerotic lesions of the vertebral arteries in the neck region. With this technique, the cervical segment of the vertebral artery can be visualized and the direction of the flow can be determined, whether antegrade or retrograde, which may be suggestive of subclavian steal. It has been reported that a reliable investigation of the prevertebral segment and the orifice of the vertebral artery is possible in more than 80% of cases (Figure 3–10 in Chapter 3). Some studies[85–87] claim more rapid identification and a higher success rate if color flow imaging is used. For detecting stenoses of ≥50% of the arch branches and at the site of the origin of the vertebral artery, duplex scanning has a high sensitivity, specificity, and overall accuracy. However, this technique still has several disadvantages, including the fact that satisfactory displays of the origin of the vertebral artery cannot be achieved in all patients. In addition, it is obvious that in those arteries in which the examination is successfully completed, only a limited spectrum of disease involvement can be identified. Accuracy of ultrasonic examination of the intradural segment of the vertebral artery can be improved by the use of simultaneous B-mode and color flow imaging. This subject will be covered in depth in another chapter in this volume.

Color Duplex Ultrasound in the Diagnosis of Temporal Arteritis

Temporal arteritis is sometimes diagnosed clinically, but a temporal artery biopsy is usually recommended to confirm the diagnosis.[88] The American College of Rheumatology requires three of the following five criteria to be met to establish the diagnosis: age ≥50 years, new onset of localized headache, temporal artery tenderness or decreased pulse, erythrocyte sedimentation rate ≥50 mm/h, and histologic findings. Schmidt *et al.*[88] examined the usefulness of color duplex ultrasonography in patients suspected of having temporal arteritis. In their prospective study, all patients seen in the departments of rheumatology and ophthalmology from January 1994 to October 1996 who had clinically suspected active temporal arteritis or polymyalgia rheumatica were examined by duplex ultrasonography. They examined both common superficial temporal arteries and the frontal and parietal rami as completely as possible in longitudinal and transverse planes to see if they were perfused, if there was a halo around the lumen, and (using simultaneous pulsed-wave Doppler ultrasonography) if there was a stenosis. Stenosis was considered to be present if blood flow velocity was more then twice the rate recorded in the area before the stenosis, perhaps with waveforms demonstrating turbulence and reduced velocity behind the area of stenosis. Two ultrasound studies were performed and read before the biopsies. Based on standard criteria, the final diagnoses were temporal arteritis in 30 patients, 21 with biopsy-confirmed disease; polymyalgia rheumatica in 37; and negative histologic findings and a diagnosis other than temporal arteritis or polymyalgia rheumatica in 15. They also studied 30 control patients matched for age and sex to the patients with arteritis.

Schmidt *et al.*[88] found that in 22 (73%) of the 30 patients with temporal arteritis, ultrasonography showed a dark halo around the lumen of the temporal arteries. The halos disappeared after a mean of 16 days (range: 7–56) of treatment with corticosteroids. Twenty-four patients (80%) had stenoses or occlusions of temporal artery segments, and 28 patients (93%) had stenoses, occlusions, or a halo. No halos were identified in the 82 patients without temporal arteritis; 6 (7%) had stenoses or occlusions. For each of the three types of abnormalities identified by ultrasonography, the interrater agreement was ≥95%.

They concluded that there are characteristic signs of temporal arteritis that can be visualized by color duplex ultrasonography. The most specific sign is a dark halo, which may be due to edema of the artery wall. In patients with typical clinical signs and a halo on ultrasonography, it may be possible to make a diagnosis of temporal arteritis and begin treatment without performing a temporal artery biopsy. This subject will be covered in depth in another chapter in this volume.

References

1. Cartier R, Cartier P, Fontaine A. Carotid endarterectomy without angiography: The reliability of Doppler ultrasonography and duplex scanning in preoperative assessment. Can J Surg 1993;36:411–421.
2. Polak JF. Noninvasive carotid evaluation: Carpe diem. Radiology 1993;186:329–331.
3. Moore WS, Ziomek S, Quinones-Baldrich WJ, *et al.* Can clinical evaluation and noninvasive testing substitute for arteriography in the evaluation of carotid artery disease? Ann Surg 1988;208:91–94.
4. Norris JW, Halliday A. Is ultrasound sufficient for vascular imaging prior to carotid endarterectomy? Stroke 2004;35:370–371.
5. Moore WS. For severe carotid stenosis found on ultrasound, further arterial evaluation is unnecessary. Stroke 2003;34:1816–1817.
6. Executive Committee for the Asymptomatic Carotid Atherosclerosis Study. Endarterectomy for asymptomatic carotid artery stenosis. JAMA 1995;273:1421–1428.
7. Dawson DL, Zierler RE, Strandness DE Jr, *et al.* The role of duplex scanning and arteriography before carotid endarterectomy: A prospective study. J Vasc Surg 1993;18:673–683.
8. Horn M, Michelini M, Greisler HP, *et al.* Carotid endarterectomy without arteriography: The preeminent role of the vascular laboratory. Ann Vasc Surg 1994;8:221–224.
9. Chervu A, Moore WS. Carotid endarterectomy without arteriography. Ann Vasc Surg 1994;8:296–302.
10. Mattos MA, Hodgson KJ, Faught WE, *et al.* Carotid endarterectomy without angiography: Is color-flow duplex scanning sufficient? Surgery 1994;116:776–783.
11. Walsh J, Markowitz I, Kerstein MD. Carotid endarterectomy for amaurosis fugax without angiography. Am J Surg 1986;152:172–174.
12. Marshall WG, Jr., Kouchoukos NT, Murphy SF, *et al.* Carotid endarterectomy based on duplex scanning without preoperative arteriography. Circulation 1988;78(Suppl I):I-1–I-5.
13. Nederkoorn PJ, Mali WPTM, Eikelboom BC, Elgersma OEH, Buskens E, Hunink MGM, Kappell LJ, Buijs PC, Wust AFJ, Lugt van der Lugt A, van der Graaf Y. Preoperative diagnosis of carotid artery stenosis: Accuracy of noninvasive testing. Stroke 2002;33:2003–2008.
14. Nederkoorn PJ, van der Graaf Y, Hunink Y. Duplex ultrasound and magnetic resonance angiography compared with digital subtraction angiography in carotid artery stenosis. Stroke 2003;34:1324–1332.
15. Westwood ME, Kelly S, Berry E, Bamford JM, Gough MJ, Airey CM, Meaney JFM, Davies LM, Cullingworth J, Smith MA. Use of magnetic resonance angiography to select candidates with recently symptomatic carotid stenosis for surgery: A systematic review. BMJ 2002;324:1–5.
16. Jackson MR, Chang AS, Robles HA, *et al.* Determination of 60% or greater carotid stenosis: A prospective comparison of magnetic resonance angiography and duplex ultrasound with conventional angiography. Ann Vasc Surg 1998;12:236–243.
17. Willinek WA, von Falkenhausen M, Born M, Gieseke J, Holler T, Klockgether T, Textor HJ, Schild HH, Urbach H. Noninvasive detection of steno-occlusive disease of the supra-aortic arteries with three-dimensional contrast-enhanced magnetic resonance angiography. A prospective, intra-individual comparative analysis with digital subtraction angiography. Stroke 2005;36:38–43.
18. Al-Kwifi O, Kim JK, Stainsby J, Huang Y, Sussman MS, Farb RI, Wright GA. Pulsatile motion effects on 3-D magnetic resonance angiography: Implications for evaluating carotid artery stenoses. Magn Reson Med 2004;52:605–611.
19. van Bemmel CM, Elgersma OE, Vonken EJ, Fiorelli M, van Leeuwen MS, Niessen WJ. Evaluation of semiautomated internal carotid artery stenosis quantification from 3-dimensional contrast-enhanced magnetic resonance angiograms. Invest Radiol 2004;39:418–426.
20. Kim DY, Park JW. Computerized quantification of carotid artery stenosis using MRA axial images. Magn Reson Imaging 2004;22:353–359.
21. U-King-Im JM, Trivedi R, Cross J, Higgins N, Graves M, Kirkpatrick P, Antoun N, Gillard JH. Conventional digital subtraction x-ray angiography versus magnetic resonance angiography in the evaluation of carotid disease: Patient satisfaction and preferences. Clin Radiol 2004;59:358–363.
22. Back MR, Rogers GA, Wilson JS, Johnson BL, Shames ML, Bandyk DF. Magnetic resonance angiography minimizes need for arteriography after inadequate carotid duplex ultrasound scanning. J Vasc Surg 2003;38:422–430.
23. Anderson GB, Ashforth R, Steinke DE, Ferdinancy R, Findlay JM. CT angiography for the detection and charac-

terization of carotid artery bifurcation disease. Stroke 2000; 31:2168–2174.
24. Koelemay MJ, Nederkoorn PJ, Reitsma JB, Majoie CB. Systematic review of computed tomographic angiography for assessment of carotid artery disease. Stroke 2004;35: 2306–2312.
25. Fell G, Breslau P, Know RA, *et al.* Importance of noninvasive ultrasonic Doppler testing in the evaluation of patients with asymptomatic carotid bruits. Am Heart J 1981;102: 221–226.
26. North American Symptomatic Carotid Endarterectomy Trial (NASCET) Investigators. Clinical alert: Benefit of carotid endarterectomy for patients with high-grade stenosis of the internal carotid artery. National Institute of Neurological Disorders and Stroke, Stroke and Trauma Division. Stroke 1991;22:816–817.
27. AbuRahma AF, Robinson PA, Boland JP, *et al.* Complications of arteriography in a recent series of 707 cases: Factors affecting outcome. Ann Vasc Surg 1993;7:122–129.
28. AbuRahma AF, Robinson PA, Stickler DL, *et al.* Proposed new duplex classification for threshold stenoses used in various symptomatic and asymptomatic carotid endarterectomy trials. Ann Vasc Surg 1998;12:349–358.
29. Sigel B, Coelho JC, Flanigan DP, *et al.* Detection of vascular defects during operation by imaging ultrasound. Ann Surg 1982;196:473–480.
30. Blaisdell FW, Lin R, Hall AD. Technical result of carotid endarterectomy—-arteriographic assessment. Am J Surg 1967;114:239–246.
31. Bandyk DF, Govostis DM. Intraoperative color flow imaging of "difficult" arterial reconstructions. Video J Color Flow Imaging 1991;1:13–20.
32. Hallett JW Jr, Berger MW, Lewis BD. Intraoperative color-flow duplex ultrasonography following carotid endarterectomy. Neurosurg Clin North Am 1996;7:733–740.
33. Baker WH, Koustas G, Burke K, *et al.* Intraoperative duplex scanning and late carotid artery stenosis. J Vasc Surg 1994;19:829–833.
34. Kinney EV, Seabrook GR, Kinney LY, *et al.* The importance of intraoperative detection of residual flow abnormalities after carotid artery endarterectomy. J Vasc Surg 1993;17: 912–922.
35. Coe DA, Towne JB, Seabrook GR, *et al.* Duplex morphologic features of the reconstructed carotid artery: Changes occurring more than five year after endarterectomy. J Vasc Surg 1997;25:850–857.
36. Cato R, Bandyk D, Karp D, *et al.* Duplex scanning after carotid reconstruction: A comparison of intraoperative and postoperative results. J Vasc Tech 1991;15:61–65.
37. Lane RJ, Ackroyd N, Appleberg M, *et al.* The application of operative ultrasound immediately following carotid endarterectomy. World J Surg 1987;11:593–597.
38. Sawchuk AP, Flanigan DP, Machi J, *et al.* The fate of unrepaired minor technical defects detected by intraoperative ultrasound during carotid endarterectomy. J Vasc Surg 1989;9:671–676.
39. Ascher E, Markevich N, Kallakuri S, Schutzer RW, Hingorani AP. Intraoperative carotid artery duplex scanning in a modern series of 650 consecutive primary endarterectomy procedures. J Vasc Surg 2004;39:416–420.
40. Halsey JH Jr. Risks and benefits of shunting in carotid endarterectomy. Stroke 1992;23:1583–1587.
41. Ackerstaff RGA, Moons KGM, van de Vlasakker CJW, Moll FL, Vermeulen FEE, Algra A, Spencer MP. Association of intraoperative transcranial Doppler monitoring variables with stroke from carotid endarterectomy. Stroke 2000;31:1817–1823.
42. Thomas M, Otis S, Rush M, *et al.* Recurrent carotid artery stenosis following endarterectomy. Ann Surg 1984;200: 74–79.
43. Mattos MA, Shamma AR, Rossi N, *et al.* Is duplex follow-up cost-effective in the first year after carotid endarterectomy? Am J Surg 1988;156:91–95.
44. Cook JM, Thompson BW, Barnes RW. Is routine duplex examination after carotid endarterectomy justified? J Vasc Surg 1990;12:334–340.
45. Mackey WC, Belkin M, Sindhi R, *et al.* Routine postendarterectomy duplex surveillance: Does it prevent late stroke? J Vasc Surg 1992;16:934–940.
46. Mattos MA, van Bemmelen PS, Barkmeier LD, *et al.* Routine surveillance after carotid endarterectomy: Does it affect clinical management? J Vasc Surg 1993;17:819–831.
47. Ouriel K, Green RM. Appropriate frequency of carotid duplex testing following carotid endarterectomy. Am J Surg 1995;170:144–147.
48. Ricotta JJ, DeWeese JA. Is route carotid ultrasound surveillance after carotid endarterectomy worthwhile? Am J Surg 1996;172:140–143.
49. Golledge J, Cuming R, Ellis M, *et al.* Clinical follow-up rather than duplex surveillance after carotid endarterectomy. J Vasc Surg 1997;25:55–63.
50. AbuRahma AF, Robinson PA, Saiedy S, *et al.* Prospective randomized trial of carotid endarterectomy with primary closure and patch angioplasty with saphenous vein, jugular vein, and polytetrafluoroethylene: Long-term follow-up. J Vasc Surg 1998;27:222–234.
51. Patel ST, Kuntz KM, Kent KG. Is routine duplex ultrasound surveillance after carotid endarterectomy cost-effective? Surgery 1998;124:343–353.
52. Roth SM, Back MR, Bandyk DF, *et al.* A rational algorithm for duplex scan surveillance after carotid endarterectomy. J Vasc Surg 1999;30:453–460.
53. Ricco JB, Camiade C, Roumy J, Neau JP. Modalities of surveillance after carotid endarterectomy: Impact of surgical technique. Ann Vasc Surg 2003;17:386–392.
54. Lovelace TD, Moneta GL, Abou-Zamzam AH, Edwards JM, Yeager RA, Landry GJ, Taylor LM, Porter JM. Optimizing duplex follow-up in patients with an asymptomatic internal carotid artery stenosis of less than 60%. J Vasc Surg 2001;33:56–61.
55. AbuRahma AF, Snodgrass KR, Robinson PA, *et al.* Safety and durability of redo carotid endarterectomy for recurrent carotid artery stenosis. Am J Surg 1994;168:175–178.
56. Kupinski AM, Khan AM, Stanton JE, Relyea W, Ford T, Mackey V, Khurana Y, Darling RC, Shah DM. Duplex ultrasound follow-up of carotid stents. J Vasc Ultrasound 2004;28:71–75.
57. Robbin ML, Lockhart ME, Weber TM, *et al.* Carotid artery stent: Early and intermediate follow-up with Doppler ultrasound. Radiology 1997;205:749–756.
58. Roederer GO, Langlois YE, Jager KA, *et al.* The natural history of carotid artery disease in asymptomatic patients with cervical bruits. Stroke 1984;15:605–613.

59. AbuRahma AF, Hannay RS, Khan JH, *et al.* Prospective randomized study of carotid endarterectomy with polytetrafluoroethylene versus collagen impregnated Dacron (Hemashield) patching: Perioperative (30-day) results. J Vasc Surg 2002;35:125–130.
60. Dawson DL, Zierler RE, Kohler TR. Role of arteriography in the preoperative evaluation of carotid artery disease. Am J Surg 1991;161:619–624.
61. Kuntz KM, Skillman JJ, Whittemore AD, *et al.* Carotid endarterectomy in asymptomatic patients: Is contrast angiography necessary? A morbidity analysis. J Vasc Surg 1995;22:706–716.
62. Kent KC, Kuntz KM, Patel MR. Perioperative imaging strategies for carotid endarterectomy: An analysis of morbidity and cost-effectiveness in symptomatic patients. JAMA 1995;274:888–893.
63. Campron H, Cartier R, Fontaine AR. Prophylactic carotid endarterectomy without arteriography in patients without hemispheric symptoms: Surgical morbidity and mortality and long-term follow-up. Ann Vasc Surg 1998;12:10–16.
64. Roederer GO, Langlois YE, Chan ARW, *et al.* Is siphon disease important in predicting outcome of carotid endarterectomy? Arch Surg 1983;118:1177–1181.
65. Mattos MA, van Bemmelen PS, Hodgson KJ, *et al.* The influence of carotid siphon stenosis on short and long-term outcome after carotid endarterectomy. J Vasc Surg 1993;17:902–911.
66. Lord RSA. Relevance of siphon stenosis and intracranial aneurysm to results of carotid endarterectomy. In: Ernst CB, Stanley JC (eds). *Current Therapy in Vascular Surgery*, 2nd ed., pp. 94–101. Philadelphia, PA: BC Decker, 1991.
67. Strandness DE Jr. Extracranial arterial disease, In: Strandness DR Jr (ed). *Duplex Scanning in Vascular Disorders*, 2nd ed., pp. 113–158. New York: Raven Press, 1993.
68. Pilcher DB, Ricci MA. Vascular ultrasound. Surg Clin North Am 1998;78:273–293.
69. AbuRahma AF, White JF III, Boland JP. Carotid endarterectomy for symptomatic carotid artery disease demonstrated by duplex ultrasound with minimal arteriographic findings. Ann Vasc Surg 1996;10:385–389.
70. AbuRahma AF, Kyer PD III, Robinson PA, *et al.* The correlation of ultrasonic carotid plaque morphology and carotid plaque hemorrhage: Clinical implications. Surgery 1998;124:721–728.
71. AbuRahma AF, Thiele SP, Wulu JT. Prospective controlled study of the natural history of asymptomatic 60% to 69% carotid stenosis according to ultrasonic plaque morphology. J Vasc Surg 2002;36:437–442.
72. AbuRahma AF, Wulu JT, Crotty B. Carotid plaque ultrasonic heterogeneity and severity of stenosis. Stroke 2002;33: 1772–1775.
73. Choo V. New imaging technology might help prevent stroke. Lancet 1998;351:809.
74. Kern R, Szabo K. Hennerici M, Meairs S. Characterization of carotid artery plaques using real-time compound B-mode ultrasound. Stroke 2004;35:870–875.
75. Biasi GM, Sampaolo A, Mingazzini P, De Amicis P. El-Barghouty N, Nicolaides AN. Computer analysis of ultrasonic plaque echolucency in identifying high-risk carotid bifurcation lesions. Eur J Vasc Endovasc Surg 1999;17:476–479.
76. Poli A, Tremoli E, Colombo A, Sirtori M, Pignoli P, Paoletti R. Ultrasonographic measurement of the common carotid artery wall thickness in hypercholesterolemic patients. A new model for the quantitation and follow-up of preclinical atherosclerosis in living human subjects. Atherosclerosis 1988;70:253–261.
77. O'Leary DH, Polak JF, Kronmal RA, *et al.* Thickening of the carotid wall. A marker for atherosclerosis in the elderly? Cardiovascular Health Study Collaborative Research Group. Stroke 1996;27:224–231.
78. Polak JF, O'Leary DH, Kronmal RA, *et al.* Sonographic evaluation of carotid artery atherosclerosis in the elderly: Relationship of disease severity to stroke and transient ischemic attack. Radiology 1993;188:363–370.
79. O'Leary DH, Polak JF, Kronmal RA, Manolio TA, Burke GL, Wolfson SK Jr. Carotid-artery intima and media thickness as a risk factor for myocardial infarction and stroke in older adults. Cardiovascular Health Study Collaborative Research Group. N Engl J Med 1999;340:14–22.
80. Fry WR, Dort JA, Smith RS, *et al.* Duplex scanning replaces arteriography and operative exploration in the diagnosis of potential cervical vascular injury. Am J Surg 1994;168:693–696.
81. Steinke W. Schwartz A, Hennerici M. Doppler color flow imaging of common carotid artery dissection. Neuroradiology 1990;32(6):502–505.
82. Sturzenegger M. Ultrasound findings in spontaneous carotid artery dissection. The value of duplex sonography. Arch Neurol 1991;48(10):1057–1063.
83. Cals N, Devuyst G, Jung DK, Afsar N, de Freitas G, Despland PA, Bogousslavsky J. Uncommon ultrasound findings in traumatic extracranial dissection. Eur J Ultrasound 2001;12:227–231.
84. Keller HM, Meier WE, Kumpe DA. Noninvasive angiography for the diagnosis of vertebral artery disease using Doppler ultrasound (vertebral artery Doppler). Stroke 1976;7:364–369.
85. Kaneda H, Irino T, Minami T, *et al.* Diagnostic reliability of the percutaneous ultrasonic Doppler technique for vertebral arterial occlusive diseases. Stroke 1977;8:571–579.
86. Bartels E, Fuchs HH, Flugel KA. Color Doppler imaging of vertebral arteries: A comparative study with duplex ultrasonography. In: Oka M, *et al.* (eds). *Recent Advantages in Neurosonology.* Amsterdam: Elsevier Science Publishers, 1992.
87. De Bray JM. Le duplex des axes verebro-sous-claviers. J Echographie Med Ultrasons 1991;12:141–151.
88. Schmidt WA, Kraft HE, Vorpahl K, *et al.* Color duplex ultrasonography in the diagnosis of temporal arteritis. N Engl J Med 1997;337:1336–1342.

Index

A.F. Aburahma, J.J. Bergan (eds.), *Noninvasive Cerebrovascular Diagnosis*, DOI 10.1007/978-1-84882-957-2,

D